Clinical Cancer Imaging

Clinical Cancer Imaging

Editor: Nadia Lilley

AMERICAN
MEDICAL PUBLISHERS
www.americanmedicalpublishers.com

AMERICAN
MEDICAL PUBLISHERS
www.americanmedicalpublishers.com

Cataloging-in-Publication Data

Clinical cancer imaging / edited by Nadia Lilley.
p. cm.
Includes bibliographical references and index.
ISBN 978-1-63927-634-9
1. Cancer--Imaging. 2. Cancer--Ultrasonic imaging. 3. Cancer--Diagnosis.
4. Diagnostic imaging. I. Lilley, Nadia.
RC270.3.D53 C55 2023
616.994 075 4--dc23

American Medical Publishers,
41 Flatbush Avenue,
1st Floor, New York,
NY 11217, USA

ISBN 978-1-63927-634-9 (Hardback)

Contents

Preface

This book was inspired by the evolution of our times; to answer the curiosity of inquisitive minds. Many developments have occurred across the globe in the recent past which has transformed the progress in the field.

Imaging is used to view inside the body for medical analysis and clinical intervention. A variety of biomedical imaging techniques are utilized for managing all stages of cancer. Imaging plays an important role in cancer clinical protocols by providing metabolic, morphological, functional and structural information. In combination with other diagnostic tools such as in vitro fluids and tissue analysis, it contributes in clinical decision-making. Hybrid imaging techniques are capable of supplying complementary information for enhanced planning of therapy and staging. Targeted minimally invasive and image guided therapy can decrease collateral impacts and improve outcome. Cancer imaging has several benefits such as minimal or no invasiveness, real time monitoring, and accessibility without tissue destruction and may help in functioning over a variety of size and time scales involved in pathological and biological processes. This book contains some path-breaking studies in clinical cancer imaging. It is a valuable compilation of topics, ranging from the basic to the most complex advancements. This book will prove to be immensely beneficial to students and researchers in this field.

This book was developed from a mere concept to drafts to chapters and finally compiled together as a complete text to benefit the readers across all nations. To ensure the quality of the content we instilled two significant steps in our procedure. The first was to appoint an editorial team that would verify the data and statistics provided in the book and also select the most appropriate and valuable contributions from the plentiful contributions we received from authors worldwide. The next step was to appoint an expert of the topic as the Editor-in-Chief, who would head the project and finally make the necessary amendments and modifications to make the text reader-friendly. I was then commissioned to examine all the material to present the topics in the most comprehensible and productive format.

I would like to take this opportunity to thank all the contributing authors who were supportive enough to contribute their time and knowledge to this project. I also wish to convey my regards to my family who have been extremely supportive during the entire project.

Editor

1

Deep Learning in Selected Cancers' Image Analysis

Taye Girma Debelee [1,2,*], Samuel Rahimeto Kebede [1,3], Friedhelm Schwenker [4] and Zemene Matewos Shewarega [1]

1 Artificial Intelligence Center, 40782 Addis Ababa, Ethiopia; samuelrahimeto@dbu.edu.et (S.R.K.); zemene.matewos@aic.et (Z.M.S.)
2 College of Electrical and Mechanical Engineering, Addis Ababa Science and Technology University, 120611 Addis Ababa, Ethiopia
3 Department of Electrical and Computer Engineering, Debreberhan University, 445 Debre Berhan, Ethiopia
4 Institute of Neural Information Processing, University of Ulm, 89081 Ulm, Germany; friedhelm.schwenker@uni-ulm.de
* Correspondence: tayegirma@gmail.com

Abstract: Deep learning algorithms have become the first choice as an approach to medical image analysis, face recognition, and emotion recognition. In this survey, several deep-learning-based approaches applied to breast cancer, cervical cancer, brain tumor, colon and lung cancers are studied and reviewed. Deep learning has been applied in almost all of the imaging modalities used for cervical and breast cancers and MRIs for the brain tumor. The result of the review process indicated that deep learning methods have achieved state-of-the-art in tumor detection, segmentation, feature extraction and classification. As presented in this paper, the deep learning approaches were used in three different modes that include training from scratch, transfer learning through freezing some layers of the deep learning network and modifying the architecture to reduce the number of parameters existing in the network. Moreover, the application of deep learning to imaging devices for the detection of various cancer cases has been studied by researchers affiliated to academic and medical institutes in economically developed countries; while, the study has not had much attention in Africa despite the dramatic soar of cancer risks in the continent.

Keywords: deep learning; medical image analysis; breast cancer; brain tumor; cervical cancer; colon cancer; lung cancer

---

1. Introduction

Over the last decades, three different approaches have been practiced to deal with medical images. The first is creating awareness among the community for a regular check-up and it was not be practiced among communities. The second approach is using medical imaging technologies for screening and it is witnessed over the last decades. However, the benefits of medical imaging technology depend on the experience of the image interpreting experts or radiologists. Then, applying a computer-aided detection (CAD) approach using machine learning techniques has brought a promising result along with the imaging technologies. Machine learning techniques have evolved rapidly in recent years to solve complex problems.

The architecture of deep convolutional neural networks (DCNNs) is composed of convolutional layers, pooling layers and fully connected layers to perform feature extraction (see Figure 1), features down sampling (see Figure 2) and classification, respectively during the process of optimization [1].

In convolutional layers, local features such as colors, end-points, corners and oriented-edges are collected in the shallow layers. These local features in the shallow layers are integrated into larger structural features like circles, ellipses, specific shapes or patterns when the layer goes deeper. Afterwards, these features of structures or patterns constitute the high-level semantic representations that describe feature abstraction for each category. In pooling layers, feature down sampling is performed either using average pooling or max-pooling layers to reduce the dimensionality of the features extracted using convolutional layers [2]. On the other hand, in fully connected layers, it takes the extracted features from the convolutional layers as inputs and works as a classifier, well known as multilayer perceptron (MLP). These fully connected layers encode the spatial correspondences of those semantic features and convey the co-occurrence properties between patterns or objects.

There have been many survey papers produced on the application of deep learning on medical image analysis and few among many produced in 2017 are considered in this survey paper. Suzuki [3] in his survey paper claimed that machine learning in deep learning form has emerged in computer vision and paved the way for many researchers to work on medical image analysis using deep learning approach. The popularity of deep learning started after the AlexNet model won the competition in 2012. Suzuki has produced an interesting survey paper that aimed to address four major points: the machine learning techniques used in the computer vision field, changes observed in machine learning after the introduction of deep learning, available machine learning models in deep learning and the impact of deep learning for medical image analysis. As claimed by Litjens et al. [4], convolutional neural network-based deep learning has become a method for medical image analysis. In their survey paper, they considered papers that were related to medical image analysis, specifically for image classification, object detection, segmentation, registration and other tasks. In addition, the areas of application of deep learning were neuro, retinal, pulmonary, digital pathology, breast, cardiac, abdominal and musculoskeletal.

Dinggang Shen et al. [5] claimed that deep learning has helped many researchers in the area of computer vision to identify, classify and quantify patterns in medical images. They specifically argued that deep learning is useful in exploiting hierarchical features from data itself than feature engineering using handcrafting using human effort. Suzuki [6] in his survey paper overviewed the area of deep learning and its application in medical imaging analysis to assess what was changed before and after the introduction of deep learning in machine learning, identifying the reasons that make deep learning powerful and their applications to medical image analysis.

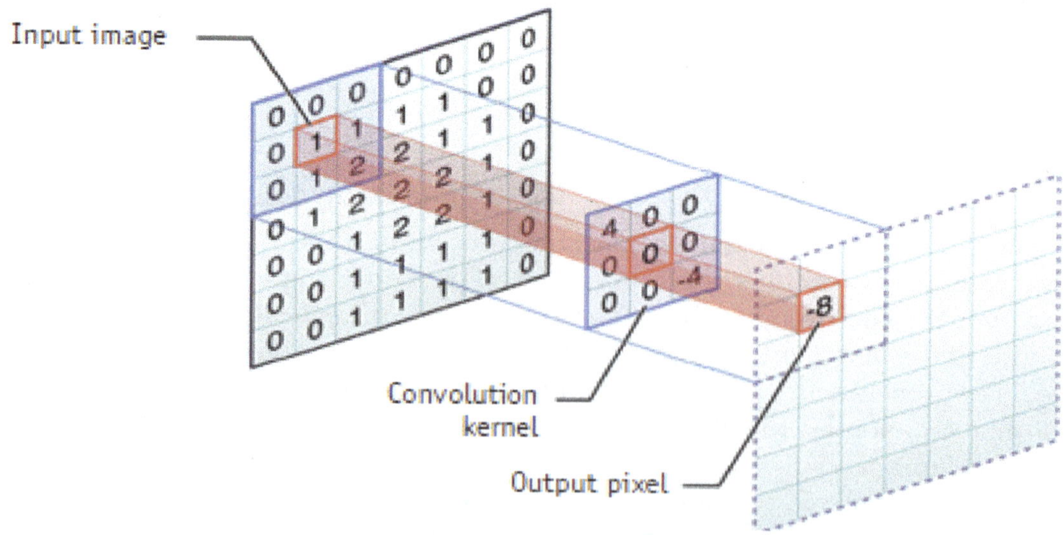

Figure 1. Example of convolution operation from [7].

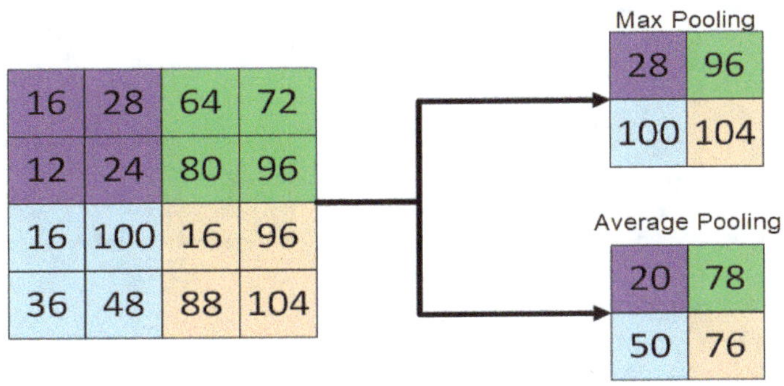

Figure 2. Example of down sampling operation using max-pooling and average-pooling.

In this survey paper, we briefly describe the breast cancer, cervical cancer, brain tumor, colon cancer and lung cancer along with their respective screening methods. Finally, we reviewed the application of deep learning for each cancer type in terms of deep learning application types like feature extraction, detection, segmentation, prediction and classification. The motivation behind selecting the cancer type for the survey was based on the cancer statistics reported in 2018 by the World Health Organization as presented in Table 1.

Table 1. World Health Organization 2018 statistical report through the global cancer observatory.

Cancer Type	New Cases (%)	Death Rate (%)
Breast Cancer	11.6	6.6
Colon Cancer	10.2	9.2
Brain Tumor	3.5	2.8
Cervical Cancer	3.2	2.5
Stomach Cancer	5.7	8.2
Liver Cancer	4.7	8.2
Lung Cancer	11.6	18.4

2. Methods

Published papers from 2016 to 2020 were considered and reviewed to (1) assess the application of deep learning for breast cancer, (2) assess the application of deep learning for cervical cancer, (3) assess the application of deep learning for a brain tumor and (4) assess the application of deep learning for colon cancer. We first defined a search criterion for the selected search databases. Our general search criteria for this survey paper are ((“colon” OR “colorectal”) AND (“cancer” OR “polyp”) AND (“deep learning”) AND (“Image”) AND (“detection” OR “classification” OR “segmentation” OR “Localization”)) OR ((“breast”) AND (“cancer” OR “mass”) AND (“deep learning”) AND (“Image”) AND (“detection” OR “classification” OR “segmentation” OR “Localization”)) OR ((“Brain”) AND (“Tumor”) AND (“deep learning”)AND (“MRI”) AND (“detection” OR “classification” OR “segmentation” OR “Localization”)) OR (“Cervix” OR “Cervical”) AND (“Deep Learning”) AND (“Classification” OR “segmentation”). The searches were carried out from four databases: (1) PubMed, (2) Science Direct, (3) IEEE Xplore Digital Library and (4) Google Scholar. The search framework of the survey paper is presented in Figure 3 and the major performance metrics used to evaluate deep learning approach applied to the selected medical images are presented in Section 2.1.

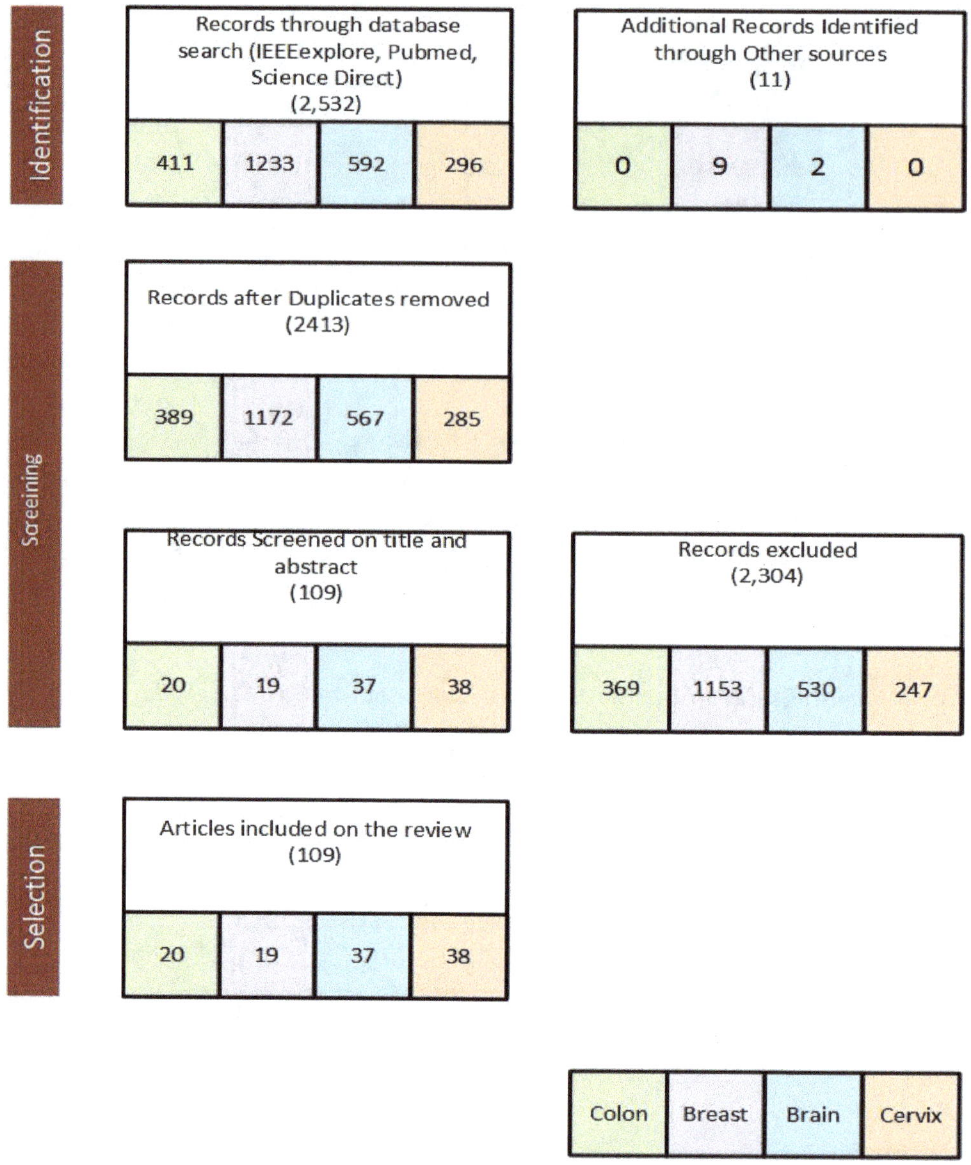

Figure 3. Search criteria framework used for IEEEexplore, PubMed, Google Scholar and Science Direct engines to select papers for review.

2.1. Segmentation and Classification Performance Metrics

Most of the performance metrics encountered in the review include area under curve (AUC), sensitivity (Sn), specificity (Sp), accuracy (Acc), precision (P), recall (R), positive predictive values (PPV), Matthews correlation coefficient (MCC), geometric mean (G-Mean), which are usually successful in describing the classification performance [8,9]. Performance measures including Dice similarity coefficient (DSC) or Zijdenbos similarity index (ZSI) or F1-score, Hausdorff distance (H) and intersection over union (IoU) are the most effective metrics for measuring system's segmentation performance [10]. Here, the true positives for the segmentation are the correctly labeled pixel while it is correctly labeled class for classification case.

3. Deep Learning in Tumor Detection, Segmentation and Classification

Region-based segmentation technique was in use in medical image analysis until the deep learning approach evolved in the field of computer vision [8]. However, Lee et al. [7] in their survey paper indicated that the existence of deep learning in the research community has become a reason to use object recognition in an image. In addition to object detection, deep learning has been applied for feature extraction, abnormality detection, cancer/tumor segmentation and classification [11].

3.1. Breast Cancer

Breast cancer occurs when there is uncontrolled growth of cells in the breast [12]. It is the most widely diagnosed type of cancer in women and the first prevalent cancer type in Ethiopia [11,13]. There are four types of breast cancer manifestation that include: mass, calcification, architectural distortion and bilateral asymmetry [11].

3.1.1. Screening Methods

As presented in Debelee et al. [11], breast cancer image analysis and breast abnormality detection start with breast cancer screening. Breast cancer screening methods include screen film mammography (SFM), digital mammography (DM), ultrasound (US), magnetic resonance imaging (MRI), digital breast tomosynthesis (DBT) and combinations of the screening methods.

3.1.2. Datasets

There are many datasets prepared for medical image analysis based on the different imaging modalities. The most common and available dataset for the breast cancer is of mammography and histopathology datasets. Some of the most common datasets are discussed in Table 2.

Table 2. Image datasets for breast cancer image analysis.

Dataset	Size	#Classes/Targets	Format	Type	Author/Repository, Year
MIAS	322	2	pgm	Mammography	Suckling, J. et al. [14]
DDSM	55,890		npy	Mammography	Scuccimarra [15]
InBreast		410	XML	Mammography	Moreira et al. [16]
Breast Cancer Wisconsin	568	3	csv	Mammography	Dua, D. and Graff, C. [17]
BreakHis	7909	2	png	Histology	Bukun [18]
BACH/ICIAR2018	400	4	tiff	Histology	G.Aresta [19]

3.1.3. Deep Learning for Detection of Breast Cancer Through Diagnostic Medical Imaging Techniques

Li Shen et al. [2] proposed a deep learning-based breast cancer detection algorithm using end-to-end training approach using mammographic images from the Digital Database for Screening Mammography (DDSM) and INbreast databases. The deep learning architectures used in their paper were ResNet-50 and VGGNet-16. The proposed approach was evaluated in terms of AUC at single model and four-model (ResNet-ResNet, ResNet-VGGNet, VGGNet-VGGNet and VGGNet-ResNet) averaging level. For the DDSM dataset, the best single model achieved a per-image AUC of 0.88, and four-model averaging improved the AUC to 0.91 with sensitivity of 86.1% and specificity of 80.1%. For INbreast database, the best single model achieved per-image AUC of 0.95, and four-model averaging achieved a better AUC value of 0.98 with sensitivity of 86.7% and specificity of 96.1%.

Wu et al. [20] proposed a DCNN architecture based on four columns of ResNet-22 to classify breast cancer screening exams using mammography. There was a total of 200,000 exams which incorporated over 1,000,000 images to train and evaluate the proposed DCNN model. The performance of their network achieved an AUC of 0.895 in predicting whether there is a cancer in the breast, when tested on the screening population and the result was compared to 14 radiologists reading results.

Alzubaidi et al. [21] transfer learning approach on their proposed 74 layer CNN. Their model was pre-trained on one same domain image dataset (erythrocytesIDB dataset, which has images of peripheral blood smears samples taken from patients with Sickle Cell Disease). They divided the original microscopy image into 12 patches and used majority voting for the classification, where the most frequent patch label is chosen to be the image label. The model achieved a patch level accuracy of 90.5% and image-level accuracy of 97.4%. The majority voting they employed seemed not a correct way since if the cells are the majority of normals and if it still has cancerous cells, the system might classify them as normal, which is not good.

Zhu et al. [22] proposed two deep learning approach to predict the occurrence of invasive cancer on MRI images. The first approach was based on transfer learning using GoogleNet pre-trained model to predict the presence of invasive cancer. As a second approach, the authors extracted features from the natural images and used SVM to predict the invasive disease. The best classification result gained in terms of AUC was 0.53 for transfer learning approach and 0.70 for extracted features.

Li et al. [23] explored the abilities of digital breast tomosynthesis (DBT) and full-field digital mammography (FFDM) in mass classification using deep neural networks equipped with or without transfer learning. They also explored an eligible combination strategy of DBT and FFDM in enhancing classification performance. They applied a 16-layer VGG network (VGG-16) and 11-layer deep convolutional neural network (DCNN) for the 2D images and extend the 11-layer DCNN to accommodate the extra dimension in 3D DBT images. The best performer from these methods, a 2D-DCNN which was trained by combining the DBT and FFDM, achieved the highest performance with average AUC, accuracy, sensitivity and specificity of 0.95, 92.13%, 83% and 93.84%, respectively on three class classification (benign, malignant, normal).

Zeiser et al. [24] explored the application of the U-Net model with different depths with or without data augmentation for the segmentation of masses on mammograms. The U-Net model trained with depth of 5 and with data augmentation was the best performer with sensitivity of 92.32%, specificity of 80.47%, accuracy of 85.95%, Dice index of 79.39% and AUC of 86.40% on the DDSM dataset.

Shen et al. [2] applied an ensemble of four best performing deep learning models which were designed based on Resnet50 and VGG16 as patch classifiers and Resnet and VGG blocks as top layer for breast cancer classification. The ensemble of these classifiers achieved the best AUC of 0.91 (sensitivity: 86.1%, specificity: 80.1%) on the detection of benign and malignant masses and classifications on the DDSM dataset.

Zhang et al. [25] used U-net architecture for the segmentation and extraction of fat tissue, fibroglandular tissue (FGT) inside the breast, and all nonbreast tissues outside the breast in breast MRI. They achieved mean DSC of 0.95 for breast and 0.91 for FGT; and mean accuracy of 0.98 for breast and 0.97 for FGT.

Zhou et al. [26] applied 3D deep convolutional neural network (CNN) based on 3D DenseNet [27] architecture with 37 layers for diagnosing breast cancer and localizing the lesions at dynamic contrast enhanced (DCE) MRI data in a weakly supervised manner. The proposed algorithm performance for breast cancer diagnosis showed 83.7% accuracy, 90.8% sensitivity, 69.3% specificity, 0.859 AUC and 0.501 Dice distance.

Summary of the performance of the above reviewed work can be summarized in Table 3.

3.1.4. Deep Learning for Breast Histopathology Image Analysis

Breast histopathology helps to confirm the presence of cancerous sales detected by other imaging modalities. Since histology slides may contain millions of cells and identifying the cancerous sales from the slides is time consuming and tedious job. Hence there are many varieties of research done in this area.

Table 3. Summary of scientific papers on detection of breast cancer using diagnostic medical imaging techniques.

Author and Citation	Dataset	AUC	Sn (%)	Sp (%)	Acc (%)	Target
	Siemens and Hologic	0.933	-	-	-	Detection
Wu et al. [20]	Personal	0.895	-	-	-	Classification/Prediction
Shen et al. [2] (Single-Model)	DDSM INbreast	0.88 0.95	- -	- -	- -	Detection Detection
Shen et al. [2] (Four-Models Average)	DDSM INbreast	0.91 0.98	86.1 86.7	80.1 96.1	- -	Detection Detection
Zhu et al. [22] (Transfer learning)	-	0.53	-	-	-	Prediction
Zhu et al. [22] (SVM)	-	0.7	-	-	-	Prediction
Li et al. [23]	-	0.95	83	93.84	92.13	Classification
Zeiser et al. [24]	DDSM	0.86	92.32	80.47	85.95	Segmentation
Zhang et al. [28]	-	-	-	-	97.5	Detection
Zhou et al. [26]	-	0.86	90.8	69.3	83.7	Classification

Sheikh et al. [29] proposed a multi-scale input and multi-feature CNN network for the classification of histopathological images. They concatenate four scales (1 ×, 0.5 ×, 0.33 × and 0.25 ×) of the original normalized image to accommodate the scale variant property of the cells and used it as an input to the CNN network. They trained their proposed model on ICIAR2018 and BreakHits datasets. The model achieved a satisfactory max accuracy of 0.83 for the ICIAR2018 dataset and 0.98 for the BreakHis dataset for binary classification. For the multiclass classification, the proposed model's accuracy was rather unsatisfactory reaching as low as 60% for the ICIAR2018 dataset.

Li et al. [30] modified the Densenet-121 architecture by removing the pooling layers of the 4th Dense-block and feeding the extracted feature maps from each Dense-block to the squeeze-and-excitation (SENet) module for breast histopathology images. The used SENet for receiving more channel-wise information. After concatenating each SENet output, they used a fully-connected layer for the classification purpose. They used a pre-trained Densenet model for their architecture using the transfer-learning approach. Using the publicly available BreakHis dataset, their algorithm achieved an average accuracy of 88% over different magnification levels for binary classification.

Yan et al. [31] used the transfer-learning approach by using Google's Inception-V3 model as patch-wise feature extraction and image-wise long short-term memory (LSTM) for classifying breast histopathological images into four classes, namely normal, benign, in situ and invasive. They fine-tuned the Inception-V3 model. Their proposed model achieved an average accuracy of 91% on the ICIAR2018 dataset.

Sharma et al. [32] studied the use of pre-trained deep learning networks as feature extractor from breast cancer histopathology images. They used transfer learning on the pre-existing networks (VGG16, VGG19 and ResNet50) for using them as feature extractor. The extracted features were then classified using SVM classifier. The VGG16 network with linear SVM achieved the highest accuracy (93.97% for 40 ×, 92.92% for 100 ×, 91.23% for 200 × and 91.79% for 400 × magnifications).

Vang et al. [33] proposed ensemble classifier and reinforcement backed deep learning approach using inception-V3 for multiclass (normal, benign, in situ and invasive) classification. The ensemble fusion approach for image level prediction involved majority voting, gradient boosting machine (GBM) and logistic regression. Their approach performed low in terms of sensitivity for the two classes (benign and normal). The sensitivity of the normal and benign predicted classes was improved by adding a dual path network (DPN) to use it as feature extractor. However, the extracted features were further sent to the next layer of ensemble prediction fusion using GBM, logistic regression and support vector machine (SVM) to refine predictions. This approach was evaluated in terms of accuracy and scored an accuracy of 87.5%.

Alzubaidi et al. [21] transfer learning approach onto their proposed 74 layer CNN. They pre-trained their model on one same domain image dataset (erythrocytesIDB dataset, which has images of peripheral blood smears samples taken from patients with Sickle Cell Disease). They divided the original microscopy image into 12 patches and used majority voting for the classification, where the most frequent patch label is chosen to be the image label. The model training was don on the ICIAR 2018 dataset. The model achieved patch level accuracy of 90.5% and image level accuracy of 97.4%. The majority voting they employed seemed not a correct way since if the cells are majority of normal and if it still has cancerous cells the system might classify them as normal, which is not good.

The summary of papers explored in classification of breast histological slides can be summarized in Table 4. From the literature reviews the algorithm proposed by Yan et al. [31] seems the best method for histopathological breast cancer detection.

Table 4. Summary of scientific papers on classification of breast cancer using histopathological images.

Author and Citation	Dataset	Acc	Sn (%)	Sp (%)
	Siemens and Hologic	0.933	-	-
Vang et al. [33]	ICIAR2018 (H & E)	87.5	-	-
Sharma and Mehra [32]	BreakHis	93.97	-	-
Sheikh et al. [29]	ICIAR2018 and BreakHis	83 98	-	-
Li et al. [30]	ICIAR2018	88	-	-
Yan et al. [31]	ICIAR2018	91	-	-
Alzubaidi et al. [21]	ICIAR 2018	97.4	-	

3.1.5. Summary

As presented in Tables 5 and 6, the deep learning architecture involved in the recently published, from 2016 to 2020, breast cancer we considered in this survey paper were ResNet, VGGNet, AlexNet, Inception V3, U-Net and DenseNet.

Table 5. Summary of breast cancer scientific papers in terms of convolutional neurla network (CNN) architecture and type of environment used in the selected papers.

Authors	Network	Pre-Training	Transfer Learning	Environment
Wu et al. [20]	ResNet-22	Yes	No	TensorFlow
Shen et al. [2]	ResNet-50, VGGNet-16	Yes	Yes	-
Vang et al. [33]	Inception V3	Yes	No	TensorFlow
Zhu et al. [22]	GoogleNet	Yes	Yes	Caffe
Li et al. [23]	VGGNet-16	Yes	Yes	-
Sharma and Mehra [32]	VGGNet-16, VGGNet-19, ResNet50	Yes	Yes	Keras, TensorFlow
Zeiser et al. [24]	U-net	No	No	-
Zhang et al. [28]	U-net	No	No	TensorFlow
Zhou et al. [26]	3D DensNet	No	No	-
Sheikh et al. [29]	MSI-MFNet	No	No	Keras
Li et al. [30]	IDSNet	Yes	Yes	Tensorflow
Yan et al. [31]	Inception-V3	Yes	Yes	Tensorflow
Alzubaidi et al. [21]	ResNet	Yes	Yes	-

Table 6. Summary of breast cancer scientific papers in terms of publication year, name of journal/conference for the selected papers and its impact factor with year of impact factor.

Authors	Publication Year	Journal/Conf.	Impact Factor	Year of Impact Factor
Wu et al. [20]	2020	ITMI	6.85	2020
Shen et al. [2]	2019	Scientific Reports	3.998	2019
Vang et al. [33]	2018	CBM	5.4	2019
Zhu et al. [22]	2019	CBM	3.434	2020
Li et al. [23]	2019	European Radiology	4.101	2019
Sharma and Mehra [32]	2020	Journal of Digital Imaging	2.99	2018
Zeiser et al. [24]	2020	Journal of Digital Imaging	2.99	2018
Zhang et al. [28]	2018	Academic Radiology	2.50	2020
Dembrower et al. [34]	2020	Radiology	7.608	2018
Zhou et al. [26]	2019	Journal of Magnetic Resonance Imaging	2.112	2018
Sheikh et al. [29]	2020	MDPI, Cancers	6.126	2019
Li et al. [30]	2020	Plos One	2.74	2019
Yan et al. [31]	2020	Elsevier, Methods	3.812	2019
Alzubaidi et al. [21]	2020	MDPI, electronics	2.412	2019

As indicated in Table 7, the result of almost all papers in this survey paper were not compared with the domain specialists and performance of the traditional machine learning algorithms.

Table 7. Summary of breast cancer scientific papers in terms of comparison to specialists and/or traditional techniques.

Author and Citation	Comparison to Specialists	Comparison to Traditional Technique (Yes/No)
Hagos et al. [35]	No	No
Wu et al. [20]	Yes	No
Shen et al. [2]	No	No
Vang et al. [33]	No	No
Zhu et al. [22]	No	No
Li et al. [23]	No	No
Sharma and Mehra [32]	No	Yes
Zeiser et al. [24]	No	Yes
Zhang et al. [28]	No	No
Zhou et al. [26]	Yes	Yes
Sheikh et al. [29]	No	Yes
Li et al. [30]	No	Yes
Yan et al. [31]	No	Yes
Alzubaidi et al. [21]	No	yes

3.2. *Cervical Cancer*

Cervical cancer is one of the most common cancers among women worldwide, especially in developing nations, and it has a relatively high incidence and mortality rates [36]. Cervical cancer usually develops slowly over time. When cervical cancer begins in the cervix, cervical cells go through changes called dysplasia, in which cells that are not normal begin to appear in the cervical tissue. In its later stage, cancer cells start to multiply and proliferate more deeply into the cervix and to surrounding areas. Fortunately, cervical cancer is mostly preventable with active screening and detection techniques.

For example, preventive screening and early detection can decrease the morbidity of cervical cancer by about 70% in the United States [37].

3.2.1. Screening Methods

Nowadays, there are a few frequently-used cervical cancer screening techniques, such as high-risk human papillomavirus (HPV) testing, Pap smear cytology testing, colposcopy and visual inspection of the cervix with acetic acid (VIA), each of which has its advantages and disadvantages.

- **Bimanual pelvic examination.** This is a visual and physical inspection by the physician. It consists of both visual inspections using a device called a speculum and physical inspection by using fingers. This test is not enough on its own and the Pap test is usually performed next.
- **Cervical cytopathology** Papanicolaou Smear (Pap smear) or liquid-based cytology is a process of gently scraping cervical cells and inspection of those cells under a microscope. It can also be analyzed digitally using computers.
- **HPV typing test.** Cervical cancer usually occurs from persistent infection of the cervix with some carcinogenic types of human papillomavirus (HPV) such as HPV16 and HPV18 [38]. It is usually performed along with a Pap test or after Pap test results show abnormal changes to the cervix. The occurrence of HPV does not confirm cancer.
- **Colposcopy.** Colposcopy is a visual inspection of the cervix using a special instrument called a colposcope. The device magnifies the cervix area under inspection like a microscope. It can be used for pregnant women.

Other types of tests were also used for cervical cancer screening such as X-ray, CT scan, MRI and PET scan but they are more expensive and used to detect advanced stages of cancer.

Cervical cytology (Pap test) is the most common test used to look for early changes in cells that can lead to cervical cancer [39]. It has been widely used for the screening of cervical cancer in developed countries and is effective in reducing the number of deaths. It is still unavailable for population-wide screening in the developing countries. This is because screening using cervical cytology is difficult, tedious, time-consuming, expensive and subjected to errors because each slide contains around three million cells with large shape and appearance variation between cells, the poor contrast of cytoplasm boundaries and the overlap between cells [40]. In developed countries like the United Kingdom, cervical cancer screening is performed every 3 years for women aged 25 to 49 years and every 5 years aged 50 to 64 years [41]. Over the past few decades, many types of research were performed in developing a computer-assisted cervical cancer screening method. Most of these researches tried to automatically identify the various stages of cancer or abnormality types by classifying cells on the Pap-smear slides. Most of these classifications consist of cell or nuclei segmentation, feature extraction and classification steps [42].

3.2.2. Datasets for Cervical Cancer

Most of the research regarding the detection and segmentation of cervical cancer used the Herlev dataset. The pap-smear benchmark database provides data for comparing classification methods. The data consists of 917 images of pap-smear cells, classified carefully by cyto-technicians and doctors [43]. The dataset is distributed unevenly into seven classes, namely superficial squamous, squamous intermediate, columnar, moderate dysplasia, moderate dysplasia, severe dysplasia and carcinoma in situ. Each image in the Herlev dataset contains only a single cell. Each slide contains many cells and cells might also overlap. Hussien [44] prepared a more realistic dataset for the classification of cervical cells. Summary of the publicly available datasets for classification and segmentation of cervical cells and cervix is given in Table 8.

Table 8. Image datasets for cervical cancer.

Dataset	Size	#Classes/Targets	Format	Type	Author, Year
Herlev	917	187	Bit Map(BMP)	Histology	Dr J. Jantzen [43]
DANS-KNAW	963	4	jpg	Histology	Hussien [44]
CRIC	400	6	png and csv	Histology	M.T. Rezende et al. [45]
Zenodo	962	4	jpg	Histology	Franco et al. [46]
ALTS	938	2	jpg	Colposcopy	Alts Group [47]
MobileODT	1448	3	jpg	Colposcopy	MobileODT [48]

3.2.3. Deep Learning for Segmentation of Cervical Cells

Traditional cytological criteria for classifying cervical cell abnormalities are based on the changes in the nucleus to cytoplasm ratio, nuclear size, irregularity of nuclear shape and membrane. In normal cells, the cytoplasm appears much larger than the nucleus with the regular shaped nuclei. Therefore numerous works are focusing on the segmentation of cell or cell components (nuclei, cytoplasm) [41]. Deep learning has been applied for the segmentation of cervical cell nuclei and the whole cell itself. The successful segmentation of each cervical cell from the slides gives a better performance for cancerous cells. Nuclei detection is only maybe helpful and is easier than segmentation of the whole cell and may be enough for the detection of cancer or help for the segmentation of the whole cell.

Song et al. [49] tried to improve cervical cell segmentation by using learning-based segmentation when overlapping cells are encountered. They include high-level shape information to guide the segmentation algorithm which is done by the convolutional neural network algorithm. They evaluated their algorithm in nuclei detection and cervical cell segmentation. By using the datasets ISBI 2015 challenge dataset, and SZU dataset they achieved a Dice similarity coefficient (DSC) of 0.95 and 0.89, respectively.

Zhao et al. [50] proposed an algorithm called Progressive Growing of U-net + (PGU-net +) for Automated Cervical Nuclei Segmentation, which tried to modify the original U-net algorithm [51], which augmented the limited medical dataset for use of deep learning. They claimed these augmentations mix the information of different scales that affect each other; hence, it limits the segmentation accuracy of the model. they proposed a progressive growing U-net (PGU-net +) model, which extracts image features at each scale independently and passing residual information with the next scale. They achieved a segmentation accuracy of 0.925 on the Herlev dataset, with precision 0.901 ± 0.13, recall 0.968 ± 0.04 and ZSI of 0.925 ± 0.09.

Sompawong et al. [52] applied a pre-trained Mask R-CNN for cervical cancer nuclei detection, segmentation and classification into normal and abnormal ones. They used liquid-based histological slides obtained from Thammasat University (TU) Hospital and obtained mean average precision (mAP) of 57.8%, the accuracy of 91.7%, the sensitivity of 91.7% and specificity of 91.7% per image. They used DeepPap as a benchmark to evaluate their algorithm. Since DeepPap used the Herlev dataset (containing images of single cells) for training and testing. It needs to be modified and retrained on the TU dataset. They showed the proposed algorithm performs better than the modified DeepPap on the TU dataset. They did not evaluate the Mask R-CNN algorithm on the Herlev dataset.

Liu et al. [53] proposed a cervical nucleus segmentation method in which pixel-level prior information was utilized to provide the supervisory information for the training of a mask regional convolutional neural network (Mask R-CNN). They added a local fully-connected conditional random field (LFCCRF) to refine the segmentation. Using the Herlev Pap smear dataset, the proposed method achieved 0.96 in both precision and recall and 0.95 in the Zijdenbos similarity index.

Liang et al. [42] used a comparison based detection which combines the decision of two CNN architectures. First reference, samples were obtained by using the ResNet50 with Feature Pyramid Network (FPN) architecture from each cell image from the dataset. At the same time features from the whole slide image, which contains many cells, were extracted through ResNet50 with FPN and region proposal network (RPN). They replaced the original parameter classifier from their baseline network, Faster R-CNN with FPN with their comparison classifier. Their proposed algorithm can detect 11 different cell types from the whole slide. The performance of the proposed algorithm achieved mean average precision (mAP) of 26.3% and average recall (AR) of 35.7%. They argue these performance measurements do not reflect how good the algorithm was since the proposed algorithm groups multiple neighboring cells with the same category into one result.

Kurnianingsih et al. [54] used deep learning methods to segment cervical cells and classify them. For the segmentation purpose, transfer learning was applied on Mask R-CNN weights trained using the COCO dataset. The pre-trained model was trained to segment cervical cell area consisting of both nuclei and cytoplasm. In the segmentation phase, when Mask R-CNN is applied to the whole cell, it outperforms the previous segmentation method in precision (0.92 $\pm$ 0.06), recall (0.91 $\pm$ 0.05) and ZSI (0.91 $\pm$ 0.04).

Deep learning-based segmentation into nuclei segmentation and cell segmentation can be summarized (see Tables 9 and 10).

Table 9. Summary of selected papers on nuclei segmentation.

Authors	Method	Dataset	Acc	P	R	F1	Sp	Sn	ZSI
Zhao et al. [50]	Progressive Growing of U-net+(PGU-net+)	Herlev	0.925	0.901	0.968				0.925
Liu et al. [53]	Mask-RCNN with LFCCRF	Herlev		0.96	0.96				0.95
Sompawong et al. [52]	Mask-RCNN	TU	89.8%				94.3%	72.5%	

Table 10. Summary of selected papers on cervical cell segmentation.

Authors	Method	Dataset	Acc	P	R	ZSI	DSC
Kurnianingsih et al. [54]	Mask R-CNN	Herlev		0.92	0.91	0.91	
Song et al. [49]	CNN with Shape information	Herlev					0.92
Liang et al. [42]	comparison based Faster R-CNN	local		26.3	35.7		

3.2.4. Deep Learning for Cervical Cell Classification

Zhang et al. [55] tried to directly classify cervical cells—without prior segmentation—based on deep features, using convolutional neural networks (ConvNets). In their algorithm (DeepPap), a pre-trained ConvNets was trained on a cervical cell dataset consisting of adaptively re-sampled image patches coarsely centered on the nuclei. Then they applied aggregation to average the prediction scores of a similar set of image patches. The proposed algorithm achieved classification accuracy (98.3%), area under the curve (AUC) (0.99) values and specificity (98.3%) on the Herlev dataset.

Hyeon et al. [56] proposed a CNN-based pre-trained model, VGGNet-16 for feature extraction, and use different classifiers namely: logistic regression, random forests, AdaBoost and SVM for classification of the pap-test images into normal and abnormal. From these classifiers, the highest scoring one is the SVM classifier with an F1-score of 0.7817 on a dataset collected locally.

LIN et al. [57] applied the transfer learning approach to fine-tune different CNN models (AlexNet, GoogLeNet, ResNet and DenseNet) which were pre-trained on ImageNet dataset [58]. The pre-trained models were fine-tuned on the Herlev cervical dataset with additional cytoplasm and nucleus morphological masks. They achieved classification accuracies of 94.5%, 71.3% and 64.5%, for two-class (abnormal versus normal), four-class (normal, low-grade squamous intraepithelial lesion (LSIL), high-grade squamous intraepithelial lesion (HSIL) and carcinoma-in-situ (CIS) [59]) and seven-class ("World Health Organization classification system") classification tasks, respectively.

Chen et al. [60] tried to combine features extracted from different types of tests. They proposed a Faster R-CNN, which is based on Faster R-CNN for fusing acetic and iodine images of the cervix.

They fuse non-image features extracted from the cervix transformation zone type, pap test, HPV test and age after they non-linearly compression of the fused image features to 29D by using one fully connected (FC) layer. They did not mention which classifier they used for normal–abnormal classification but achieved an accuracy of 87.4% (88.6% sensitivity and 86.1% specificity) on a locally collected dataset.

Kurnianingsih et al. [54] trained a compact VGG network based on their Mask R-CNN based segmentation algorithm. For the classification, a compact VGG Net classifier yields a sensitivity score of more than 96% with a low standard deviation (± 2.8%) for the binary classification problem and yields a higher result of more than 95% with low standard deviation (maximum 4.2%) for the 7-class problem.

Performance comparison of different pre-trained deep learning models on Pap smear classification was done by Promworn et al. [61]. They compared the performance of CNN models namely resnet101, densenet161, AlexNet, vgg19_bn and squeeznet1_1, which are the top five models based on accuracy in ImageNet. The models are retrained on the Herlev dataset. Based on accuracy, densenet161 was the best performer on both binary classification (94.38%) and multiclass classification (68.54). Based on sensitivity, AlexNet and resnet have achieved 100% on binary classification. Whereas densenet161 was the best performer on multiclass classification with 68.18%. Again, based on specificity, densenet161 was superior with values 82.61% for binary and 69.57% for multiclass classification.

Yutao Ma et al. [62] developed a CADx system by using a convolutional neural network (CNN) for feature extraction and support vector machines (SVM) for classifying the optical coherence microscopy (OCM) images into five classes namely normal, ectropion, low-grade and high-grade squamous intraepithelial lesions (LSIL and HSIL) and cancer. They also used HPV test results for the classification in conjunction with features extracted from the OCM images by the CNN. An 88.3 ± 4.9% classification accuracy was achieved for all five classes. In the binary classification task (low-risk (normal, ectropion and LSIL) vs. high-risk (HSIL and cancer)), the CADx method achieved an area under the curve (AUC) value of 0.959 with 86.7 ± 11.4% sensitivity and 93.5 ± 3.8% specificity.

Ahmed et al. [63] proposed transfer learning-based approaches for the classification of cervical cells. They explored six different methods for the classification of cervical cells by combining three pre-trained models as features, shallow CNN, which consisted of only two convolutional layers and two max-pooling layers, VGG-16 Net and CaffeNet as a feature extraction technique and two classifiers, extreme learning machine (ELM) and auto encoder (AE) for the classification purpose. They used the Herlev dataset for training and testing their system. The best performer from these combinations is the CaffeNet+ELM which achieved a binary classification accuracy of 99.7 and 97.2 for the 7 class classification.

Dong et al. [64] used artificially extracted features such as color, texture and morphology along with the Inception-V3 model for the classification of cervical cells. They used features extracted manually since the features extracted from the CNN architecture since the knowledge of cervical cells is lacking there. Nine artificial features were combined with features extracted from the Inception-V3 architecture joined on the fully connected layer and used the Softmax function for the classification. They keep the aspect ratio of the cells when resizing for the Inception-V3 network will harm the morphological features. The proposed algorithm achieved an overall accuracy of 98.2%, the sensitivity of 99.4% and specificity of 96.73% for normal abnormal classification on the Herlev dataset.

Martinez-Mias et al. [65] tried to improve and make it realistic the cervical classification from PAP smears using a cell merger approach. They used CNN for PAP smear image classification, and optimize and integrate the cell fusion approach since most PAP smear slides contain overlapping cells. They used a local PAP smear dataset collected from ten patients and labeled using biopsy results. Hence, it was used as a gold standard. They trained the CaffeNet model using data prepared using a cell merger to reflect the reality of the PAP smear examination. For classifying the cervical cells into four classes the CaffeNet with the cell merger dataset achieved an average accuracy of just 55.6% with the performance as low as just 16.7% for LSIL class. For the normal/abnormal classification, their proposed algorithm achieved an accuracy, sensitivity and specificity of 88.8%, 0.92 and 0.83, respectively. This performance is satisfactory considering the classification was done on overlapping cell regions.

Xiang et al. [66] used YOLOv3 as a cell detector and Inception-V3-based classifier for cervical cell classification into ten classes that could be present on the slide namely, normal cells (NORMAL), atypical squamous cells-undetermined significance (ASC-US), atypical squamous cells-cannot exclude HSIL(ASC-H), low-grade squamous intraepithelial lesion (LSIL), high-grade squamous intraepithelial lesion (HSIL), atypical glandular cells (AGC), adenocarcinoma (ADE), vaginalis trichomoniasis (VAG), monilia (MON) and dysbacteriosis (DYS). The model achieves 97.5% sensitivity (Sens) and 67.8% specificity (Spec) on cervical cell image-level screening.

The cervical cell classification algorithms can be categorized into two categories, binary and multiclass. In the binary classification cervical cells are classified into normal and abnormal cells (see Table 11). Multiclass classification describing the severity of the cancer including the normal ones (see Table 12).

Table 11. Summary of selected papers on cervical cell binary classification.

Authors	Method	Dataset	Acc(%)	Sn(%)	Sp(%)	AUC	F1	P	R
Zhang et al. [55]	DeepPap	Herlev	98.3	-	98.3	0.99	-	-	-
Hyeon et al. [56]	VGG16	SVM	local	-	-	-	0.78	0.78	0.78
Lin et al. [57]	GoogleNet5C	Herlev	94.5	-	-	-	-	-	-
Chen et al. [60]	Mask R-CNN 7 class	local-	87.4	88.6	86.1	-	-	-	-
Kurnianingsih et al. [54]	Mask R-CNN	Herlev	98.1	96.7	98.6	96.5	-	-	-
Promworn et al. [61]	densenet161	Herlev	94.38	100	-	-	-	-	-
Yutao Ma et al. [62]	CNN and SVM	OCM image	-	86.7	93.5	0.96	-	-	-
Ahmed et al. [63]	CaffNet+ELM	Herlev	99.5	-	-	-	-	-	-
Dong et al. [64]	Inception-V3	Herlev	98.23	99.4	96.7	-	-	-	-
Martinez-Mias et al. [65]	CaffeNet	Local	88.8	92	83	-	-	-	-

Table 12. Summary of selected papers on cervical cell multiclass classification.

Authors	Method	Dataset	Acc	Sn	Sp	Others
	regressor 7 classes					
Yutao Ma et al. [62]	CNN and SVM 5 classes	OCM image	88.3			
Lin et al. [57]	GoogleNet5C 4 classes	Herlev Dataset	71.3			
Lin et al. [57]	GoogleNet5C seven classes	Herlev Dataset	64.5			
Kurnianingsih et al. [54]	Mask R-CNN 7 class	Herlev	95.9	96.2	99.3	
Promworn et al. [61]	densenet161 7 classes	Herlev dataset	68.54	68.18	69.57	
Ahmed et al. [63]	CaffNet+ELM	Herlev	91.2	-	-	-
Martinez-Mias et al. [65]	CaffeNet	Local	55.6	-	-	-
Xiang et al. [66]	YOLOv3+InceptionV3	local	89.3	97.5	67.8	-

3.2.5. Deep Learning for Cervix Classification

Colposcopic images are also used for cervical cancer detection using deep learning methods. A colposcopy helps to observe the cervix at up to ×10 magnification [67]. Cervical intraepithelial lesions are easily recognized when treated with acetic acid solutions using colposcopy.

Cervix type classification from smartphone camera was tried in [68] using capsule networks which achieves an accuracy of 94%. A more advanced approach called CervixNet [69] which is designed based on a novel hierarchical convolutional mixture of experts (HCME) method achieved an accuracy of 96.77%.

M. Arora et al. [70] used the transfer learning approach from a pre-trained CNN, Inception V3 model [71] by modifying the output layer. The output layer was replaced by a pooling layer and a fully connected layer for the classification of the cervix based on its image. A cervical image dataset from Kaggle was used here, which has three types of cervix based on the location of the transformation layer. The type of cervix will help the physician whether further tests are needed or not. They obtained an average accuracy of just 54.54%.

Guo et al. [72] explored the application of two versions of regions with convolutional neural networks (R-CNN), Mask R-CNN and Mask^X R-CNN, on three different dataset for cervix classification for automatic segmentation of cervix region. Mask R-CNN is effective on datasets with annotations having the exact boundaries. The Mask^X R-CNN can also trained the bounding box annotation. The highest performance was achieved using Mask R-CNN with Dice and IoU of 0.947 and 0.901, respectively. Mask^X R-CNN also achieved a very good performance with Dice and IoU of 0.92 and 0.86 respectively. These colposcopy images suffer from presense of many distractors such as pubic hair, intra-uterine devices (IUDs), the speculum and even parts of human hand. The main problem in cervix classification from cervix photos is the presence of out of focus images [73].

Guo et al. [74] used an ensemble of three deep learning architectures, RetinaNet, Deep SVDD and a customized CNN for the detection of cervix on smarthphone captured images. They achieved an average accuracy and F1-score of 91.6% and 0.890, respectively.

3.2.6. Summary

Screening through a Pap test for cervical cancer can take days for the final analysis to complete since the pathologist needs to go through millions of cells. A deep learning-based system can detect those cells in minutes if it is accurate enough to be trusted. One of the main challenges of deep learning methods is the presence of other types of cells and other materials present in the image and the overlapping between two adjacent cervical cells. To solve these problems, a large and carefully annotated dataset needs to be built for the algorithms to learn. Building this many datasets for medical images is very difficult. The most commonly used dataset for cervical cancer screening is the Herlev dataset as shown in Table 10.

Deep learning has been applied for cervical cancer screening in many of its screening methods. Most of the successful deep learning-based cervical cancer detection methods were based on a dataset using pap smear histology images. Colposcopic images are also taking more attention since they are easy to take and not invasive. Their accuracies on the detection of cervical cancers is not as good as that of the histology images. Cervical cancer detection using the deep learning methods based on the colposcopic images are becoming common since a large dataset can be collected and annotated easily. Colposcopic screening could be applied for mass screening purposes with the aid of deep learning, since taking samples are easy. As we can see from Tables 9–12, the Herlev dataset is the most used dataset for cervical cell classification and segmentation works. Most of the coloscopic datasets used for cervix classifications are locally collected. We can also see that the deep learning methods for nuclei segmentation are more accurate than that of cell segmentations since cell boundaries might overlap between adjacent cells. For the classification case, binary classifiers are more accurate than that of multiclass classifiers which can detect the type of abnormalities in the cells.

From Tables 11–13, we can see those deep learning methods with pre-trained networks and those with transfer learning mechanisms are more accurate than networks trained from scratch with TensorFlow the widely used software.

Most of the reviewed papers on the application of deep learning on cervical cancer screening were published in 2019 with an average impact factor of 3.4 (see Table 14). And, as shown in Table 15, only one of the papers compares the algorithm performance with that of the specialist.

Table 13. Summary of cervical cancer scientific papers in terms of CNN architecture, and type of environment used in the selected papers.

Author and Citation	Network	Pre-Training	Transfer Learning	Environment
Zhao et al. [50]	U-Net	No	No	-
Liu Y. et al. [53]	Mask-RCNN	Yes	No	Tensorflow
Sompawong et al. [52]	Mask-RCNN	Yes	Yes	-
Kurnianingsih et al. [54]	Mask-RCNN and VGGNet	Yes	Yes	-
Song et al. [49]	CNN-Custom	No	No	-
Lianget al. [42]	ResNet50	Yes	Yes	Tensorflow
Zhang et al. [55]	ConvNet	Yes	Yes	Caffe
Hyeon et al. [56]	CNN	Yes	Yes	-
Yutao Ma et al. [62]	VGG-16	Yes	Yes	Tensorflow
Lin et al. [57]	GoogLeNet	Yes	Yes	Caffe
Promworn et al. [61]	DenseNet161	No	No	PytTorch
Wimpy and Suyanto [68]	Capsule Network	Yes	No	Tensorflow
Gorantla et al. [69]	ResNet101	yes	Yes	-
Arora et al. [70]	CNN-Custom	No	No	-
Ahmed et al. [63]	CaffeNet	yes	yes	Caffe
Martinez-Mias et al. [65]	CaffeNet	yes	yes	Caffe

Table 14. Summary of cervical cancer scientific papers in terms of article publication year, name of the journal for the selected papers and its impact factor with year of impact factor.

Author and Citation	Publication Year	Journal/Conference	Impact Factor	Impact Assigned Year
Zhao et al. [50]	2019	MMMI 2019	-	-
Liu Y. et al. [53]	2018	IEEE Access	4.098	2018
Sompawong et al. [52]	2019	Conference ACEMBS	0.54	2019
Kurnianingsih et al. [54]	2019	IEEE Access	4.098	2018
Song et al. [49]	2016	Conference ISBI	1.51	2019
Liang et al. [42]	2019	Neurocomputing	3.317	2016
Zhang et al. [55]	2017	JBHI	5.223	2020
Hyeon etal. [56]	2017	Conference ICMDM	-	-
Yutao Ma et al. [62]	2019	IEEE Transaction on Biomedical Engineering	4.78	2019
Lin et al. [57]	2019	IEEE Access	4.098	2018
Promworn et al. [61]	2019	Conference ICNEMS	0.312	2019
Wimpy and S. Suyanto [68]	2019	Conference ISRITI	-	-
Gorantla et al. [69]	2019	BIBE	0.392	2012
Arora et al. [70]	2018	Conference ICSCCC	0.91	2019
Ahmed et al. [63]	2019	Future Generation computer systems	6.125	2019
Dong et al. [64]	2020	ASCJ	5.5	2020
Martinez-Mias et al. [65]	2020	ESWA	5.45	2020

Table 15. Summary of cervical cancer scientific papers in terms of comparison to specialists and/or traditional techniques.

Author and Citation	Comparison to Specialists	Comparison to Traditional Technique (Yes/No)
Zhao et al. [50]	No	Yes
Liu Y. et al. [53]	No	Yes
Sompawong et al. [52]	No	Yes
Kurnianingsih et al. [54]	No	Yes
Song et al. [49]	No	Yes
Lianget al. [42]	No	Yes
Zhang et al. [55]	Yes	No
Hyeon et al. [56]	No	No
Yutao Ma et al. [62]	Yes	No
Lin et al. [57]	No	Yes
Promworn et al. [61]	No	Yes
Wimpy and S. Suyanto [68]	No	Yes
Gorantla et al. [69]	No	Yes
Arora et al. [70]	No	No
Ahmed et al. [63]	No	Yes
Dong et al. [64]	No	Yes
Martinez-Mias et al. [65]	No	No

3.3. Brain Tumor

Brain tumor is a group of abnormal cells around or inside the brain due to the uncontrolled division of cells with a serious effect of deterring the normal functionality of the brain activity and destroying the healthy cells[75].

Brain tumor is classified into benign or low-grade (grade I and II) and malignant or high-grade (grade III and IV). Benign is a non-cancerous tumor that does not exhibit any progression and cannot spread to other parts of the body; it started in the brain with a very low growth rate. On the other hand, a malignant tumor is cancerous with an attribute of growing rapidly and spreading to other parts of the body. Malignant tumors can further be categorized as primary and secondary. Primary malignant tumor originates in the brain itself; whereas, the secondary type begins from somewhere else in the body and spreads to the brain. Cancerous cells that spread to the brain commonly originate from the lung, kidney, breast, skin and colon. A metastatic brain tumor is another expression for this type of brain tumor. Glioblastoma multiform (GBM) is the most common type of primary brain tumor that grows fast from glial cells. An intense clinical treatment plan is required for high-grade gliomas (HGG) as they have a higher spreading rate than the low-grade gliomas (LCG) [76]. It is evidenced that patients with GBMs decease in less than a year. Early detection helps a therapeutic plan of patients and improves the overall survival rate [77]. The most prevalent brain cancer is high-grade glioma with 85% of new cases of malignant primary tumor diagnosed every year [78].

3.3.1. Screening Methods

Magnetic resonance imaging is the most common brain tumor diagnosis and has a great role in treatment planning strategies [79]. These images have an important contribution towards an automatic medical image analysis field as they provide quite a lot of information about the brain structure and abnormalities [80].

This is the reason why MRI images have a great impact on the automatic medical image analysis field. There are various steps taken in the course of brain tumor treatment. The first step is determining if the tumor does exist in the brain or not. Then, the infected region in the brain tissues must be extracted from an MRI image in a process called segmentation [81]. Segmentation is not an easy task as MRI images may not help human readers easily discern regions of concern for various technical reasons. However, segmentation is a very important task in properly conducting the diagnosis, treatment and appraisal of treatment outcomes. A great number of automatic segmentation methods with varying degrees of accuracy have been developed as applications of the computational science for utilization of imaging devices advance.

There are different modalities of the MRI including T1-weighted (T1), T2-weighted contrast-enhanced (T1c), T2-weighted (T2) and T2-weighted fluid attenuated inversion recovery (FLAIR) for segmenting the brain tumor [82]. Moreover, features of the MRI like textures, local histograms and structure tensor eigenvalues have been used in brain tumor segmentation [83]. Deep learning-based methods have become state-of-the-art as they score superior performance in image analysis fields [84].

3.3.2. Datasets

Most of the researchers have applied publicly available brain tumor image datasets to test their methods. Summary of publicly available datasets for brain tumor segmentation and classification is summarized in Table 16.

Table 16. Image datasets for brain tumor (N—normal, AB—abnormal).

Dataset	Size	#Classes	Format/Targets	Type	Author, Year
LBPA40	288	2	html	MRI	Shattuck et al. [85]
BRATS 2015	43,708	2	.mha	MRI	Menze et al. [86]
BRATS2013	1799	2	.mha	MRI	Menze et al. [86]
RIDER_NEURO_MRI	29	2	.tcia	MRI	Barboriak et al. [87]
SUH	49	2	-	MRI	Fabelo et al. [88]
HMS	66	2	.gif	MRI	Keith A. Johnson
FBT	3064	2	.mat	MRI	C. Jun [89]
NHTM	3064	2	.png	MRI	C. Jun [89]
GCE	150	2	.png	MRI	Jun Cheng [90]

3.3.3. Deep Learning in Brain Tumor Segmentation

Alkassar et al. [91] proposed transfer learning and fully convolution network (FCN) to achieve robust tumor segmentation using VGG-16 networks. The proposed method achieved a global accuracy of 0.97785 and a 0.89 Dice score in terms of whole tumor segmentation on MRI images from the BRATS2015 dataset.

Amiri et al. [92] proposed a simple and reliable brain segmentation method in MRI images through recursively and deeply transferring a learned random forest (RF) to guide an SVM classifier for segmenting tumor lesions while capturing the complex characteristics of brain tumor appearance. They tested this method on 20 patients with high-grade gliomas from the Brain Tumor Image Segmentation Challenge (BRATS) dataset. Their method outperforms both SVM and RF with a high statistical significance using paired t-test; i.e., a mean Dice index of 72% compared to SVM (59%) and RF (63%).

Chahal et al. [93] proposed a novel approach using deep learning which utilizes both global and local brain image datasets for precise segmentation. Their proposed deep learning model combines two-pathway and cascade architectures to analyze and implement brain segmentation. The results are evaluated over Input Cascade and the outcomes showed better performance—that is, a metrics of Dice score for high grade and low-grade image with values 0.943 and 0.950, respectively—than existing MFC cascade.

Ding et al. [94] proposed deep residual dilate network with middle supervision (RDM-Net) which combines the residual network with dilated convolution. By evaluating their framework on the BRATS 2015 challenge, their framework proved to achieve better performance than other state-of-the-art methods incomplete tumor (Dice score of 0.86) and core tumor segmentation (Dice score of 0.78). However, the Dice score for enhancing tumors only achieves 0.63 which is not as good as the other counterpart methods. The reason for this could be the focus on the 2D slices segmentation by the proposed framework which pays less attention to the context information within slices by comparing with 3D segmentation. The loss of context information may lead to worse performance on the enhancing tumor segmentation.

Mallick et al. [95] have used a deep wavelet autoencoder (DWA) for an image compression technique which blends the basic feature reduction property of autoencoder along with image decomposition property of wavelet transform for further classification task by using DNN. The performance of the DWA-DNN classifier was compared with other existing classifiers like autoencoder-DNN or DNN and the proposed method surpasses them all with an overall accuracy of 96% where that of AE-DNN is 93% and DNN is 91%.

Ramirez et al. [96] proposed a new variational model for saliency detection in images and its application to brain tumor segmentation. The model works by incorporating a saliency term to a classical total variation-based restoration functional and hence discriminates what is relevant (salient) from the background. They have, therefore, introduced a deep learning framework for using available knowledge from a specific application to optimize the parameters of the energy functional. The proposed framework achieved a Dice score of 0.857, precision 0.845 and recall 0.882.

Sajid et al. [97] proposed a deep learning-based method that uses different modalities of MRI for the segmentation of brain tumors. The proposed hybrid convolutional neural network architecture uses a patch-based approach and deals with the over-fitting problems by utilizing dropout regularize alongside batch normalization, whereas the data imbalance problem is dealt with by using a two-phase training procedure. The proposed method contains a preprocessing step, in which images are normalized and bias field corrected, a feed-forward pass through a CNN and a post-processing step as a means of removing remnant false positives in the skull portion. The proposed method is validated on the BRATS 2013 dataset, where it achieves scores of 0.86, 0.86 and 0.91 in terms of Dice score, sensitivity and specificity for whole tumor region, improving results compared to existing state-of-the-art techniques.

Wang et al. [98] proposed an automatic method named residual and pyramid pool network (WRN-PPNet) to segment brain tumor by first obtaining 2D slices from 3D MRI brain tumor images and then normalizing the 2D slices and putting them in the model. The model will output the tumor segmentation results. The experimental results show that the proposed method is simple and robust compared to the other state-of-the-art methods with an average Dice, sensitivity and PPV values on randomly selected datasets 0.94, 0.92 and 0.97, respectively.

Zhao et al. [99] proposed a new method for brain segmentation which is an integration of fully convolutional neural networks (FCNNs) and conditional random fields (CRFs) in a unified framework. The result helps to obtain segmentation results with the appearance and spatial consistency. The following steps are taken to for training the deep learning model using 2D image patches and image slices: (1) training FCNNs using image patches; (2) training CRFs as recurrent neural networks (CTF-RNN) using image slices with parameters of FCNNs fixed; and (3) fine-tuning the FCNNs and the CRF-RNN using image slices. In the model, 3 segmentation models are particularly trained using 2D image patches and slices obtained in axial, coronal, and sagittal views respectively are combined to segment brain tumors using a voting-based fusion strategy. The method used BRTS 2013, BRATS 2015 and BRATS 2016 with an experimental result of a competitive score. The method achieved a promising performance on the BRATS 2013 and BRATS 2015 testing dataset. The method could also achieve competitive performance with only 3 imaging modalities (FLAIR, T1c and T2) rather than 4(FLAIR, T1, T1c and T2). In BRATS 2016, the method ranked first on its multi-temporal evaluation.

Kuzina et al. [100] proposed a knowledge transfer method between diseases via the generative Bayesian prior network to mitigate the common challenge of obtaining large image datasets for automatic segmentation. They have applied deep weight prior; hence the name UNet-DWP for their method, to incorporate information about the structure of previously learned convolutional filters during the training of a new model. A comparison between a pre-trained approach and random initialization to this approach proves that this method yields the best results in terms of the Dice similarity coefficient metric on a small subset of the BRATS2018 dataset. The performance of the model was rated by taking subsets containing 5, 10, 15 or 20 randomly selected images from the dataset and comparing them with the fixed test sample size of 50 images. They have also used a blend of binary cross-entropy and Dice losses to train U-Net in the non-Bayesian setting. The results indicate that the model outperforms both pre-trained and randomly initialized U-Nets for all the training sizes.

Zeineldin et al. [101] proposed a new generic deep learning architecture named DeepSeg to address the challenge of distinguishing tumor boundaries from healthy cells in the brain tumor diagnosis. This method helps to wholly automate detection and segmentation of the brain lesion using FLAIR MRI data. The developed system is a decoupling framework interacting encoding and decoding relationship where the encoder part performs spatial information using a convolutional neural network and the decoder provides the full-resolution probability map from the resulting semantic map. The study has employed different CNN models such as residual neural network (ResNet), dense convolutional network (DenseNet) and NASNet using modified U-Net architecture. The proposed architecture has been tested on MRI datasets of brain tumor segmentation (BRATS2019) challenge which includes s336 cases as training data and 125 cases for validation data yielding Dice and Hausdorff distance scored of about 0.81 to 0.84 and 9.8 to 19.7, respectively. The proposed DeepSeg is open source and freely available at https://github.com/razeineldin/DeepSeg/.

Fabelo et al. [102] suggested a deep learning-based hyperspectral image (HSI) processing modality to be used as a reliable support in real-time neurosurgical procedure for carrying out accurate resection of the tumor without affecting much of the normal brain tissue. The study employed a number of deep learning techniques for the detection of brain tumors using HSI. The HS image database was obtained during the course of operation and the system employed a highly sophisticated and specialized visible and near-infrared (VNIR) push broom camera. Classification methods with 2D-CNN and pixel-wise classification with 1D-DNN have been found to yield a very good result. Despite the challenge in obtaining sufficient number of training samples and the anomalies incurred due to brain movement during scanning, the overall average accuracy for the proposed method was 80%. The method has also achieved a very high specificity for both binary and multiclass classification schemes with values of 100% and 90%, respectively.

The summary of researches on deep learning methods for brain tumor segmentation is presented in Table 17.

3.3.4. Deep Learning in Brain Tumor Classification

Like in the segmentation, deep learning-based methods have performed fairly well in image classification of brain tumors. Yet, variation in the shape, size, location and contrast of tumor tissue cells is the major factor that impacts the accurate classification of brain tumors from MRI images [103].

Deep learning techniques involving different enhancement methods are used to classify different types of brain tumors—glioma, meningioma and pituitary. The classification is further categorized into axial, coronal and sagittal planes that are used by various algorithms to minimize the error rate of neural networks in identifying the brain tumor [104].

Mohsen et al. [80] employed a DNN classifier where a 7-fold cross-validation technique was applied for building and training the DNN of 7-hidden layers structure for classifying a dataset of brain MRIs into four classes, i.e., normal, glioblastoma, sarcoma and metastatic bronchogenic carcinoma.

They have combined the classifier with the discrete wavelet transform (DWT)—a powerful feature extraction tool—and principal components analysis (PCA). They achieved a classification rate of 96.97%, recall 0.97, precision 0.97, F-measure 0.97 and AUC (ROC) 0.984.

Table 17. Summary of selected papers on brain tumor segmentation.

Authors	Method Learning	Dataset	Acc.	P	R	F	Sp	Sn	Dice	PPV
Alkassar et al. [91]	DNN+FCN+VGG-16	BRATS2015	0.98						0.89	
Amiri et al. [92]	RF-SVM	BRATS							0.72	
Chahal et al. [93]	CNN	BRATS2013		0.96				0.93	0.95	
Ding et al. [94]	RDM-Net	BRATS2015							0.86	
Mallick et al. [95]	DWA-DNN	RIDER_NEURO_MRI	0.93			0.93	0.92	0.94		
Ramirez et al. [96]	CNN+TVS	Flair-MRI Brats2015		0.84	0.88				0.86	
Sajid et al.[97]	hybrid CNN	BRATS 2013					0.91	0.86	0.86	
Wang et al. [98]	WRN-PPNet	BRATS2015						0.92	0.94	0.97
Zhao et al. [99]	FCNNs and CRF-RNN	BRATS 2013–16						0.82	0.84	0.89
Kuzina et al. [100]	UNet-DWP	BRATS2018							0.76	
Zeineldin et al. [101]	DeepSeg	BRATS 2019							0.81–0.84	
Fabelo et al. [102]	HSI+2D-CNN	SUH	80					80–100		

Alqudah et al. [105] used a convolutional neural network (CNN) for classifying a dataset of 3064 T1 weighted contrast-enhanced brain MR images for grading the brain tumors into three classes called glioma, meningioma and pituitary. The research has used T1-weighted contrast-enhanced brain MR images for classifying brain tumor grades. They have used a free online available dataset at [90] which contains images having the above-mentioned attributes. A total of 18 layers in the proposed CNN architecture would enable the classifier to rate the brain tumor effectively. In their work they proved that the proposed CNN classifier is a powerful tool with an accuracy of 98.93% and sensitivity 98.18% for cropped lesions; for the uncropped lesions, they have obtained an accuracy of 99% and 98.52% sensitivity; for segmented lesion images, the result is 97.62 accuracy and 97.40% sensitivity.

Ucuzal et al. [106] developed a deep learning free web-based software that can be utilized in the detection and diagnosis of the three types of brain tumors (glioma/meningioma/pituitary) on T1-weighted magnetic resonance imaging. In the research, 3064 T1-weighted MR image scans for the three types of brain tumors have been used. Out of which, 2599 instances were used in the training phase; whereas, the remaining 465 were used in the testing phase. A python programming language library called Auto Keras was used in image pre-processing (image rotation, changing width and length, truncating images, rescaling, etc). Furthermore, a Bayesian optimization technique was used to tune the hyperparameters of the model. With this, they have verified that all the calculated performance metrics—i.e., accuracy, precision, sensitivity, specificity, F1-score, MCC, G-Mean of the experimental results are higher than 98% for classifying the types of brain tumors on the testing dataset obtained from Nanfang Hospital and Tianjin Medical University General Hospital which is an open-source dataset downloaded from [107]. This data set consists of 3064 T1-weighted contrast-enhanced MR images from 233 patients: 708 meningiomas, 1426 glioma and 930 pituitary tumors. The developed web-based software can be publicly available at [108].

Selvy et al. [109] developed a model that makes use of an image processing technique and artificial neural network for successful detection of the brain tumor. To enhance the contrast of the original image in its analysis and manipulation, they have used histogram equalization (HE) technique where gray level co-occurrence matrix (GLCM) would be used on the feature extraction. A probabilistic neural network (PNN) classifier is applied to the obtained feature to accurately determine tumor location in brain MRI images. The PNN classifier has produced an accuracy of 90.9%, specificity of 100% and sensitivity 85.75%.

Sultan et al. [110] proposed a deep learning (DL) model to classify different brain tumor types. The model which bases a convolutional neural network has employed two publicly available datasets acquired from Nanfang Hospital and General Hospital, Tianjing Medical University, China from 2005 to 2010. The two datasets entail 233 and 73 patients with a total of 3064 and 516 images on T1-weighted contrast-enhanced images, respectively. The overall accuracy of the proposed network is 96.13% for the first and 98.7% for the second dataset. The result inferred that the model has the ability to perform brain tumor multi-classification. The network training and performance computations are finally presented. The system parameters used to train the neural network structure are Intel i7-7700HQ CPU (2.8 GHz), NVIDIA GTX 1060 (6 GB) GPU, 16GB RAM, Matlab 2018b and Python 3. The network is constructed from 16 layers where the input layer holds the pre-processed images passing through the convolution layers and their activation functions (3 convolution, 3 ReLU, normalization and 3 max-pooling layers). Additionally, two dropout layers are used to prevent overfitting followed by a fully connected layer and a softmax layer to predict the output and finally a classification layer that produces the predicted class. Although the dataset is relatively not big (due to the variety of imaging views), data augmentation helped well to show better results and hence, overcome this problem.

Badža and Barjaktarovic [111] presented a new CNN architecture for Brain Tumor Image Segmentation and classification for three tumor types. The study has employed an image database that contains 3064 T1-weighted contrast-enhanced MRI images acquired from Nanfang Hospital and General Hospital, Tianjin Medical University, China from 2005 to 2010. The input layer of the proposed network was represented by MRI images of the database after being normalized to 256 × 256 pixels. The network architecture having consisted of input, two main blocks, classification block and output was employed to perform tumor classification. The blocks consist of the rectified linear unit (ReLU) activation layer, the dropout layer and the max-pooling layer engaged in fine-tuning and resizing the images. A CNN developed in Matlab R2018a (The MathWorks) was employed for the tumor classification. The evaluation of the network was assessed using four approaches: combinations of two 10-fold cross-validation methods and the two databases mentioned above. The generalization capability of the network was tested with one of the 10-fold methods, subject-wise cross-validation, and the improvement was tested by using an augmented image database. The best result for the 10-fold cross-validation method was obtained for the record-wise cross-validation for the augmented data set, and, in that case, the accuracy was 96.56%. With good generalization capability and good execution speed, the new developed CNN architecture could be used as an effective decision-support tool for radiologists in medical diagnostics.

The summary of the papers reviewed is presented in Table 18.

Table 18. Summary of selected papers on brain tumor classification.

Authors	Method	Dataset	Acc.	P	R	F	Sp	Sn	MCC	G-Mean
Mohsen et al. [80]	DWT-DNN	Harvard		0.97	0.97	0.97				
Alqudah et al. [105]	CNN	Online	98.40	98.19			99.19	98.18		
Ucuzal et al. [106]	CNN Multiclass	NHTM	99.74	99.58		99.59	99.81	99.60	99.39	99.70
Selvy et al. [109]	PNN	GCE	90			100	85.75			
Sultan et al. [110]	CNN	NHTM	96.13–98.7							
Badža and Barjaktarovic [111]	CNN	NHTM	96.56							

3.3.5. Summary

As shown in Table 19, papers from 2016,2018, 2019, and 2020 were reviewed here. Unlike other cancer type papers, reviewed papers on brain tumors consist of a significant number of papers that compared the performance of their model with that of the domain expert(see Table 20).

As indicated in Tables 17 and 18, Brain Tumor Image Segmentation Challenge (BRATS) of various versions is the most widely used dataset among the researchers and appeared in ten out of the seventeen papers reviewed.

From Table 21 it was found that a Tensor flow-based framework run by a high-speed core processor or a GPU was widely used, seven out of seventeen, followed by PyTorch, two out of seventeen, to implement the experiments and conducting the deep learning training. However, the rest of the papers have not explicitly indicated which software platform they have applied. On the other hand, VGGNet is the most frequently applied network to achieve robust tumor segmentation 52.9% of the papers have made a comparison with domain experts; on the other hand, 94.1% of the paper has made a comparison with the traditional method.

Table 19. Summary of brain tumor scientific papers in terms of article publication year, name of journal for the selected papers and its impact factor with year of impact factor.

Author and Citation	Publication Year	Journal	Impact Factor	Impact Assigned Year
Alkassar et al. [91]	2019	ICECCPCE19 Conference	0.627	2019
Amiri et al. [92]	2016	ATSIP 2016 Conference	0.17	2019
Chahal et al. [93]	2019	RDCAPE Conference	-	-
Ding et al. [94]	2019	IEEE Access	3.745	2019
Mallick et al. [95]	2019	IEEE Access	3.745	2019
Ramirez et al. [96]	2018	ISBI Conference	1.51	2019
Sajid et al.[97]	2019	Arabian Journal for Science and Engineering	0.33	2019
Wang et al. [98]	2019	IJCNN Conference	0.37	2019
Zhao et al. [99]	2018	Medical Image Analysis	3.88	2019
Kuzina et al. [100]	2019	Frontiers in Neuroscince	3.7	2020
Mohsen et al. [80]	2018	Future Computing and Informatics	3.88	2019
Alqudah et al. [105]	2019	IJATCSE	0.2	2019
Ucuzal et al. [106]	2019	ISMSIT	0.84	2019
Zeineldin et al. [101]	2020	IJCARS	1.961	2017
Fabelo et al. [102]	2019	MDPI	3.275	2019
Selvy et al. [109]	2019	IJSRCSEIT	1.638	2016
Sultan et al. [110]	2019	IEEE Access	3.745	2019
Badža and Barjaktarovic [111]	2020	MDPI	2.474	2019

Table 20. Summary of brain tumor scientific papers in terms of comparison to specialists and/or traditional techniques.

Author and Citation	Comparison to Specialists (Yes/No)	Comparison to Traditional Technique (Yes/No)
Alkassar et al. [91]	Yes	Yes
Amiri et al. [92]	No	Yes
Chahal et al. [93]	No	Yes
Ding et al. [94]	No	Yes
Mallick et al. [95]	No	Yes
Ramirez et al. [96]	Yes	Yes
Sajid et al.[97]	No	Yes
Wang et al. [98]	Yes	Yes
Zhao et al. [99]	Yes	Yes
Kuzina et al. [100]	No	Yes
Mohsen et al. [80]	No	Yes
Alqudah et al. [105]	No	Yes
Ucuzal et al. [106]	Yes	No
Zeineldin et al. [101]	Yes	Yes
Fabelo et al. [102]	Yes	Yes
Selvy et al. [109]	No	No
Sultan et al. [110]	Yes	Yes
Badža and Barjaktarovic [111]	No	Yes

Table 21. Summary of brain tumor scientific papers in terms of CNN architecture, and type of environment used in the selected papers.

Author and Citation	Network	Pre-Training	Transfer Learning	Environment
Alkassar et al. [91]	VGGNet-16	Yes	Yes	
Amiri et al. [92]	RF+SVM	Yes	Yes	
Chahal et al. [93]	CNN	Yes	Yes	
Ding et al. [94]	RDM-Net	Yes	Yes	
Mallick et al. [95]	DWA-DNN	Yes	Yes	Tensor flow
Ramirez et al. [96]	CNN+TVS	Yes	Yes	Tensor flow
Sajid et al.[97]	hybrid CNN	Yes	Yes	Tensor Flow
Wang et al. [98]	WRN-PPNet	Yes	Yes	Tensor flow
Zhao et al. [99]	FCNNs and CRF-RNN	Yes	Yes	Tensor flow
Kuzina et al. [100]	UNet-DWP	Yes	Yes	
Mohsen et al. [80]	DWT-DNN	Yes	Yes	
Alqudah et al. [105]	VGGNet-19	Yes	Yes	
Ucuzal et al. [106]	UNet-DWP	Yes	Yes	Tensor flow and Keras
Zeineldin et al. [101]	ResNet+DenseNet+NasNet	Yes	Yes	Keras, Tensor Flow
Fabelo et al. [102]	UNet	Yes	Yes	Tensor Flow
Selvy et al. [109]	GLCM+PNN	Yes	Yes	
Sultan et al. [110]	CNN	Yes	Yes	Matlab 2018b and Python
Badža and Barjaktarovic [111]	CNN	Yes	Yes	Matlab 2018b

3.4. Colorectal Cancer (CRC)

Worldwide in 2018, more than 1,849,518 (which accounts for 10.2% of overall cancer cases) new cases of colorectal cancer (CRC) are diagnosed and nearly 880,792 people died which is 9.2% of all cancer-related deaths [112]. It is the third most common cancer worldwide and the second most deadly [112]. Since colorectal cancer takes a long time before it becomes invasive, it is often curable if found early. Hence, casual screening for colorectal cancer can substantially reduce its mortality. Approximately 95% of all colorectal cancers are adenocarcinomas [113]. Colorectal adenocarcinomas develop in the lining of the colon or rectum and are characterized by glandular formation.

3.4.1. Screening Methods

There are three common screening methods for colorectal cancer: fecal occult blood test (FOBt), flexible sigmoidoscopy (FS) and total colonoscopy (TC) [114]. FOBt reveals traces of blood in stool samples which is an early sign of colorectal cancer. FS involves visual inspection of the distal bowel for polyps and cancers. TC visualizes the entire bowel and therefore is a more invasive examination. The advancement of whole slide imaging (WSI) scanners has opened new opportunities in automating pathology image analysis by digitizing the slides [115]. Histological examination of the glands, most frequently with the hematoxylin & eosin (H & E) stain, is routine practice for assessing the differentiation of cancer within colorectal adenocarcinoma [113]. Pathologists use the degree of glandular formation as an important factor in deciding the grade of the tumor. Accurate segmentation of structures of the glandular formations such as glands and nuclei have crucial importance, because their morphological properties can assist the pathologist in screening the malignancy [113].

3.4.2. Datasets

In Table 22, we present some of the publicly available and widely used datasets for colorectal cancer detection and segmentation.

Table 22. Publicly available datasets for colorectal cancer (CRC), UMCM—University Medical Center Mannheim, CVC—computer vision center.

Dataset	Size	#Classes/Targets	Format	Type	Author, Year
CVC-EndoSceneStill	912	4	bmp	Colonoscopy	Vázquez et al. [116], 2017
CVC-ColonDB	300	4	bmp	Colonoscopy	J. Bernal et al. [117], 2012
CVC-ClinicDB	612	4	tiff	Colonoscopy	J. Bernal et al. [118], 2015
UMCM	500	8	mat	histology	Kather et al. [119], 2016

3.4.3. Deep Learning for Cell Detection and Classification on Histological Slides

Kainz et al. [120] applied deep learning methods to segment and classify colon glands into benign and malignant types for GlaS@MICCAI2015 challenge. They first pre-processed the stained RGB by taking the Red channel and ignoring the others. Then contrast enhancement was performed using contrast limited adaptive histogram equalization (CLAHE) technique. Two CNN classifiers were trained: Object-Net, Separator-Net. Object-Net is for the detection of benign and malignant glands from their respective backgrounds. Separator-Net is for classifying gland-separating structures since the Object-Net architecture segment two neighboring glands as one. These to classifiers are then regularized using a figure-ground segmentation based on weighted total variation to produce the final segmentation result. They have achieved 96% average accuracy on the two tests provided by the challenge.

Sirinukunwattana et al. [121] proposed a spatially constrained convolutional neural network (SC-CNN) that includes parameter estimation layer and spatially constrained layer for spatial regression to predict the probability of a pixel being the center of a nucleus in hematoxylin and eosin (H & E) stained histopathology images. For classifying the detected nuclei they combine neighboring ensemble predictor (NEP) with a standard softmax CNN (s-CNN). For the nuclei detection using SC-CNN, they achieved 0.77 precision, 0.82 recall, and 0.8 F1-score. The NEP&s-CNN classifier achieved an F1-score of 0.784 and the overall nuclei detection and classification (SC-CNN+NEP&s-CNN) achieved an F1-score of 0.69.

Graham et al. [113] used a fully convolutional neural network that counters the loss of information caused by the max-pooling layer by introducing original down-sampled image into the residual unit using the minimal information loss (MIL) units. They applied atrous spatial pyramid pooling for multi-level aggregation and preserving the resolution. They achieved an F1-score of 0.92 for gland segmentation using the GlaS challenge dataset.

Chamanzar et al. [122] develop a deep learning method that can detect and segment a single cell using only point labeled dataset. They combined Voronoi transformation, Local pixel clustering and Repel encoding methods with U net with Resnet encoder by feeding them to a multi-task scheduler for training the system. They achieved an accuracy of 93% for cell segmentation and 94.1% for detection of adenocarcinoma.

Sari et al. [123] proposed a novel approach for feature extraction, which defines the features by considering only the salient subregions of the image. The salient subregions were detected by the detection of nuclear and non-nuclear pixels using an algorithm presented in [124]. Then a deep belief network of restricted Boltzmann machines (RBMs) re-characterizes these regions and extract features. These features are clustered using the k-means clustering algorithm and SVM classifier for categorizing those regions. They achieved an average precision, recall, and F1-score of 82.3%, 89.9% and 85.1, respectively at the detection of colon adenocarcinoma.

Shapcott et al. [125] proposed a deep learning-based cell identification on histological images of the colon with a systematic random sampling of the WSI slides. Their proposed system consists of two CNNs in series in which the first one detects cells on the WSI slide while the second one classifies those cells into epithelial, inflammatory, a fibroblast or "other". The training was performed on a local dataset and Evaluated using the "The Cancer Genome Atlas (TCGA)" dataset. Using five patients' slides, they achieved an average accuracy of 65% in the detection of cells and 76% in the classification.

Tang et al. [126] proposed Segnet based gland segmentation on the histology image of the colon. Augmented MICCAI2015 challenge dataset was used to train the SegNet network which is a CNN with encode-decoder architecture for pixel-wise segmentation. SegNet achieved an average Dice similarity index of 0.872 and Hausdorff distance of 104.61.

Vuong et al. [127] proposed an algorithm based on DenseNet121 that can perform both classification and regression tasks on WSI images, for improving the overall performance of the system. They designed this multi-task deep learning model by adding two fully connected layers, one for classification and one for regression, after the DenseNet121 network. The classifier classifies the tissue image into four distinctive pathologies and the regressor considers these four pathological categories as continuous values. They achieved 85.1% accuracy in classifying colon tissues into four categories.

Sabol et al. [128] proposed a semantically explainable fuzzy classifier called cumulative fuzzy class membership criterion (CFCMC) for classifying WSI of colorectal cancer tissue into eight different tissue types. They compared many CNN architectures as feature extraction for the CFCMC classifier with the Xception architecture performance being the best feature extractor for the CFCMC. The explainability of the system is its ability to provide a degree of confidence for each of its predictions. The proposed method achieved an accuracy of 92.78% for the classification of the different tissue samples. The explainability was evaluated by pathologists based on its objectivity, level of details, reliability and quality. Based on these measures, they confirmed that the explainability of the system is better than the traditional CNN architectures.

3.4.4. Deep Learning for Classification of Polyps on Endoscopic Images

Colorectal polyps are abnormalities in the colon tissues that can develop into colorectal cancer. The survival rate for patients is higher when the disease is detected at an early stage and polyps can be removed before they develop into malignant tumors. These tests are usually performed using endoscopic analysis of the colon. During this study, the endoscopist explores the colon cavity looking for abnormal growths of tissue, polyps. However, polyp detection is a challenging problem given its high variation in appearance, size, shape and in many cases its high similarity with the surrounding tissue.

The application of CTs for the screening of colorectal cancer suffers from false positives due to the similarity between polyps and colorectal tubes on the CT image. Approaches in [129] can help to distinguish between colorectal tubes and polyps in CT scans of the colon area using a three dimensional massive-training artificial neural network (3D-MTANN). The proposed model manages to reduce false positives by 33% while keeping a sensitivity of 96%.

Ornela Bardhi et al. [130] used CNNs with auto-encoders for the automatic detection of colon polyp. They used the SegNet architecture from the TensorFlow to build the model and train it from scratch using three datasets: CVC-ColonDB, CVC-ClinicDB and ETIS-LaribPolypDB. They achieved a maximum accuracy of 96.7% on the EITS dataset for the detection of colon polyps.

Bour et al. [131] trained different architectures: ResNet50, ResNet101, Xception, VGG19 and Inception V3 for classification of polyps. ResNet50 achieved the highest accuracy of 87.1 % with precision 87.1%, recall 87.1%, F1-score 87.1% and specificity 93%.

Liu et al. [132] used a deep learning network, faster_rcnn_inception_resnet_v2 model for localization and classification of endoscopic images of the colon. They achieved 90.645% mean average precision and 0.5 for the intersection over union (IoU).

Ozawa et al. [133] used deep convolutional neural network (CNN) architecture called single shot multibox detector (SSD) for the detection of colorectal polyps. All layers were fine-tuned using stochastic gradient descent with a global learning rate of 0.0001. The trained SSD detected the trained CNN detected 1246 colorectal polyps from a dataset collected at Tada Tomohiro Institute of Gastroenterology and Proctology with a sensitivity of 92% and a positive predictive value (PPV) of 86%.

Nadimi et al. [134] used a modified version of ZF-net, a CNN architecture proposed by Matthew D. Zeiler and Rob Fergus [135], as the basis for a Faster R-CNN to localize regions of images containing colorectal polyps. They trained their architectures using a locally collected dataset labeled as colorectal polyps (N = 4800) and normal mucosa (N = 6500). The proposed architecture achieved an accuracy, sensitivity and specificity of 98.0%, 98.1% and 96.3%, respectively. The proposed approach produces the bounding box annotation of the polyp.

3.4.5. Summary

The most common colorectal cancer screening methods use endoscopic images to find abnormal colon tissues, polyps and locating cancerous cells or glands on WSI images. Hence most of the application of deep learning for detecting colorectal cancer is either finding adenocarcinoma on WSI or detection of polyps on colonoscopic images. Most of the research shows promising results in both polyp detection and adenocarcinoma or glands detection as seen in Tables 23 and 24.

Table 23. Summary of selected papers on detection and classification for colorectal cancer histological slides.

Authors	Method	Dataset	Acc	P	R	F1	DSC	H
Kainz et al. [120]	Separator-Net and Object-Net	MICCAI2015	96	59	74	62	-	-
Graham et al. [113]	MILD-Net	$GlaS^{+}$	-	-	-	87	88	142
Chamanzar et al. [122]	WSMTL	local	93	-	-	79.1	78.4	-
Sari et al. [123]	DeepFeature	local	-	82.3	89.9	85.1	-	-
Shapcott et al. [125]	CNNs	local and TCGA	65	-	-	-	-	-
Sirinukunwattana et al. [121]	SC-CNN+NEP & s-CNN	MICCAI2015	-	-	-	-	69	-
Tang et al. [126]	Segnet	MICCAI2015	-	-	-	-	87.2	104.61
Vuong et al. [127]	Multitask DensNet121	local	85.1	-	-	-	-	-
Sabol et al. [128]	CFSCMC	UMCM	92.78	-	-	-	-	-

The main challenge for the analysis of colposcopic images is most of the dataset suffers from out of focus problems. Detection of polyps from endoscopic images presents a big opportunity for deep learning methods to shine since most of the physicians may miss smaller polyps. Still, challenges are there due to low-quality samples and the operator might miss some areas.

Papers who used pre-trained models and applied transfer learning approaches discuss their findings in detail and are from reputable journals (see Tables 25 and 26). From Table 27, only two of the papers measure the performance of their proposed model against expert physicians.

Table 24. Summary of selected papers on colorectal cancer polyp detection.

Authors	Method	Dataset	Acc	P	R	F1	Sp	Sn	PPV
Ornela Bardhi et al. [130]	SegNet	EITs	96.7	-	-	-	-	-	-
Bour et al. [131]	Resnet50	local	87.1	87.1	87.1	87.1	93	-	-
Liu et al. [132]	faster_rcnn_inception_resnet_v2	local	90.6	-	-	-	-	-	-
Ozawa et al. [133]	SSD	local	-	-	-	-	-	92	86
Nadimi et al. [134]	mZF-net+ResNet	local	98	-	-	-	98.1	96	-

Table 25. Summary of colorectal cancer in terms of article publication year, name of journal for the selected papers and its impact factor with year impact factor has been assigned.

Author and Citation	Publication Year	Journal/Conference	Impact Factor	Impact Assigned Year
Kainz et al. [120]	2017	PeerJ	2.38	2019
Graham et al. [113]	2018	Medical Image Analysis	8.79	2018
Chamanzar et al. [122]	2020	ISBI conference	2.283	2019
Sari et al. [123]	2019	IEEE Transactions on Medical Imaging	9.71	2019
Shapcott et al. [125]	2019	Frontiers in bioengineering and biotechnology	3.644	2020
Sirinukunwattana et al. [121]	2016	IEEE transactions on medical imaging	9.71	2019
Tang et al. [126]	2018	Conference YAC	1.461	2019
Vuong et al. [127]	2020	Conference ICEIC	0.76	2019
Ornela Bardhi et al. [130]	2017	Conference ISSPIT	1.393	2019
Bour et al. [131]	2017	Conference ISSPIT	1.393	2019
Liu et al. [132]	2019	Conference ISNE	0.152	2019
Ozawa et al. [133]	2020	Therapeutic advances in gastroenterology	4.08	2020
Nadimi et al. [134]	2020	CEE	2.663	2020
Sabol et al. [128]	2020	YJBIN	3.526	2020

Table 26. Summary of colorectal cancer in terms of CNN architecture and type of environment used in the selected papers.

Author and Citation	Network	Pre-Training	Transfer Learning	Environment
Kainz et al. [120]	Object-Net and SeparatorNet—custom	No	No	Matlab
Graham et al. [113]	MILD-Net—custom	No	No	Tensorflow
Chamanzar et al. [122]	U-net and Resnet	Yes	Yes	PyTorch
Sari et al. [123]	DeepBelief	Yes	Yes	-
Shapcott et al. [125]	-	No	No	Tensorflow
Sirinukunwattana et al. [121]	-	No	No	Matlab
Tang et al. [126]	SegNet	No	No	Caffe
Vuong et al. [127]	DensNet121	No	No	PyTorch
Ornela Bardhi et al. [130]	SegNet	No	No	Tensorflow
Bour et al. [131]	ResNet50	Yes	Yes	Tensorflow
Liu et al. [132]	faster_rcnn_inception_resnet_v2	No	No	Tensorflow
Ozawa et al. [133]	Single Shot MultiBox Detector (SSD)	No	No	Caffe
Nadimi et al. [134]	mZF-Net+ResNet	Yes	Yes	Matlab 2018a
Sabol et al. [128]	Xception+CFCMC	Yes	Yes	-

Table 27. Summary of colorectal cancer papers in terms of comparison to specialists and/or traditional techniques.

Author and Citation	Comparison to Specialists	Comparison to Traditional Technique (Yes/No)
Kainz et al. [120]	No	No
Graham et al. [113]	No	Yes
Chamanzar et al. [122]	No	Yes
Sari et al. [123]	No	No
Shapcott et al. [125]	No	No
Sirinukunwattana et al. [121]	No	Yes
Tang et al. [126]	No	Yes
Vuong et al. [127]	No	No
Ornela Bardhi et al. [130]	No	No
Bour et al. [131]	Yes (Approval)	No
Liu et al. [132]	No	Yes
Ozawa et al. [133]	No	No
Nadimi et al. [134]	No	No
Sabol et al. [128]	Yes	Yes

3.5. Lung Cancer

Lung cancer is the deadliest cancer worldwide with the highest incidence rate [112]. The death rate is so high because the majority of the cases are discovered at an advanced stage, where curative treatment is no longer feasible. Hence, screening for early detection is significant enough for decreasing mortality.

3.5.1. Screening Methods

The recommended screening test for lung cancer is low-dose computed tomography (LDCT), which uses a low dose of X-ray radiation to get detailed images of the lungs. Physicians will study different slices of the LDCT to determine the presence of an abnormal area called lung nodule (or mass) [136]. Other approaches also exist like chest X-ray(the usual X-ray image), sputum cytology (microscopic analysis of mucus from the lungs). According to a study performed in [136], these approaches do not seem to decrease the mortality rate.

3.5.2. Datasets

In Table 28, some of the publicly available and widely used datasets for lung cancer detection and segmentation are listed.

Table 28. Publicly available datasets for CRC, UMCM—University Medical Center Mannheim, CVC—computer vision center.

Dataset	Size	#Classes/Targets	Format	Type	Author, Year
UCI ML repository	32	3		CSV	Hong and Yang [137], 1991
SPIE-AAPM-NCI	22489	2	dicom	CT	Armato et al. [138], 2015
Lung Nodule Malignancy	6690	2	hdf5	CT	Scott Mader [139], 2017
LUNA2016	888	2	mhd.zip	CT	Consortium for Open Medical Image Computing [119], 2016

3.5.3. Deep Learning for Lung Nodules Detection

Before the introduction of convolution-based deep learning methods, Suzuki [140] uses massive training artificial neural networks (MTANN) for the detection and decreasing false positives in lobules detection using extracted subregions from LDCT images. MTANNs are designed based on the concepts of artificial neural network filters, where MTANN will classify each subregion (kernel) independently. Hence, the convolution process is external. They used Multiple MTANNs in parallel to distinguish between nodules and non-nodules by training each MTANN with the same nodules but different types of non-nodules. multi-MTANN was applied to differentiate between benign and malignant nodules from LDCT images in [141].

Tajbakhsh and Suzuki [142] compared the performances of the two widely studied deep learning models, CNNs and MTANNs, for the detection and classification of lung nodules. The proposed MTANN-based architecture outperforms the best performing CNN (AlexNet in their experiment) insensitivity and false-positive rates achieving 100% sensitivity and 2.7 false positives per patient. In the classifications of the nodules into benign and malignant the MTANNs achieved an AUC of 0.88.

Gu et al. [143] proposed a novel CAD system for the detection of lung nodules using a 3D-CNN. They implemented a multiscale approach for making the system more efficient at the detection of various sizes of nodules. The proposed CAD system considers the preprocessing step, which is usually essential in building a standalone CAD system. It has a volume segmentation step for generating ROI cubes for the 3D-CNN to classify them. After the classification, DBSCAN was used to merge neighboring regions into one since they might be different parts of the same nodule. Using the LUNA16 dataset, they found out that small scale cubes are efficient in the detection of smaller nodules (92% sensitivity and four false positives per patient), but larger ones have lower sensitivity (88%), but with an average of one false positive per patient.

Sahu et al. [144] proposed a multiple view sampling-based multi-section CNN model for nodule classification and malignancy estimation from CT scans. Their proposed model is computationally lighter than the widely used and relatively efficient 3D-CNNs. They used sample slices extracted at different orientations, with spherical sampling performing the best, and a pre-trained MobileNet network to build their system. On the classification task, the proposed model achieved a sensitivity of 96% and AUC of 98% on the LUNA2016 dataset. They measure the severity of malignancy by training the logistic regression model to estimate the class probability of malignancy. It achieved an accuracy of 93.79% on malignancy estimation. Since it is a lightweight model, the model can work on smaller devices such as smart-phones, tablets, etc.

Ozdemir et al. [145] proposed an efficient end-to-end CAD system by coupling nodule detection with malignancy ranking step. They called the nodule detection system as CAD_e (detection) whose output is an input for malignancy ranking step, CAD_x (diagnosis) step in the complete CAD system. Training and evaluation were performed on the LUNA16 and Kaggle Bowl datasets [146]. The proposed model includes model uncertainty in its decision, making it relatively trustworthy in a real-world application. The proposed CAD_e system achieved a sensitivity of 96.5%+ and 19.7 false positives per patient without using false positive reduction techniques. The CAD_x system also achieves an AUC of 98%. The combination of the two systems was further tuned to build the full CAD system.

Bansal et al. [147] proposed Deep3DSCan for lung cancer segmentation and classification. They used a deep 3D segmentation algorithm to extract a 3D volume of interest from CTs. A combination of features extracted using a deep fine-tuned residual network and morphological features were used to train the ResNet based model. Training and testing used the publicly available LUNA16 dataset. The proposed architecture achieved an accuracy of 88% in segmentation and classification tasks with an F1-score of 0.88.

3.5.4. Summary

Many of the papers discussed here studied the detection and classification of lung nodules from the LDCT images. The end-to-end papers covered in these reviews ([142,145,147]) can help to build an effective CAD system to assist the radiologist.Bansal et al. [147] seems to work better than the other works reviewed here since its performance covers both the detection and classification tasks (see Table 29). We must also consider MTANN-based papers since they deliver a satisfactory result with smaller data sizes. Papers reviewed here can be summarized in Tables 30 and 31. Here we did not consider to create a table for domain expert approval since none was participated in the papers we reviewed.

Table 29. Summary of selected papers on lung cancer detection and classification.

Authors	Method	Dataset	Acc	FPR	Sp	Sn	AUC
Tajbakhsh and Suzuki [142]	MTANN, detection	local	-	2.7	-	100	
Tajbakhsh and Suzuki [142]	MTANN, classification	local	-	-	-	-	0.88
Gu et al. [143]	3D-CNN, detection	LUNA16	-	2.5	-	90	
Sahu et al. [144]	multi-section MobileNet	LUNA16	93.8	-	-	96	0.98
Ozdemir et al. [145]	V-Net, classification	LUNA16	-	19	-	96.5	0.98
Bansal et al. [147]	ResNet	LUNA16	88	-	89.7	87	0.88

Table 30. Summary of lung cancer in terms of article publication year, name of journal for the selected papers and its impact factor with the year impact factor has been assigned.

Author and Citation	Publication Year	Journal/Conference	Impact Factor	Impact Assigned Year
Tajbakhsh and Suzuki [142]	2017	Pattern Recognition	7.196	2019
Gu et al. [143]	2018	CBM	3.43	2019
Sahu et al. [144]	2019	IEEE-JBHI	5.180	2020
Ozdemir et al. [145]	2020	IEEE Transactions on Medical Imaging	9.71	2020
Bansal et al. [147]	2020	IET Image Processing	2.61	2020

Table 31. Summary of Colorectal cancer in terms of CNN architecture and type of environment used in the selected papers.

Author and Citation	Network	Pre-Training	Transfer Learning	Environment
Tajbakhsh and Suzuki [142]	MTANN	-	-	Caffe
Gu et al. [143]	3D-CNN	-	-	Keras
Sahu et al. [144]	Mobile-Net	Yes	Yes	Keras
Ozdemir et al. [145]	Vnet	-	-	-
Bansal et al. [147]	Resnet	-	-	Pythorch

3.5.5. Deep Learning for Other Cancer Detection and Segmentation

In this sub-section, we included the application of deep learning on skin, liver and stomach cancer detection. Melanoma is skin cancer which is the deadliest cancer in its nature. In a normal diagnosis distinguishing melanoma lesions from nonmelanoma, lesions are very challenging [148]. For such difficulties, researchers have introduced an automatic skin cancer diagnosis system for detection and segmentation. As a result of uneasy visual characteristics of skin lesion that include inhomogeneous features and fuzzy boundaries. To overcome the challenges, Adegun and Viriri [148] proposed a deep learning-based automatic melanoma lesion detection and segmentation algorithm. They evaluated their approach in terms of Dice coefficient and accuracy 92% and 95% on ISIC 2017 dataset and accuracy and Dice coefficient of 95% and 93% on PH2 datasets.

Another deadly cancer with high morbidity is liver cancer. There are no widely recommended methods for early detection of liver cancer. For patients at higher risk, an imaging test such as CT, MRI, ultrasound and angiography can be used to test for liver cancer. If the physician believes in the need, a biopsy may be used to confirm the diagnosis. Hence, deep learning methods have been proposed in assisting physicians in the diagnosis of liver cancers, including hepatocellular carcinoma (HCC), liver metastasis, cysts, hemangioma and other masses [149]. A custom CNN for classifying HCC in liver cancer from MRI images, which achieved 92% sensitivity (Sn), 98% specificity (Sp) and 92% accuracy was proposed in [150]. In [151], VGGNet was used to develop a CAD system that identifies four types of liver cancers, cysts, hemangiomas, HCC and metastatic liver cancer from ultrasound images. The developed CAD system achieved an average accuracy of 88%. A hybridized fully convolutional neural network (HFCNN) was applied in the detection of liver cancer from abdominal CT images in [64]. HFCNN accurately segments 94.7% of the tumor volume.

Stomach (gastric) cancer is also another common cancer with the fourth-highest incidence rate and the third-highest mortality rate in the world [112]. The most common screening methods for stomach cancer are UGI series, serum pepsinogen (PG) testing, Hpylori serology and endoscopy [152]. Endoscopy is the most accurate of these methods, but it is highly invasive [152]. Some popular deep learning architectures, the inception, ResNet and VGGNet that were pre-trained on ImageNet were applied using transfer learning methods has been applied to identify benign ulcer and cancer from gastrointestinal endoscopic color images in [153]. The ResNet model achieved the highest performance with normal versus abnormal accuracies of 90% and ulcer versus cancer accuracy of 77%.

A pre-trained Inception-Resnet-v2 model was trained and compared with endoscopists in classifying classification of gastric neoplasms in [154]. The Inception-Resnet-v2 model performance was lower in five-class (advanced gastric cancer, early gastric cancer, high-grade dysplasia, low-grade dysplasia and no neoplasm) classification, i.e., 76.4% vs. 87.6%. The Inception-Resnet-v2 model performance is comparable with endoscopist in the differentiation of gastric cancer and neoplasm (accuracy 76.0% vs. 82.0%).

4. Conclusions

The paper review indicates that deep learning methods have achieved state-of-the-art breast cancer, cervical cancer, brain tumor. colon cancer and lung cancer detection, feature extraction, classification and segmentation. In this article, a good number of deep learning-based methods for breast cancer, cervical cancer, brain tumor and colon cancer image analysis are studied. The developed and implemented methods employed a CNN approach combined with other techniques to mitigate the existing challenge arising from a large dataset demand for such systems to learn. Problems related to noise and corrupted images have been properly addressed in some of the works as they suggest utilizing normal images and limited dataset size in modes that encompass a combination of two or more architectures to discern breast, cervical, brain and colon abnormalities.

The use of enhanced activation functions have also been recommended to improve the overall performance of deep learning-based systems in medical image analysis. Moreover, many researchers have added multiple layers in the CNN architecture to increase the performance of the system. Some researchers worked on designing unique architectures for specific task properties instead of using CNN as it is. Subsequently, most of the methods are proved to produce a successful performance in terms of specificity, sensitivity and Dice score when tested on renowned datasets and BRATS challenges. The lack of sufficient datasets can be considered a challenge for many of the deep learning-based researches. All of the reviewed papers have not used different medical images other than MRI for brain and in most cases mammograms for breast.

Author Contributions: Conceptualization, T.G.D. and S.R.K.; Methodology, T.G.D., S.R.K. and F.S.; Validation, F.S., and T.G.D.; Writing—original draft preparation, T.G.D., S.R.K. and Z.M.S.; Writing—review and editing, S.R.K., Z.M.S.and T.G.D. All authors have read and agreed to the published version of the manuscript.

References

1. Afework, Y.K.; Debelee, T.G. Detection of Bacterial Wilt on Enset Crop Using Deep Learning Approach. *Int. J. Eng. Res. Afr.* **2020**, *51*, 1–17.
2. Shen, L.; Margolies, L.R.; Rothstein, J.H.; Fluder, E.; McBride, R.; Sieh, W. Deep Learning to Improve Breast Cancer Detection on Screening Mammography. *Sci. Rep.* **2019**, *9*. [CrossRef] [PubMed]
3. Suzuki, K. Survey of Deep Learning Applications to Medical Image Analysis. *Med. Imaging Technol.* **2017**, *35*, 212–226.
4. Litjens, G.; Kooi, T.; Bejnordi, B.E.; Setio, A.A.A.; Ciompi, F.; Ghafoorian, M.; van der Laak, J.A.W.M.; van Ginneken, B.; Sánchez, C.I. A survey on deep learning in medical image analysis. *Med. Image Anal.* **2017**, *42*, 60–88. [CrossRef] [PubMed]
5. Shen, D.; Wu, G.; Suk, H.I. Deep Learning in Medical Image Analysis. *Annu. Rev. Biomed. Eng.* **2017**, *19*, 221–248. [CrossRef] [PubMed]
6. Suzuki, K. Overview of deep learning in medical imaging. *Radiol. Phys. Technol.* **2017**, *10*, 257–273. [CrossRef] [PubMed]
7. Lee, J.; Jun, S.; Cho, Y.; Lee, H.; Kim, G.B.; Seo, J.B.; Kim, N. Deep Learning in Medical Imaging: General Overview. *Korean J. Radiol.* **2017**, *18*, 570–584. [CrossRef]
8. Debelee, T.G.; Schwenker1, F.; Rahimeto, S.; Yohannes, D. Evaluation of modified adaptive k-means segmentation algorithm. *Comput. Vis. Media* **2019**. [CrossRef]

9. Kebede, S.R.; Debelee, T.G.; Schwenker, F.; Yohannes, D. Classifier Based Breast Cancer Segmentation. *J. Biomim. Biomater. Biomed. Eng.* **2020**, *47*, 1–21.
10. Rahimeto, S.; Debelee, T.; Yohannes, D.; Schwenker, F. Automatic pectoral muscle removal in mammograms. *Evol. Syst.* **2019**. [CrossRef]
11. Debelee, T.G.; Schwenker, F.; Ibenthal, A.; Yohannes, D. Survey of deep learning in breast cancer image analysis. *Evol. Syst.* **2019**. [CrossRef]
12. Debelee, T.G.; Gebreselasie, A.; Schwenker, F.; Amirian, M.; Yohannes, D. Classification of Mammograms Using Texture and CNN Based Extracted Features. *J. Biomim. Biomater. Biomed. Eng.* **2019**, *42*, 79–97. [CrossRef]
13. Debelee, T.G.; Amirian, M.; Ibenthal, A.; Palm, G.; Schwenker, F. Classification of Mammograms Using Convolutional Neural Network Based Feature Extraction. *LNICST* **2018**, *244*, 89–98.
14. Suckling, J.; Parker, J.; Dance, D.; Astley, S.; Hutt, I.; Boggis, C.; Ricketts, I. *Mammographic Image Analysis Society (MIAS) Database v1.21 [Dataset]*; Dataset; Digital Mammogram Database Exerpta Medica: Dordrecht, The Netherland, 2015.
15. Scuccimarra, E.A. *DDSM Mammography [Dataset]*; Dataset; Digital Mammogram Database Exerpta Medica: Dordrecht, The Netherland, 2018.
16. Moreira, I.C.; Amaral, I.; Domingues, I.; Cardoso, A.; Cardoso, M.J.; Cardoso, J.S. INbreast. *Acad. Radiol.* **2012**, *19*, 236–248. [CrossRef]
17. Dua, D.; Graff, C. *UCI Machine Learning Repository*; University of California, Irvine, School of Information and Computer Sciences: Newport Beach, CA, USA, 2017.
18. Bukun. *Breast Cancer Histopathological Database (BreakHis)*; Dataset; P and D Laboratory—Pathological Anatomy and Cytopathology: Parana, Brazil, 2019.
19. Aresta, G.; Araújo, T.; Kwok, S.; Chennamsetty, S.S.; Safwan, M.; Alex, V.; Marami, B.; Prastawa, M.; Chan, M.; Donovan, M.; et al. BACH: Grand challenge on breast cancer histology images. *Med. Image Anal.* **2019**, *56*, 122–139. [CrossRef]
20. Wu, N.; Phang, J.; Park, J.; Shen, Y.; Huang, Z.; Zorin, M.; Jastrzebski, S.; Fevry, T.; Katsnelson, J.; Kim, E.; et al. Deep Neural Networks Improve Radiologists' Performance in Breast Cancer Screening. *IEEE Trans. Med. Imaging* **2020**, *39*, 1184–1194. [CrossRef]
21. Alzubaidi, L.; Al-Shamma, O.; Fadhel, M.A.; Farhan, L.; Zhang, J.; Duan, Y. Optimizing the Performance of Breast Cancer Classification by Employing the Same Domain Transfer Learning from Hybrid Deep Convolutional Neural Network Model. *Electronics* **2020**, *9*, 445. [CrossRef]
22. Zhu, Z.; Harowicz, M.; Zhang, J.; Saha, A.; Grimm, L.J.; Hwang, E.S.; Mazurowski, M.A. Deep learning analysis of breast MRIs for prediction of occult invasive disease in ductal carcinoma in situ. *Comput. Biol. Med.* **2019**, *115*, 103498. [CrossRef]
23. Li, X.; Qin, G.; He, Q.; Sun, L.; Zeng, H.; He, Z.; Chen, W.; Zhen, X.; Zhou, L. Digital breast tomosynthesis versus digital mammography: Integration of image modalities enhances deep learning-based breast mass classification. *Eur. Radiol.* **2019**, *30*, 778–788. [CrossRef]
24. Zeiser, F.A.; da Costa, C.A.; Zonta, T.; Marques, N.M.C.; Roehe, A.V.; Moreno, M.; da Rosa Righi, R. Segmentation of Masses on Mammograms Using Data Augmentation and Deep Learning. *J. Digit. Imaging* **2020**. [CrossRef]
25. Zhang, Y.; Chen, J.H.; Chang, K.T.; Park, V.Y.; Kim, M.J.; Chan, S.; Chang, P.; Chow, D.; Luk, A.; Kwong, T.; et al. Automatic Breast and Fibroglandular Tissue Segmentation in Breast MRI Using Deep Learning by a Fully-Convolutional Residual Neural Network U-Net. *Acad. Radiol.* **2019**, *26*, 1526–1535. [CrossRef]
26. Zhou, J.; Luo, L.Y.; Dou, Q.; Chen, H.; Chen, C.; Li, G.J.; Jiang, Z.F.; Heng, P.A. Weakly supervised 3D deep learning for breast cancer classification and localization of the lesions in MR images. *J. Magn. Reson. Imaging* **2019**, *50*, 1144–1151. [CrossRef]
27. Huang, G.; Liu, Z.; Maaten, L.V.D.; Weinberger, K.Q. Densely Connected Convolutional Networks. In Proceedings of the 2017 IEEE Conference on Computer Vision and Pattern Recognition (CVPR), Honolulu, HI, USA, 21–26 July 2017. [CrossRef]
28. Zhang, J.; Saha, A.; Soher, B.J.; Mazurowski, M.A. Automatic deep learning-based normalization of breast dynamic contrast-enhanced magnetic resonance images. *arXiv* **2018**, arXiv:1807.02152v1.

29. Sheikh, T.S.; Lee, Y.; Cho, M. Histopathological Classification of Breast Cancer Images Using a Multi-Scale Input and Multi-Feature Network. *Cancers* **2020**, *12*, 2031. [CrossRef] [PubMed]
30. Li, X.; Shen, X.; Zhou, Y.; Wang, X.; Li, T.Q. Classification of breast cancer histopathological images using interleaved DenseNet with SENet (IDSNet). *PLoS ONE* **2020**, *15*, e0232127. [CrossRef]
31. Yan, R.; Ren, F.; Wang, Z.; Wang, L.; Zhang, T.; Liu, Y.; Rao, X.; Zheng, C.; Zhang, F. Breast cancer histopathological image classification using a hybrid deep neural network. *Methods* **2020**, *173*, 52–60. [CrossRef]
32. Sharma, S.; Mehra, R. Conventional Machine Learning and Deep Learning Approach for Multi-Classification of Breast Cancer Histopathology Images—a Comparative Insight. *J. Digit. Imaging* **2020**, *33*, 632–654. [CrossRef]
33. Vang, Y.S.; Chen, Z.; Xie, X. Deep Learning Framework for Multi-class Breast Cancer Histology Image Classification. In *Lecture Notes in Computer Science*; Springer International Publishing: Berlin/Heidelberg, Germany, 2018; pp. 914–922. [CrossRef]
34. Dembrower, K.; Liu, Y.; Azizpour, H.; Eklund, M.; Smith, K.; Lindholm, P.; Strand, F. Comparison of a Deep Learning Risk Score and Standard Mammographic Density Score for Breast Cancer Risk Prediction. *Radiology* **2020**, *294*, 265–272. [CrossRef]
35. Hagos, Y.B.; Merida, A.G.; Teuwen, J. Improving Breast Cancer Detection using Symmetry Information with Deep Learning. *arXiv* **2018**, arXiv:1808.08273v1.
36. Ferlay, J.; Shin, H.R.; Bray, F.; Forman, D.; Mathers, C.; Parkin, D.M. Estimates of worldwide burden of cancer in 2008: GLOBOCAN 2008. *Int. J. Cancer* **2010**, *127*, 2893–2917. [CrossRef]
37. Wingo, P.A.; Cardinez, C.J.; Landis, S.H.; Greenlee, R.T.; Ries, L.A.G.; Anderson, R.N.; Thun, M.J. Long-term trends in cancer mortality in the United States, 1930–1998. *Cancer* **2003**, *97*, 3133–3275. [CrossRef] [PubMed]
38. Schiffman, M.; Doorbar, J.; Wentzensen, N.; De Sanjosé, S.; Fakhry, C.; Monk, B.J.; Stanley, M.A.; Franceschi, S. Carcinogenic human papillomavirus infection. *Nat. Rev. Dis. Prim.* **2016**, *2*, 1–20. [CrossRef]
39. Patten, J. (Ed.) *Comprehensive Cervical Cancer Control: A Guide to Essential Practice*; World Health Organization: Geneva, Switzerland, 2014.
40. GençTav, A.; Aksoy, S.; ÖNder, S. Unsupervised segmentation andclassification of cervical cell images. *Pattern Recognit.* **2012**, *45*, 4151–4168. [CrossRef]
41. Tang, G.Y.; Parekh, J. Methods of Screening for Cervical Cancer. *JAMA* **2018**, *320*, 1938. [CrossRef]
42. Liang, Y.; Tang, Z.; Yan, M.; Chen, J.; Liu, Q.; Xiang, Y. Comparison-Based Convolutional Neural Networks for Cervical Cell/ClumpsDetection in the Limited Data Scenario. *arXiv* **2019**, arXiv:1810.05952.
43. Jantzen, J.; Norup, J.; Dounias, G.; Bjerregaard, B. Pap-smear benchmark data for pattern classification. In Proceedings of the Nature Inspired Smart Information Systems (NiSIS 2005), Albufeira, Portugal, 3–5 October 2005.
44. Hussain, E. Liquid based cytology pap smear images for multi-class diagnosis of cervical cancer. *Data Brief* **2019**. [CrossRef]
45. Rezende, M.T.; Tobias, A.H.G.; Silva, R.; Oliveira, P.; Medeiros, F.S.D.; Ushizima, D.; Carneiro, C.M.; Bianchi, A.G.C. CRIC Cervix Cell Classification. 2020. Available online: https://figshare.com/collections/CRIC_Cervix_Cell_Classification/4960286 (accessed on 11 August 2020). [CrossRef]
46. Franco, R.A.S.; Carvalho, M.A.G.; Coelho, G.P.; Martins, P.; Enciso, J.L. Dataset of Cervical Cell Images for the Study of Changes Associated with Malignancy in Conventional Pap Test. *ZENODO* **2018**. [CrossRef]
47. Group, A. Human Papillomavirus Testing for Triage of Women With Cytologic Evidence of Low-Grade Squamous Intraepithelial Lesions: Baseline Data From a Randomized Trial. *J. Natl. Cancer Inst.* **2000**, *92*, 397–402. [CrossRef] [PubMed]
48. MobileODT. Intel & Mobile ODT Cervical Cancer Screening. 2017. Available online: https://www.kaggle.com/c/intel-mobileodt-cervical-cancer-screening (accessed on 14 August 2020).
49. Song, Y.; Cheng, J.Z.; Ni, D.; Chen, S.; Lei, B.; Wang, T. Segmenting overlapping cervical cell in Pap smear images. In Proceedings of the 2016 IEEE 13th International Symposium on Biomedical Imaging (ISBI), Prague, Czech Republic, 13–16 April 2016. [CrossRef]
50. Zhao, J.; Dai, L.; Zhang, M.; Yu, F.; Li, M.; Li, H.; Wang, W.; Zhang, L. PGU-net+: Progressive Growing of U-net+ for Automated Cervical Nuclei Segmentation. In *Multiscale Multimodal Medical Imaging*; Springer International Publishing: Berlin/Heidelberg, Germany, 2019; pp. 51–58. [CrossRef]

51. Ronneberger, O.; Fischer, P.; Brox, T. U-Net: Convolutional Networks for Biomedical Image Segmentation. In *Lecture Notes in Computer Science*; Springer International Publishing: Berlin/Heidelberg, Germany, 2015; pp. 234–241. [CrossRef]
52. Sompawong, N.; Mopan, J.; Pooprasert, P.; Himakhun, W.; Suwannarurk, K.; Ngamvirojcharoen, J.; Vachiramon, T.; Tantibundhit, C. Automated Pap Smear Cervical Cancer Screening Using Deep Learning. In Proceedings of the 2019 41st Annual International Conference of the IEEE Engineering in Medicine and Biology Society (EMBC), Berlin, Germany, 23–27 July 2019. [CrossRef]
53. Liu, Y.; Zhang, P.; Song, Q.; Li, A.; Zhang, P.; Gui, Z. Automatic Segmentation of Cervical Nuclei Based on Deep Learning and a Conditional Random Field. *IEEE Access* **2018**, *6*, 53709–53721. [CrossRef]
54. Kurnianingsih, A.K.H.S.; Nugroho, L.E.; Widyawan; Lazuardi, L.; Prabuwono, A.S.; Mantoro, T. Segmentation and Classification of Cervical Cells Using Deep Learning. *IEEE Access* **2019**, *7*, 116925–116941. [CrossRef]
55. Zhang, L.; Lu, L.; Nogues, I.; Summers, R.M.; Liu, S.; Yao, J. DeepPap: Deep Convolutional Networks for Cervical Cell Classification. *IEEE J. Biomed. Health Inform.* **2017**, *21*, 1633–1643. [CrossRef]
56. Hyeon, J.; Choi, H.J.; Lee, K.N.; Lee, B.D. Automating Papanicolaou Test Using Deep Convolutional Activation Feature. In Proceedings of the 2017 18th IEEE International Conference on Mobile Data Management (MDM), Daejeon, Korea, 29 May–1 June 2017. [CrossRef]
57. Lin, H.; Hu, Y.; Chen, S.; Yao, J.; Zhang, L. Fine-Grained Classification of Cervical Cells Using Morphological and Appearance Based Convolutional Neural Networks. *IEEE Access* **2019**, *7*, 71541–71549. [CrossRef]
58. Deng, J.; Dong, W.; Socher, R.; Li, L.J.; Li, K.; Fei-Fei, L. Imagenet: A large-scale hierarchical image database. In Proceedings of the 2009 IEEE Conference on Computer Vision and Pattern Recognition, Miami, FL, USA, 20–25 June 2009; pp. 248–255.
59. Nayar, R.; Wilbur, D.C. The Pap test and Bethesda 2014. *Cancer Cytopathol.* **2015**, *123*, 271–281. [CrossRef]
60. Chen, T.; Ma, X.; Ying, X.; Wang, W.; Yuan, C.; Lu, W.; Chen, D.Z.; Wu, J. Multi-Modal Fusion Learning For Cervical Dysplasia Diagnosis. In Proceedings of the 2019 IEEE 16th International Symposium on Biomedical Imaging (ISBI 2019), Venice, Italy, 8–11 April 2019. [CrossRef]
61. Promworn, Y.; Pattanasak, S.; Pintavirooj, C.; Piyawattanametha, W. Comparisons of PAP-Smear Classification with Deep Learning Models. In Proceedings of the 14th annual IEEE International Conference on Nano/Micro Engineering and Molecular Systems, Bangkok, Thailand, 11–14 April 2019.
62. Ma, Y.; Xu, T.; Huang, X.; Wang, X.; Li, C.; Jerwick, J.; Ning, Y.; Zeng, X.; Wang, B.; Wang, Y.; et al. Computer-Aided Diagnosis of Label-Free 3-D Optical Coherence Microscopy Images of Human Cervical Tissue. *IEEE Trans. Biomed. Eng.* **2019**, *66*, 2447–2456. [CrossRef] [PubMed]
63. Ghoneim, A.; Muhammad, G.; Hossain, M.S. Cervical cancer classification using convolutional neural networks and extreme learning machines. *Future Gener. Comput. Syst.* **2020**, *102*, 643–649. [CrossRef]
64. Dong, N.; Zhao, L.; Wu, C.; Chang, J. Inception v3 based cervical cell classification combined with artificially extracted features. *Appl. Soft Comput.* **2020**, *93*, 106311. [CrossRef]
65. Martínez-Más, J.; Bueno-Crespo, A.; Martínez-España, R.; Remezal-Solano, M.; Ortiz-González, A.; Ortiz-Reina, S.; Martínez-Cendán, J.P. Classifying Papanicolaou cervical smears through a cell merger approach by deep learning technique. *Expert Syst. Appl.* **2020**, *160*, 113707. [CrossRef]
66. Xiang, Y.; Sun, W.; Pan, C.; Yan, M.; Yin, Z.; Liang, Y. A novel automation-assisted cervical cancer reading method based on convolutional neural network. *Biocybern. Biomed. Eng.* **2020**, *40*, 611–623. [CrossRef]
67. Garcia-Arteaga, J.; Kybic, J.; Li, W. Automatic colposcopyvideo tissue classification using higher order entropy-basedimage registration. *Comput. Biol. Med.* **2011**, *41*, 960–970. [CrossRef]
68. Wimpy, B.; Suyanto, S. Classification of Cervical and Type Image and Using and Capsule Networks. In Proceedings of the 2019 International Seminar on Research of Information Technology and Intelligent Systems (ISRITI), Yogyakarta, Indonesia, 5–6 December 2019.
69. Gorantla, R.; Singh, R.K.; Pandey, R.; Jain, M. Cervical Cancer Diagnosis using CervixNet—A Deep Learning Approach. In Proceedings of the 2019 IEEE 19th International Conference on Bioinformatics and Bioengineering (BIBE), Athens, Greece, 28–30 October 2019. [CrossRef]
70. Arora, M.; Dhawan, S.; Singh, K. Deep Neural Network for Transformation Zone Classification. In Proceedings of the 2018 First International Conference on Secure Cyber Computing and Communication (ICSCCC), Jalandhar, India, 15–17 December 2018.

71. Tang, J. *Intelligent Mobile Projects with TensorFlow: Build 10+ Artificial Intelligence Apps Using TensorFlow Mobile and Lite for iOS, Android, and Raspberry Pi*; Packt Publishing: Birmingham, UK, 2018.
72. Guo, P.; Xue, Z.; Long, L.R.; Antani, S. Cross-Dataset Evaluation of Deep Learning Networks for Uterine Cervix Segmentation. *Diagnostics* **2020**, *10*, 44. [CrossRef]
73. Guo, P.; Singh, S.; Xue, Z.; Long, R.; Antani, S. Deep Learning for Assessing Image Focus for Automated Cervical Cancer Screening. In Proceedings of the 2019 IEEE EMBS International Conference on Biomedical & Health Informatics (BHI), Chicago, IL, USA, 19–22 May 2019. [CrossRef]
74. Guo, P.; Xue, Z.; Mtema, Z.; Yeates, K.; Ginsburg, O.; Demarco, M.; Long, L.R.; Schiffman, M.; Antani, S. Ensemble Deep Learning for Cervix Image Selection toward Improving Reliability in Automated Cervical Precancer Screening. *Diagnostics* **2020**, *10*, 451. [CrossRef]
75. Sharma, M.; Mukharjee, S. Brain Tumor Segmentation Using Genetic Algorithm and Artificial Neural Network Fuzzy Inference System (ANFIS). In *Advances in Computing and Information Technology*; Springer: Berlin/Heidelberg, Germany, 2013; pp. 329–339. [CrossRef]
76. Hanif, F.; Muzaffar, K.; Perveen, K.; Malhi, S.M.; Simjee, S.U. Glioblastoma Multiforme: A Review of its Epidemiology and Pathogenesis through Clinical Presentation and Treatment. *Asian Pac. J. Cancer Prev. APJCP* **2017**, *18*, 3–9. [CrossRef]
77. Rees, J.H. Diagnosis and treatment in neuro-oncology: An oncological perspective. *Br. J. Radiol.* **2011**, *84*, S82–S89. [CrossRef]
78. Rasmussen, B.K.; Hansen, S.; Laursen, R.J.; Kosteljanetz, M.; Schultz, H.; Nørgård, B.M.; Guldberg, R.; Gradel, K.O. Epidemiology of glioma: Clinical characteristics, symptoms, and predictors of glioma patients grade I–IV in the the Danish Neuro-Oncology Registry. *J. Neuro Oncol.* **2017**, *135*, 571–579. [CrossRef]
79. Kalpathy-Cramer, J.; Gerstner, E.R.; Emblem, K.E.; Andronesi, O.; Rosen, B. Advanced magnetic resonance imaging of the physical processes in human glioblastoma. *Cancer Res.* **2014**, *74*, 4622–4637. [CrossRef] [PubMed]
80. Mohsen, H.; El-Dahshan, E.S.A.; El-Horbaty, E.S.M.; Salem, A.B.M. Classification using deep learning neural networks for brain tumors. *Future Comput. Inform. J.* **2018**, *3*, 68–71. [CrossRef]
81. Bahadure, N.B.; Ray, A.K.; Thethi, H.P. Image Analysis for MRI Based Brain Tumor Detection and Feature Extraction Using Biologically Inspired BWT and SVM. *Int. J. Biomed. Imaging* **2017**, *2017*, 1–12. [CrossRef] [PubMed]
82. Srinivas, B.; Rao, G.S. Segmentation of Multi-Modal MRI Brain Tumor Sub-Regions Using Deep Learning. *J. Electr. Eng. Technol.* **2020**, *15*, 1899–1909. [CrossRef]
83. Nadeem, M.W.; Ghamdi, M.A.A.; Hussain, M.; Khan, M.A.; Khan, K.M.; Almotiri, S.H.; Butt, S.A. Brain Tumor Analysis Empowered with Deep Learning: A Review, Taxonomy, and Future Challenges. *Brain Sci.* **2020**, *10*, 118. [CrossRef] [PubMed]
84. Akkus, Z.; Galimzianova, A.; Hoogi, A.; Rubin, D.L.; Erickson, B.J. Deep Learning for Brain MRI Segmentation: State of the Art and Future Directions. *J. Digit. Imaging* **2017**, *30*, 449–459. [CrossRef]
85. Shattuck, D.W.; Prasad, G.; Mirza, M.; Narr, K.L.; Toga, A.W. Online resource for validation of brain segmentation methods. *NeuroImage* **2009**, *45*, 431–439. [CrossRef] [PubMed]
86. Menze, B.H.; Jakab, A.; Bauer, S.; Kalpathy-Cramer, J.; Farahani, K.; Kirby, J.; Burren, Y.; Porz, N.; Slotboom, J.; Wiest, R.; et al. The Multimodal Brain Tumor Image Segmentation Benchmark (BRATS). *IEEE Trans. Med. Imaging* **2015**, *34*, 1993–2024. [CrossRef]
87. Barboriak, D. Data From RIDER_NEURO_MRI. 2015. Available online: https://wiki.cancerimagingarchive.net/display/Public/RIDER+NEURO+MRI (accessed on 15 August 2020). [CrossRef]
88. Fabelo, H.; Ortega, S.; Szolna, A.; Bulters, D.; Pineiro, J.F.; Kabwama, S.; J-O'Shanahan, A.; Bulstrode, H.; Bisshopp, S.; Kiran, B.R.; et al. In-Vivo Hyperspectral Human Brain Image Database for Brain Cancer Detection. *IEEE Access* **2019**, *7*, 39098–39116. [CrossRef]
89. Cheng, J.; Huang, W.; Cao, S.; Yang, R.; Yang, W.; Yun, Z.; Wang, Z.; Feng, Q. Enhanced Performance of Brain Tumor Classification via Tumor Region Augmentation and Partition. *PLoS ONE* **2015**, *10*, e0140381. [CrossRef]
90. Cheng, J. Brain Tumor Dataset. 2017. Available online: https://doi.org/10.6084/m9.figshare.1512427.v5 (accessed on 26 October 2020).

91. Alkassar, S.; Abdullah, M.A.M.; Jebur, B.A. Automatic Brain Tumour Segmentation using fully Convolution Network and Transfer Learning. In Proceedings of the 2019 2nd International Conference on Electrical, Communication, Computer, Power and Control Engineering (ICECCPCE), Mosul, Iraq, 13–14 February 2019. [CrossRef]
92. Amiri, S.; Rekik, I.; Mahjoub, M.A. Deep random forest-based learning transfer to SVM for brain tumor segmentation. In Proceedings of the 2016 2nd International Conference on Advanced Technologies for Signal and Image Processing (ATSIP), Monastir, Tunisia, 21–23 March 2016. [CrossRef]
93. Chahal, E.S.; Haritosh, A.; Gupta, A.; Gupta, K.; Sinha, A. Deep Learning Model for Brain Tumor Segmentation & Analysis. In Proceedings of the 2019 3rd International Conference on Recent Developments in Control, Automation & Power Engineering (RDCAPE), Noida, India, 10–11 October 2019. [CrossRef]
94. Ding, Y.; Li, C.; Yang, Q.; Qin, Z.; Qin, Z. How to Improve the Deep Residual Network to Segment Multi-Modal Brain Tumor Images. *IEEE Access* **2019**, *7*, 152821–152831. [CrossRef]
95. Mallick, P.K.; Ryu, S.H.; Satapathy, S.K.; Mishra, S.; Nguyen, G.N.; Tiwari, P. Brain MRI Image Classification for Cancer Detection Using Deep Wavelet Autoencoder-Based Deep Neural Network. *IEEE Access* **2019**, *7*, 46278–46287. [CrossRef]
96. Ramirez, I.; Martin, A.; Schiavi, E. Optimization of a variational model using deep learning: An application to brain tumor segmentation. In Proceedings of the 2018 IEEE 15th International Symposium on Biomedical Imaging (ISBI 2018), Washington, DC, USA, 4–7 April 2018. [CrossRef]
97. Sajid, S.; Hussain, S.; Sarwar, A. Brain Tumor Detection and Segmentation in MR Images Using Deep Learning. *Arab. J. Sci. Eng.* **2019**, *44*, 9249–9261. [CrossRef]
98. Wang, Y.; Li, C.; Zhu, T.; Yu, C. A Deep Learning Algorithm for Fully Automatic Brain Tumor Segmentation. In Proceedings of the 2019 International Joint Conference on Neural Networks (IJCNN), Budapest, Hungary, 14–19 July 2019. [CrossRef]
99. Zhao, X.; Wu, Y.; Song, G.; Li, Z.; Zhang, Y.; Fan, Y. A deep learning model integrating FCNNs and CRFs for brain tumor segmentation. *Med. Image Anal.* **2018**, *43*, 98–111. [CrossRef] [PubMed]
100. Kuzina, A.; Egorov, E.; Burnaev, E. Bayesian Generative Models for Knowledge Transfer in MRI Semantic Segmentation Problems. *Front. Neurosci.* **2019**, *13*. [CrossRef] [PubMed]
101. Zeineldin, R.A.; Karar, M.E.; Coburger, J.; Wirtz, C.R.; Burgert, O. DeepSeg: Deep neural network framework for automatic brain tumor segmentation using magnetic resonance FLAIR images. *Int. J. Comput. Assist. Radiol. Surg.* **2020**, *15*, 909–920. [CrossRef]
102. Fabelo, H.; Halicek, M.; Ortega, S.; Shahedi, M.; Szolna, A.; Piñeiro, J.; Sosa, C.; O'Shanahan, A.; Bisshopp, S.; Espino, C.; et al. Deep Learning-Based Framework for In Vivo Identification of Glioblastoma Tumor using Hyperspectral Images of Human Brain. *Sensors* **2019**, *19*, 920. [CrossRef]
103. Shree, N.V.; Kumar, T.N.R. Identification and classification of brain tumor MRI images with feature extraction using DWT and probabilistic neural network. *Brain Inform.* **2018**, *5*, 23–30. [CrossRef]
104. Tandel, G.S.; Biswas, M.; Kakde, O.G.; Tiwari, A.; Suri, H.S.; Turk, M.; Laird, J.; Asare, C.; Ankrah, A.A.; Khanna, N.N.; et al. A Review on a Deep Learning Perspective in Brain Cancer Classification. *Cancers* **2019**, *11*, 111. [CrossRef] [PubMed]
105. Alqudah, A.M. Brain Tumor Classification Using Deep Learning Technique—A Comparison between Cropped, Uncropped, and Segmented Lesion Images with Different Sizes. *Int. J. Adv. Trends Comput. Sci. Eng.* **2019**, *8*, 3684–3691. [CrossRef]
106. Ucuzal, H.; Yasar, S.; Colak, C. Classification of brain tumor types by deep learning with convolutional neural network on magnetic resonance images using a developed web-based interface. In Proceedings of the 2019 3rd International Symposium on Multidisciplinary Studies and Innovative Technologies (ISMSIT), Ankara Turkey, 11–13 October 2019. [CrossRef]
107. Bazin, P. Example MP2RAGEME Data Set. 2019. Available online: https://uvaauas.figshare.com/articles/Example_MP2RAGEME_data_set/7938326 (accessed on 15 August 2020). [CrossRef]
108. Tetik, B.; Ucuzal, H.; Yasar, S.; Colak, C. Brain Tumor Classification Software[Web-Based Software]. Available online: http://biostatapps.inonu.edu.tr/BTSY (accessed on 17 August 2020)
109. Selvy, P.T.; Dharani, V.P.; Indhuja, A. Brain Tumour Detection Using Deep Learning Techniques. *Int. J. Sci. Res. Comput. Sci. Eng. Inf. Technol.* **2019**, 169–175. [CrossRef]
110. Sultan, H.H.; Salem, N.M.; Al-Atabany, W. Multi-Classification of Brain Tumor Images Using Deep Neural Network. *IEEE Access* **2019**, *7*, 69215–69225. [CrossRef]

111. Badža, M.M.; Barjaktarović, M.Č. Classification of Brain Tumors from MRI Images Using a Convolutional Neural Network. *Appl. Sci.* **2020**, *10*, 1999. [CrossRef]
112. WHO. Global Cancer Observatory (GCO). 2018. Available online: https://gco.iarc.fr/ (accessed on 1 July 2020).
113. Graham, S.; Chen, H.; Gamper, J.; Dou, Q.; Heng, P.A.; Snead, D.; Tsang, Y.W.; Rajpoot, N. MILD-Net: Minimal Information Loss Dilated Network for Gland Instance Segmentation in Colon Histology Images. *Med. Image Anal.* **2018**. [CrossRef]
114. Benson, V.S.; Patnick, J.; Davies, A.K.; Nadel, M.R.; Smith, R.A.; Atkin, W.S. Colorectal cancer screening: A comparison of 35 initiatives in 17 countries. *Int. J. Cancer* **2007**, *122*, 1357–1367. [CrossRef] [PubMed]
115. Rony, J.; Belharbi, S.; Dolz, J.; Ayed, I.B.; McCaffrey, L.; Granger, E. Deep weakly-supervised learning methods for classification and localization in histology images: A survey. *arXiv* **2019**, arXiv:1909.03354v3.
116. Vázquez, D.; Bernal, J.; Sánchez, F.J.; Fernández-Esparrach, G.; López, A.M.; Romero, A.; Drozdzal, M.; Courville, A. A Benchmark for Endoluminal Scene Segmentation of Colonoscopy Images. *J. Healthc. Eng.* **2017**, *2017*, 1–9. [CrossRef] [PubMed]
117. Bernal, J.; Sánchez, J.; Vilariño, F. Towards automatic polyp detection with a polyp appearance model. *Pattern Recognit.* **2012**, *45*, 3166–3182. [CrossRef]
118. Bernal, J.; Sánchez, F.J.; Fernández-Esparrach, G.; Gil, D.; Rodríguez, C.; Vilariño, F. WM-DOVA maps for accurate polyp highlighting in colonoscopy: Validation vs. saliency maps from physicians. *Comput. Med. Imaging Graph.* **2015**, *43*, 99–111. [CrossRef]
119. Kather, J.N.; Weis, C.A.; Bianconi, F.; Melchers, S.M.; Schad, L.R.; Gaiser, T.; Marx, A.; Zöllner, F.G. Multi-class texture analysis in colorectal cancer histology. *Sci. Rep.* **2016**, *6*. [CrossRef]
120. Kainz, P.; Pfeiffer, M.; Urschler, M. Segmentation and classification of colon glands with deep convolutional neural networks and total variation regularization. *PeerJ* **2017**, *5*, e3874. [CrossRef]
121. Sirinukunwattana, K.; Ahmed Raza, S.E.; Tsang, Y.W.; Snead, D.R.J.; Cree, I.A.; Rajpoot, N.M. Locality Sensitive Deep Learning for Detection and Classification of Nuclei in Routine Colon Cancer Histology Images. *IEEE Trans. Med. Imaging* **2016**, *35*, 1196–1206. [CrossRef]
122. Chamanzar, A.; Nie, Y. Weakly Supervised Multi-Task Learning for Cell Detection and Segmentation. In Proceedings of the 2020 IEEE 17th International Symposium on Biomedical Imaging (ISBI), Iowa City, IA, USA, 4 April 2020. [CrossRef]
123. Sari, C.T.; Gunduz-Demir, C. Unsupervised Feature Extraction via Deep Learning for Histopathological Classification of Colon Tissue Images. *IEEE Trans. Med. Imaging* **2019**, *38*, 1139–1149. [CrossRef] [PubMed]
124. Ozdemir, E.; Gunduz-Demir, C. A Hybrid Classification Model for Digital Pathology Using Structural and Statistical Pattern Recognition. *IEEE Trans. Med. Imaging* **2013**, *32*, 474–483. [CrossRef]
125. Shapcott, M.; Hewitt, K.J.; Rajpoot, N. Deep Learning With Sampling in Colon Cancer Histology. *Front. Bioeng. Biotechnol.* **2019**, *7*, 52. [CrossRef]
126. Tang, J.; Li, J.; Xu, X. Segnet-based gland segmentation from colon cancer histology images. In Proceedings of the 2018 33rd Youth Academic Annual Conference of Chinese Association of Automation (YAC), Nanjing, China, 18 May 2018. [CrossRef]
127. Vuong, T.L.T.; Lee, D.; Kwak, J.T.; Kim, K. Multi-task Deep Learning for Colon Cancer Grading. In Proceedings of the 2020 International Conference on Electronics, Information, and Communication (ICEIC), Fukuoka, Kapan, 5–7 September 2020. [CrossRef]
128. Sabol, P.; Sinčák, P.; Hartono, P.; Kočan, P.; Benetinová, Z.; Blichárová, A.; Verbóová, Ľ.; Štammová, E.; Sabolová-Fabianová, A.; Jašková, A. Explainable classifier for improving the accountability in decision-making for colorectal cancer diagnosis from histopathological images. *J. Biomed. Inform.* **2020**, *109*, 103523. [CrossRef]
129. Suzuki, K.; Yoshida, H.; Näppi, J.; Dachman, A.H. Massive-training artificial neural network (MTANN) for reduction of false positives in computer-aided detection of polyps: Suppression of rectal tubes. *Med. Phys.* **2006**, *33*, 3814–3824. [CrossRef] [PubMed]
130. Bardhi, O.; Sierra-Sosa, D.; Garcia-Zapirain, B.; Elmaghraby, A. Automatic colon polyp detection using Convolutional encoder-decoder model. In Proceedings of the 2017 IEEE International Symposium on Signal Processing and Information Technology (ISSPIT), Bilbao, Spain, 18–20 December 2017. [CrossRef]

131. Bour, A.; Castillo-Olea, C.; Garcia-Zapirain, B.; Zahia, S. Automatic colon polyp classification using Convolutional Neural Network: A Case Study at Basque Country. In Proceedings of the 2019 IEEE International Symposium on Signal Processing and Information Technology (ISSPIT), Ajman, UAE, 10–12 December 2019. [CrossRef]
132. Liu, X.; Li, Y.; Yao, J.; Chen, B.; Song, J.; Yang, X. Classification of Polyps and Adenomas Using Deep Learning Model in Screening Colonoscopy. In Proceedings of the 2019 8th International Symposium on Next Generation Electronics (ISNE), Zhengzhou, China, 9–10 October 2019. [CrossRef]
133. Ozawa, T.; Ishihara, S.; Fujishiro, M.; Kumagai, Y.; Shichijo, S.; Tada, T. Automated endoscopic detection and classification of colorectal polyps using convolutional neural networks. *Ther. Adv. Gastroenterol.* **2020**, *13*, 1756284820910659. [CrossRef]
134. Nadimi, E.S.; Buijs, M.M.; Herp, J.; Kroijer, R.; Kobaek-Larsen, M.; Nielsen, E.; Pedersen, C.D.; Blanes-Vidal, V.; Baatrup, G. Application of deep learning for autonomous detection and localization of colorectal polyps in wireless colon capsule endoscopy. *Comput. Electr. Eng.* **2020**, *81*, 106531. [CrossRef]
135. Zeiler, M.D.; Fergus, R. Visualizing and Understanding Convolutional Networks. In *Computer Vision—ECCV 2014*; Springer International Publishing: Berlin/Heidelberg, Germany, 2014; pp. 818–833. [CrossRef]
136. Lung Cancer Screening (PDQ®): Patient Version. 2020. Available online: https://www.cancer.gov/types/lung/hp/lung-screening-pdq (accessed on 11 October 2020).
137. Hong, Z.Q.; Yang, J.Y. Optimal discriminant plane for a small number of samples and design method of classifier on the plane. *Pattern Recognit.* **1991**, *24*, 317–324. [CrossRef]
138. Armato, S.G., III; Hadjiiski, L.; Tourassi, G.D.; Drukker, K.; Giger, M.L.; Li, F.; Redmond, G.; Farahani, K.; Kirby, J.S.; Clarke, L.P. SPIE-AAPM-NCI Lung Nodule Classification Challenge Dataset. *Cancer Imaging Arch.* **2015**. [CrossRef]
139. Mader, S. Lung Nodule Malignancy. Data available at Kaggle. 2017. Available online: https://www.kaggle.com/kmader/lungnodemalignancy (accessed on 14 August 2020).
140. Suzuki, K.; Armato, S.G.; Li, F.; Sone, S.; Doi, K. Massive training artificial neural network (MTANN) for reduction of false positives in computerized detection of lung nodules in low-dose computed tomography. *Med. Phys.* **2003**, *30*, 1602–1617. [CrossRef]
141. Suzuki, K.; Li, F.; Sone, S.; Doi, K. Computer-aided diagnostic scheme for distinction between benign and malignant nodules in thoracic low-dose CT by use of massive training artificial neural network. *IEEE Trans. Med. Imaging* **2005**, *24*, 1138–1150. [CrossRef]
142. Tajbakhsh, N.; Suzuki, K. Comparing two classes of end-to-end machine-learning models in lung nodule detection and classification: MTANNs vs. CNNs. *Pattern Recognit.* **2017**, *63*, 476–486. [CrossRef]
143. Gu, Y.; Lu, X.; Yang, L.; Zhang, B.; Yu, D.; Zhao, Y.; Gao, L.; Wu, L.; Zhou, T. Automatic lung nodule detection using a 3D deep convolutional neural network combined with a multi-scale prediction strategy in chest CTs. *Comput. Biol. Med.* **2018**, *103*, 220–231. [CrossRef]
144. Sahu, P.; Yu, D.; Dasari, M.; Hou, F.; Qin, H. A Lightweight Multi-Section CNN for Lung Nodule Classification and Malignancy Estimation. *IEEE J. Biomed. Health Inform.* **2019**, *23*, 960–968. [CrossRef] [PubMed]
145. Ozdemir, O.; Russell, R.L.; Berlin, A.A. A 3D Probabilistic Deep Learning System for Detection and Diagnosis of Lung Cancer Using Low-Dose CT Scans. *IEEE Trans. Med. Imaging* **2020**, *39*, 1419–1429. [CrossRef] [PubMed]
146. Hamilton, B.A. Data Science Bowl 2017. Data Available at Kaggle. 2017. Available online: https://www.kaggle.com/c/data-science-bowl-2017 (accessed on 1 August 2020).
147. Bansal, G.; Chamola, V.; Narang, P.; Kumar, S.; Raman, S. Deep3DSCan: Deep residual network and morphological descriptor based framework for lung cancer classification and 3D segmentation. *IET Image Process.* **2020**, *14*, 1240–1247. [CrossRef]
148. Adegun, A.A.; Viriri, S. Deep Learning-Based System for Automatic Melanoma Detection. *IEEE Access* **2020**, *8*, 7160–7172. [CrossRef]
149. Azer, S.A. Challenges Facing the Detection of Colonic Polyps: What Can Deep Learning Do? *Medicina* **2019**, *55*, 473. [CrossRef]
150. Hamm, C.A.; Wang, C.J.; Savic, L.J.; Ferrante, M.; Schobert, I.; Schlachter, T.; Lin, M.; Duncan, J.S.; Weinreb, J.C.; Chapiro, J.; et al. Deep learning for liver tumor diagnosis part I: Development of a convolutional neural network classifier for multi-phasic MRI. *Eur. Radiol.* **2019**, *29*, 3338–3347. [CrossRef]

151. Yamakawa, M.; Shiina, T.; Nishida, N.; Kudo, M. Computer aided diagnosis system developed for ultrasound diagnosis of liver lesions using deep learning. In Proceedings of the 2019 IEEE International Ultrasonics Symposium (IUS), Glasgow, UK, 6–9 October 2019; pp. 2330–2333.
152. Kim, G.H.; Liang, P.S.; Bang, S.J.; Hwang, J.H. Screening and surveillance for gastric cancer in the United States: Is it needed? *Gastrointest. Endosc.* **2016**, *84*, 18–28. [CrossRef]
153. Lee, J.H.; Kim, Y.J.; Kim, Y.W.; Park, S.; Choi, Y.I.; Kim, Y.J.; Park, D.K.; Kim, K.G.; Chung, J.W. Spotting malignancies from gastric endoscopic images using deep learning. *Surg. Endosc.* **2019**, *33*, 3790–3797. [CrossRef]
154. Cho, B.J.; Bang, C.S.; Park, S.W.; Yang, Y.J.; Seo, S.I.; Lim, H.; Shin, W.G.; Hong, J.T.; Yoo, Y.T.; Hong, S.H.; et al. Automated classification of gastric neoplasms in endoscopic images using a convolutional neural network. *Endoscopy* **2019**, *51*, 1121–1129. [CrossRef] [PubMed]

2

Detection of Glioblastoma Subclinical Recurrence Using Serial Diffusion Tensor Imaging

Yan Jin [1], James W. Randall [1,2], Hesham Elhalawani [1], Karine A. Al Feghali [1], Andrew M. Elliott [1], Brian M. Anderson [3], Lara Lacerda [1], Benjamin L. Tran [1], Abdallah S. Mohamed [1], Kristy K. Brock [3], Clifton D. Fuller [1] and Caroline Chung [1,*]

1 Department of Radiation Oncology, the University of Texas MD Anderson Cancer Center, Houston, TX 77030, USA; yjinz@ucla.edu (Y.J.); jamesran92@gmail.com (J.W.R.); elhalawani.hesham@gmail.com (H.E.); kal1@mdanderson.org (K.A.A.F.); andrew.elliott@mdanderson.org (A.M.E.); lcalvarez@mdanderson.org (L.L.); bltran@mdanderson.org (B.L.T.); asmohamed@mdanderson.org (A.S.M.); cdfuller@mdanderson.org (C.D.F.)

2 The University of Texas Medical Branch, Galveston, TX 77555, USA

3 Department of Imaging Physics, the University of Texas MD Anderson Cancer Center, Houston, TX 77030, USA; bmanderson@mdanderson.org (B.M.A.); kkbrock@mdanderson.org (K.K.B.)

* Correspondence: cchung3@mdanderson.org

Abstract: Glioblastoma is an aggressive brain tumor with a propensity for intracranial recurrence. We hypothesized that tumors can be visualized with diffusion tensor imaging (DTI) before they are detected on anatomical magnetic resonance (MR) images. We retrospectively analyzed serial MR images from 30 patients, including the DTI and T1-weighted images at recurrence, at 2 months and 4 months before recurrence, and at 1 month after radiation therapy. The diffusion maps and T1 images were deformably registered longitudinally. The recurrent tumor was manually segmented on the T1-weighted image and then applied to the diffusion maps at each time point to collect mean FA, diffusivities, and neurite density index (NDI) values, respectively. Group analysis of variance showed significant changes in FA ($p = 0.01$) and NDI ($p = 0.0015$) over time. Pairwise t tests also revealed that FA and NDI at 2 months before recurrence were 11.2% and 6.4% lower than those at 1 month after radiation therapy ($p < 0.05$), respectively. Changes in FA and NDI were observed 2 months before recurrence, suggesting that progressive microstructural changes and neurite density loss may be detectable before tumor detection in anatomical MR images. FA and NDI may serve as non-contrast MR-based biomarkers for detecting subclinical tumors.

Keywords: glioblastoma; radiation therapy; recurrence; MRI; diffusion tensor imaging

---

1. Introduction

Glioblastoma (GBM) is the most common primary malignant brain tumor among adults [1]. Despite treatment with surgical resection, radiation therapy (RT), chemotherapy, and temozolomide, many patients experience intracranial tumor recurrence, and prognosis remains poor, with a median survival time of only 12–15 months [2–4]. In current clinical practice, the onset of recurrence is defined in terms of changes in traditional images, such as contrast-enhanced computed tomography or structural T1-weighted post-contrast magnetic resonance imaging (T1 MRI), followed if possible by histologic verification. However, given the high frequency of recurrence in GBM and the poor survival rate thereafter, early detection of recurrence is key to facilitating timely medical treatment and prolonging survival.

Glioma cells have been shown to migrate into healthy brain tissues along white matter (WM) tracts [5,6]. The molecular mechanism underlying this phenomenon is complex and contains multiple steps, including tumor cell adhesion to components of the extracellular matrix and modification to their compositions, migration by breaking adherence attachments to the matrix, and the degradation of matrix proteins by secreting enzymes [7]. This suggests that examining the integrity of WM tracts within the potential recurrent regions before visible, enhancing tumor recurrence may help further elucidate the mechanism of recurrence.

Diffusion-weighted imaging is a noninvasive MRI technique in which measurements of water diffusion in tissues [8] provide biological and clinically relevant information about the integrity of WM that cannot be provided by other imaging modalities. Diffusion tensor imaging (DTI) applies a mathematical elliptical model to represent the diffusion characteristics at each voxel [9]. A variety of diffusion-derived feature maps, such as fractional anisotropy (FA), mean diffusivity (MD), axial diffusivity (AD), and radial diffusivity (RD), can be extracted from DTI images and have provided complementary information about the integrity of WM in several neurologic diseases, such as multiple sclerosis [10], Parkinson disease [11], and Alzheimer disease [12].

In brain tumors, DTI has previously been used to assess WM disruptions to identify tumor grades [13,14], distinguish tumor tissue from peritumoral tissue [15], and study the patterns of shape (isotropic versus anisotropic) in recurrence [16]. Reduced FA has been linked with decreased fiber density index near tumors in patients with GBM [17]. However, details of how WM tracts are disrupted during the clinical course of recurrence are yet to be elucidated. We hypothesized that tumor cells in the recurrent regions cause microstructural disruptions in WM integrity and these disruptions can be visualized by DTI before tumors can be detected on conventional anatomical MRI. To test this hypothesis, we conducted a retrospective longitudinal study to evaluate whether changes in a series of DTI feature maps precede the clinical onset of recurrence. We also used an advanced diffusion analysis technique, neurite orientation dispersion and density imaging (NODDI) [18], to provide further details on how microstructures in WM are affected at the microscale level.

2. Materials and Methods

2.1. Patients and Image Acquisition

Under an institutional review board-approved protocol (PA18-1113), we extracted MRI data from 30 patients treated for GBM at the University of Texas MD Anderson Cancer Center who had experienced recurrence after RT. All patients had anatomical T1 and DTI brain imaging at four time points: at 1 month after RT (baseline), 4 months before recurrence, 2 months before recurrence, and at recurrence. The average time between baseline and recurrence was 13 months with a standard deviation of 12 months.

All scans were obtained according to a standard protocol developed for GBM follow-up at the University of Texas MD Anderson Cancer Center and were acquired on 1.5 T/3T MRI scanners (GE Medical Systems) with axial orientation. T1 images had a 256 × 256/512 × 512 in-plane acquisition matrix and a voxel resolution of 0.86 × 0.86 × 6.5 mm^3 (TR/TE = 550/8 ms)/0.43 × 0.43 × 5 mm^3 (TR/TE = 967/12 ms). DTI images consisted of 28 volumes with a 256 × 256 in-plane acquisition matrix and a voxel resolution of 0.86 × 0.86 × 6.5 mm^3 (TR/TE = 1000/99 ms)/0.86 × 0.86 × 5 mm^3 (TR/TE = 10,250/94 ms), including one non-diffusion sensitization volume, i.e., T2-weighted b0 volume, and 27 diffusion-weighted volumes (b = 1200 s/mm^2).

2.2. Image Preprocessing

T1 images were first skull-stripped with the open source skull stripping toolkit LABEL [19]. DTI images were also skull-stripped with Brain Extraction Tool in the Functional Magnetic Resonance Imaging of the Brain (FMRIB) Software Library (FSL; https://fsl.fmrib.ox.ac.uk/fsl/fslwiki) [20,21] and then corrected for eddy current-induced distortions and subject movements using EDDY [22] in FSL.

2.3. Microstructural Features with NODDI

We used NODDI, an advanced diffusion analysis technique, to provide additional details about the microstructural features the images represent. Dendrites and axons, known as neural processes or neurites, are the basic units for brain circuits. Using NODDI to investigate variations in branching complexity (i.e., density and orientation) allowed us to characterize changes in microstructural integrity in terms of recurrence. Specifically, NODDI provides three indices to describe such changes: neurite density index (NDI), orientation dispersion index (ODI), and free water fraction (FWF) [23]. NDI and ODI quantify the density and angular variation of neurites, and FWF describes the contamination of tissues by free water at the microstructural level [23].

2.4. Longitudinal Image Processing Pipeline

Our longitudinal image processing pipeline consisted of the following six steps: Step 1. Diffusion Feature Extraction: The following diffusion-derived feature maps were extracted from the DTI images of each patient at each time point by using DTIFIT in FSL: fractional anisotropy (FA), mean diffusivity (MD), axial diffusivity (AD), and radial diffusivity (RD). Next, we calculated the microstructural indices (NDI, ODI, and FWF) at each voxel of the DTI images with the NODDI Matlab Toolbox (http://mig.cs.ucl.ac.uk/index.php?n=Tutorial.NODDImatlab). Step 2. Longitudinal Image Alignment: We applied advanced normalization tools (http://stnava.github.io/ANTs/) [24] to register each patient's T1 images at 1 month after RT, 4 months before recurrence, and 2 months before recurrence to the T1 image obtained at recurrence. Because these T1 images had been acquired at different times, a nonlinear (warping) registration algorithm was used to ensure the best alignment effect. Step 3. Multi-Modality Image Alignment: At each time point, each patient's DTI images were co-registered using linear (rigid) registration with the corresponding T1 images, as both images were acquired during the same imaging session. Step 4. GTV Manual Segmentation: An experienced radiation oncologist manually segmented the tumor recurrence volume on the T1 images at the time of recurrence. Step 5. GTV Transfer: For each patient, the recurrent tumor volume was applied to the T1 images at the previous three time points with the deformation fields generated by nonlinear registrations in step 2. The recurrent tumor volume was then transferred to the corresponding DTI images with the affine matrix generated by linear registrations in step 3. The quality of registration and GTV transfer at steps 2–5 was manually inspected. Step 6. Mean Feature Calculation: The mean values of all diffusion features (FA, MD, AD, and RD) and microstructural features (NDI, ODI, and FFW) within the transferred and original recurrent GTV regions at the four time points were calculated.

2.5. Statistical Analysis

We compared all mean DTI features at the four time points using analysis of variance (ANOVA) to examine potential changes between these time points. Findings are reported as F ratios, i.e., the ratio of the between-group variance to the within-group variance. If any changes were detected, *t* tests were applied to further investigate changes occurring at each pair of time points.

3. Results

3.1. Diffusion Feature Maps

Mean FA values inside the regions of recurrence over the four time points are shown in box plots in Figure 1a. The ANOVA revealed statistically significant differences between time points ($F = 3.4$, $p = 0.01$), with a downward trend over time. To further examine which groups were different from one another, we used pairwise t tests to compare the four time points. After Bonferroni correction, the mean FA value at recurrence was significantly lower than those at the three prior time points ($p < 0.05$), with a decrease of 30.8% (95% confidence interval-CI: (18.2%, 43.0%)), 22.9% (95% CI: (11.0%, 38.9%)), and 19.2% (95% CI: (8.7%, 35.4%)) from the farthest to the nearest time point, respectively. Moreover, the mean FA value at 2 months before recurrence was also 11.2% lower than that at 1 month after RT, i.e., the baseline ($p < 0.05$). At the individual level, 14 and 18 out of 30 patients showed a lower mean FA value at 4 months before recurrence and 2 months before recurrence, compared to baseline, respectively.

Findings from the ANOVA of the mean values of the other feature maps (MD, AD, and RD) over time are shown in Figure 1b–d. No statistically significant differences were detected in these feature maps between time points: for MD, F = 1.38, $p = 0.25$; for AD, F = 0.99, $p = 0.40$; and for RD, F = 1.57, $p = 0.20$. Although these values were not statistically different, they demonstrated a trend of increasing values over time, as is evident in those figures. Further pairwise t tests showed that the mean values of MD, AD, and RD at 2 months before recurrence were 9.5% (95% CI: (4.0%, 15.4%)), 7.8% (95% CI: (2.5%, 13.0%)), and 10.9% (95% CI: (4.8%, 17.1%)) higher than those at baseline, respectively ($p < 0.05$ after Bonferroni correction). At the individual level, 18, 16, and 18 patients had a higher mean MD, AD, and RD value at 2 months before recurrence, compared to baseline, respectively.

Changes in these features (FA, MD, AD, and RD) may indicate that WM degeneration occurred at recurrent tumor regions before the tumor became visible on T1.

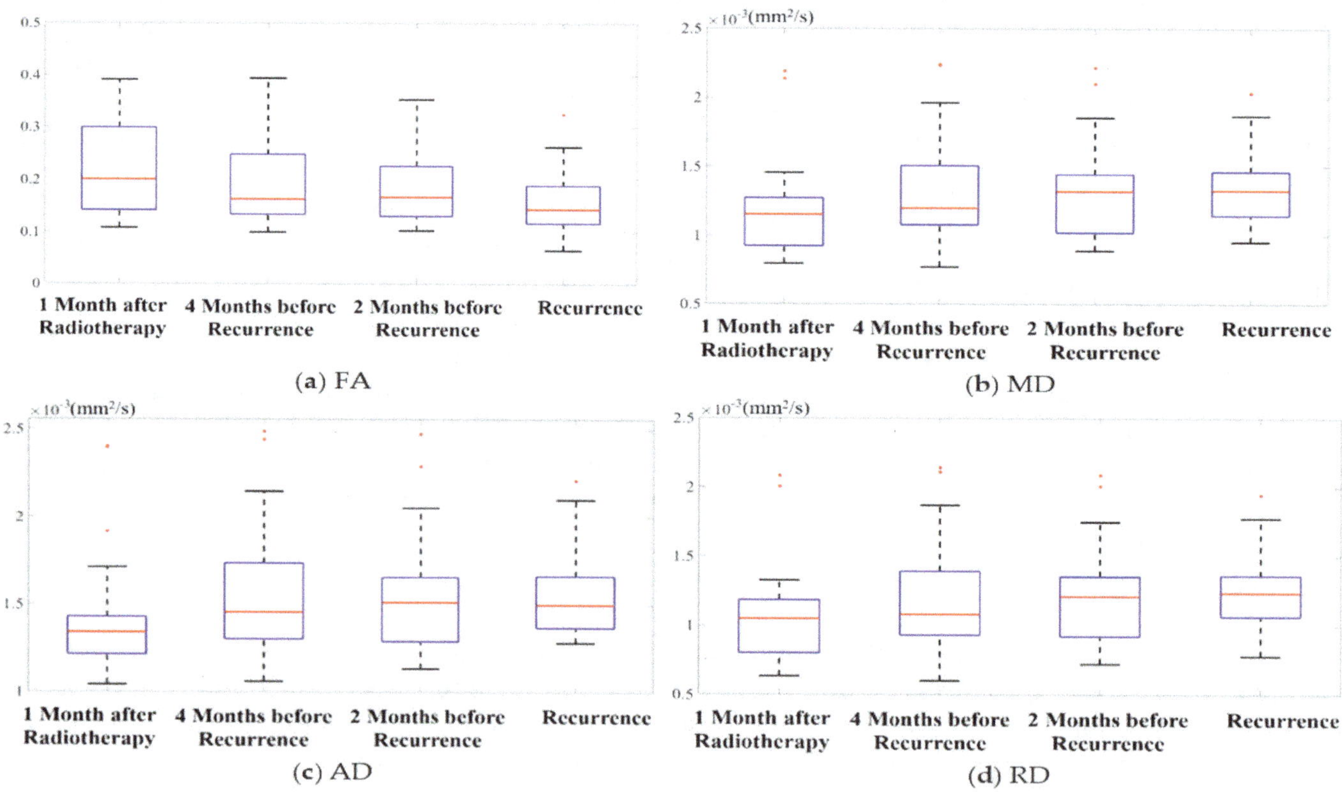

Figure 1. Box plots of the mean values of (**a**) fractional anisotropy (FA), (**b**) mean diffusivity (MD), (**c**) axial diffusivity (AD), and (**d**) radial diffusivity (RD) within recurrent tumor regions over the four time points. The five bars in the box plots indicate, from bottom to top, the minimum, first quartile, median, third quartile, and the maximum. The red dots indicate outliers.

3.2. Microstructural Features

To investigate which WM microstructural components were affected by tumor recurrence, we used the same statistical tests of the mean values of NDI, ODI, and FFW (obtained with the NODDI toolbox) at the regions of recurrence over time. The NDI results were similar to those of the FA findings (Figure 2a). ANOVA revealed differences among the four time points (F = 5.47, p = 0.0015), with a downward trend over time. Pairwise t tests showed that the mean NDI value at recurrence was significantly lower than baseline and 4 months before recurrence, a relative change of 11.9% (95% CI: (4.3%, 19.5%)), and 7.2% (95% CI: (0.4%, 15.6%)), respectively ($p < 0.05$ after Bonferroni correction). Furthermore, compared to baseline, the mean NDI values at 4 months before recurrence were 4.2% (95% CI: (1.5%, 6.9%)) lower and the mean NDI values at 2 months before recurrence were 6.4% (95% CI: (3.4%, 9.5%)) lower ($p < 0.05$ after Bonferroni correction). At the individual level, 21 and 20 patients demonstrated a reduced mean NDI value at 4 months before recurrence and 2 months before recurrence, compared to baseline, respectively.

The ANOVA showed no differences in ODI over time (F = 1.16, p = 0.33) (Figure 2b). Similarly, FWF did not change over time according to the ANOVA (F = 0.93, p = 0.43) (Figure 2c).

The observation of a change in NDI but not in ODI before recurrence suggests that microstructural changes in WM due to tumor recurrence may have resulted from a reduction in neurite density rather than a disruption in orientation distribution.

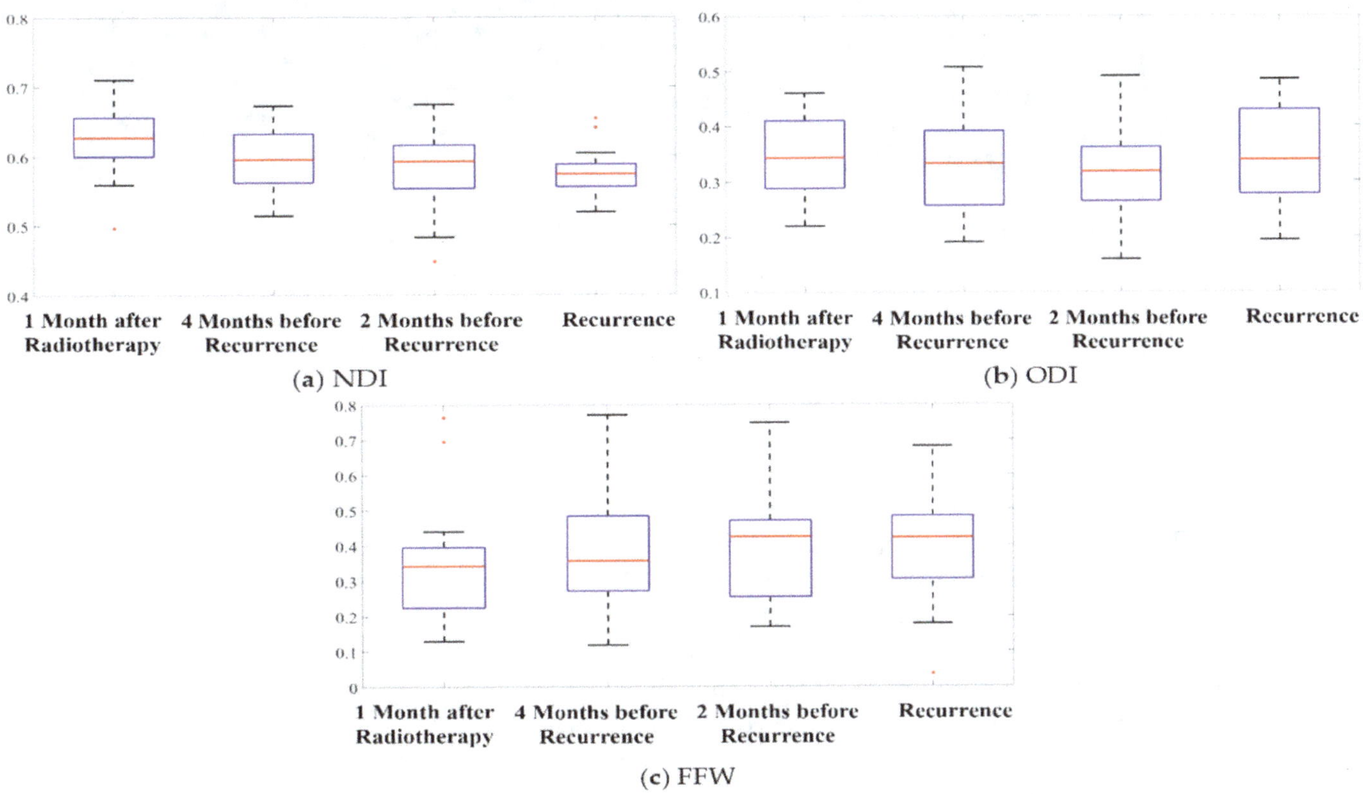

Figure 2. Box plots of the mean values of (**a**) neurite density index (NDI), (**b**) orientation dispersion index (ODI), and (**c**) free water fraction [FWF] within recurrent tumor regions over the four time points. The five bars in the box plots indicate, from bottom to top, the minimum, first quartile, median, third quartile, and the maximum. The red dots indicate outliers.

3.3. *Qualitative Comparison*

T1 MRI and FA images of a representative patient at each of the four time points are shown in Figure 3. The recurrent tumor (circled in red) was not visible on the three conventional T1 images before the evident time point of recurrence, but WM deterioration at the recurrent region was visibly appreciable on the FA images at 4 months and 2 months before recurrence. Notably, this recurrence appeared at the intersection of the internal capsule and geniculocalcarine tract (optic radiation), which are major WM tracts in the brain. These images corroborate our hypothesis that tumor cells may cause WM disruptions that may be evident on DTI images before the actual tumor is visible in T1 images.

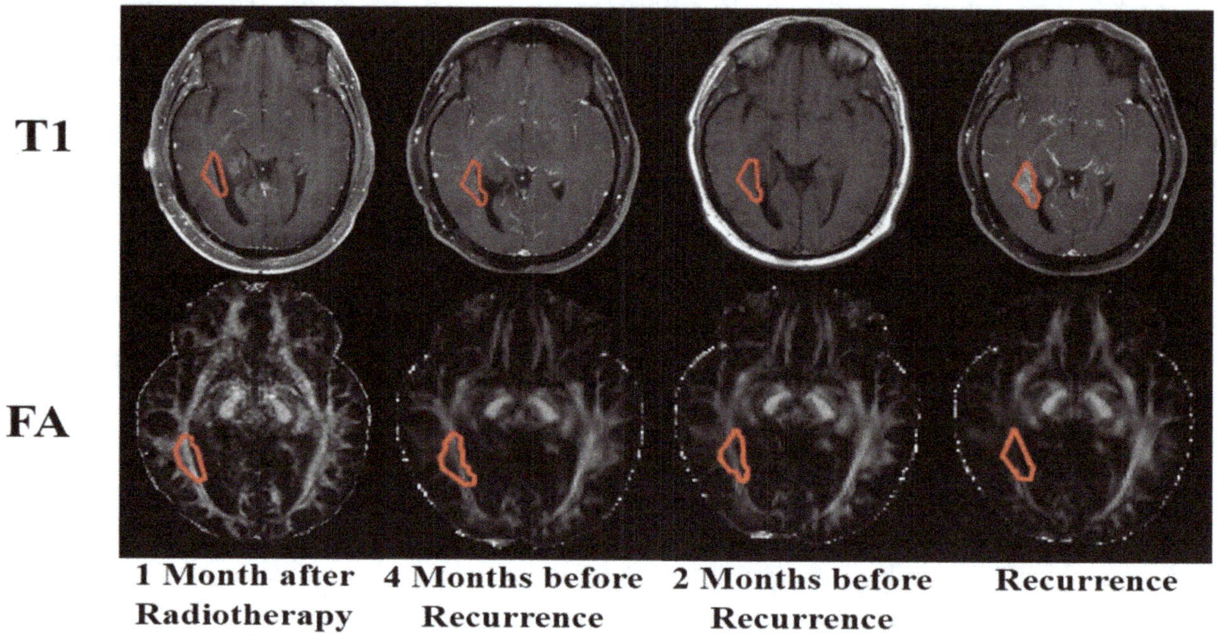

Figure 3. Serial T1 and fractional anisotropy (FA) images of a representative patient. Red outlines indicate the location of the recurrent tumor.

3.4. Radiation Therapy versus Recurrence

It is known that RT would cause dose-dependent white matter damage around treatment areas [25,26]. Therefore, the values of diffusion parameters such as FA would be affected after treatment. In order to distinguish the longitudinal reduction of FA in the study was caused by recurrence or RT, we selected 9 patients from our dataset whose recurrent intervals were longer than 12 months. And we calculated the mean FA values of the recurrence regions at an additional time point—6 months after RT. We performed pairwise t tests at between 6 months after RT and 1 month after RT, 4 months before recurrence, 2 months before recurrence, and recurrence, respectively.

There was no statistically significant change in the mean FA values between 1 month after RT and 6 months after RT ($p = 0.80$, 95% CI: (−12.7%, 12.7%)). However, compared with those at 6 months after RT, the mean FA values were significantly lower at 2 months before recurrence ($p = 0.04$, 95% CI: (0.8%, 28.3%)) and at recurrence ($p = 0.008$, 95% CI: (12.7%, 63.4%)). The mean FA values inside the regions of recurrence over the five time points are shown in box plots in Figure 4. Qualitatively, we showed the FA images at 1 month after RT, 6 months after RT, 2 months before recurrence, and recurrence from two representative patients in Figure 5. The red contours outlined the recurrent tumor regions. White matter inside the contours seemed to be intact at 1 month and 6 months after RT, whereas degeneration could be observed at 2 months before recurrence and at recurrence. Both quantitative and qualitative results indicate that the change in FA in our study may result from tumor recurrence instead of radiation-induced damage.

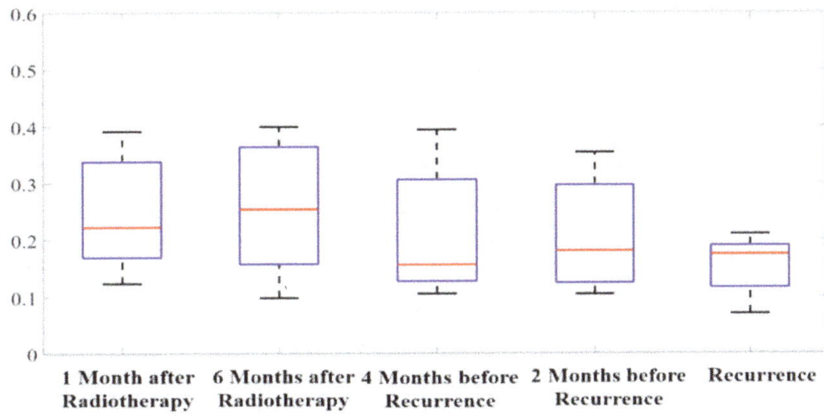

Figure 4. Box plots of the mean values of fractional anisotropy (FA) within recurrent tumor regions over the five time points for selected 9 patients. The five bars in the box plots indicate, from bottom to top, the minimum, first quartile, median, third quartile, and the maximum.

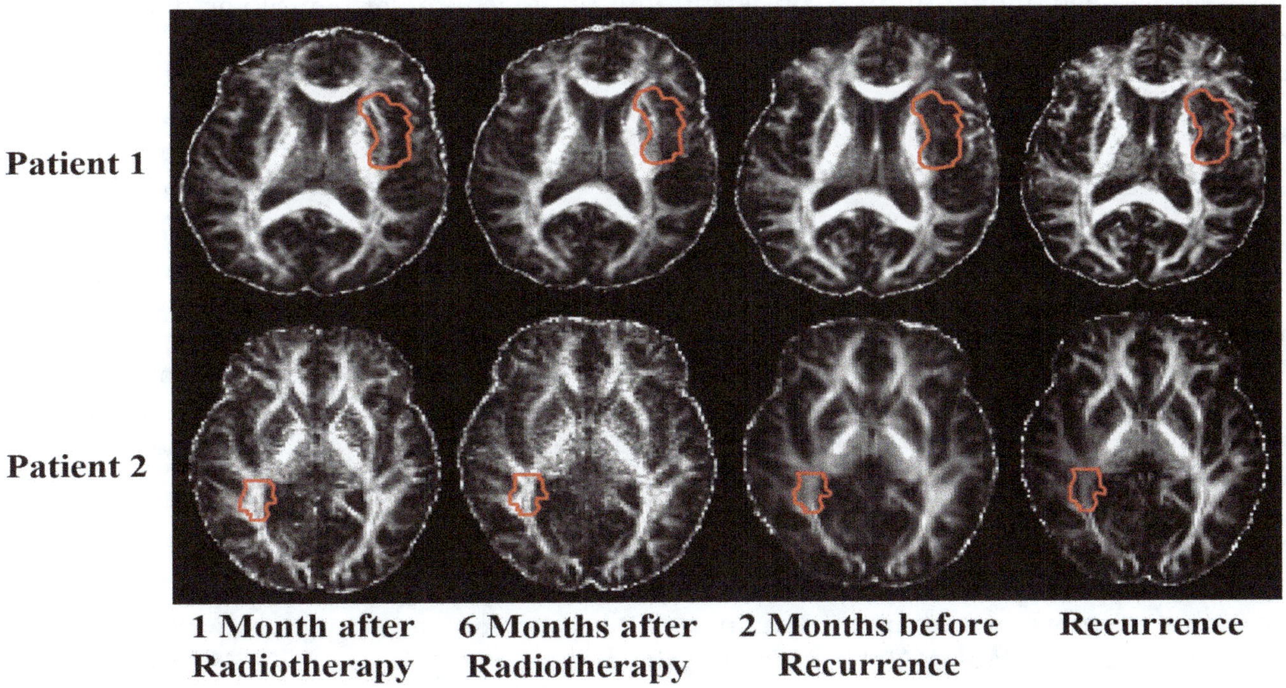

Figure 5. Serial fractional anisotropy (FA) images of two representative patients at four time points, including 6 months after radiation therapy. Red outlines indicate the location of the recurrent tumor.

4. Discussion

Although T1 weighted post contrast MRI remains the gold standard for predicting GBM recurrence, other imaging modalities such as positron emission tomography (PET) and perfusion MRI have been utilized to assist and improve the diagnostic accuracy of tumor recurrence [27,28]. In particular, DTI has the unique capability of displaying information on tissue cellularity, microstructures, and microvasculature by means of noninvasive images [29–31] and thus is increasingly investigated for cancer diagnosis [32] and the prediction of treatment response [33]. Numerous feature maps can be generated from DTI to measure changes in different diffusion properties. For example, FA represents the directionality or the degree of diffusion anisotropy, whereas MD reflects the overall diffusion properties. AD describes the diffusion properties along a particular direction (the principal axis), whereas RD accounts for the diffusion in the other two directions perpendicular to the principal direction [12].

Although DTI has been studied in several types of cancer [34], there are limited studies in GBM. For example, Chang et al. [35] compared the MD values in post-surgical images with those of post-recurrence images in tumor and surrounding tissues to predict tumor recurrence. The current study is one of the first to investigate the utility of DTI for detecting possible changes in WM microstructure before the appearance of a recurrent tumor on conventional MRI.

Our results support our hypothesis that the disruption of WM integrity near the site of recurrence in patients with GBM can precede the appearance of an enhancing tumor on structural MRI. When WM degenerates, the diffusion directionality decreases. When fiber tracts disassociate, water molecules can move freely without obstruction in any direction, and diffusivity usually increases. In general, FA and MD usually move in opposite directions. In our study, we expected that FA values would be lower at recurrence than that at baseline, and that MD would increase as a result of WM degeneration caused by underlying tumor growth. Our findings reflect these expectations, and we found similar trends of increasing values for AD and RD over time. Chang et al. [35] found that MD values were lower inside the tumor than in the surrounding peritumoral region, whereas we found that MD values tended to increase within the tumor region from baseline to recurrence. The pattern of rising MD values, as seen in our study, is consistent with findings in other neurologic diseases, such as Alzheimer disease, where MD values increased in the regions of WM degeneration [12]. Other studies of diffusion MRI brain tumors have speculated that MD is an important marker for tumor response assessment as it is negatively associated with cell density or cellularity, which is a critical measure for tumor progression [34,36,37]. However, our results suggest that the directionality feature (FA) was more sensitive to changes in WM that predicted for GBM recurrence than the other diffusivity features (MD, AD, and RD) suggesting that FA may also be a useful non-contrast imaging biomarker of GBM recurrence.

To further explore changes at the microstructural level and possibly provide more insight into tumor invasion along WM tracts, we used NODDI, a recently developed imaging technique that provides information on specific voxel-wise microstructural substrates via three components, each with values ranging from 0 to 1: NDI describes relative neurite density, ODI quantifies relative angular or morphologic variations, and FWF defines the aggregated free water portion. In the current study, NDI could distinguish recurrence at different stages of development, but the other two components could not. Because changes in FA can result from a combination of NDI and ODI [16], we suspect that the decrease in FA in our study may have been caused by a decrease in NDI rather than in ODI. This in turn suggests that neurite loss (as opposed to neurite morphologic change) may be the main pathologic process for tumor invasion in GBM recurrence, a finding that warrants histologic confirmation in future studies. Not surprisingly, similar patterns of change have also been observed in other neurodegenerative diseases, such as frontotemporal lobar degeneration and amyotrophic lateral sclerosis [23].

In previous studies, diffusion parameters demonstrated significant changes from their baseline values in the areas affected by RT at 6 months after RT [25,26]. In our study, the mean FA values of the region of interest did not show obvious changes between 6 months after RT and baseline (i.e. 1 month after RT) whereas they did show changes between 6 months after RT and 2 months before recurrence in the region of tumor recurrence. Although the small sample size may limit the statistical power, it does imply that the changes we observed from our dataset may be due to white matter deterioration caused by early tumor recurrence rather than radiation.

Despite its promising findings, the current study had several limitations. Our sample size was limited by the difficulty of retrospectively identifying patients treated with concurrent RT and temozolomide with complete sets of serial imaging data at the proposed study time points. With regards to the imaging consistency, the serial DTI images for patients included in this retrospective review were acquired at varying magnet strengths, both 1.5T and 3T without any consistent pattern over time. Although the pattern of image acquisition at varying magnet strengths was random, it may have impacted our results. Additionally, although all the registration results were manually checked after the automated, deformable image registration algorithm, any residual errors in the registration of the GTV to the diffusion images across all four time points have the potential to affect the quantitative measures within these GTV regions before recurrence.

As this is a small retrospective study, the intent of the study was to investigate whether there were suggestive findings that DTI changes may help detect earlier pathological changes prior to traditional anatomical imaging in areas of GBM recurrence based on the hypothesis that an active tumor in a region may lead to the disruption of white matter integrity. For the purpose of this early signal finding study, group analysis enabled statistical analysis. At the individual patient level, we provide several examples of patients with demonstrated changes in DTI at a time point sooner than the clinical onset of recurrence. In our patient cohort, 18 patients of the 30 total group demonstrated changes in FA 2 months prior to confirmed tumor recurrence. Based on these findings, we conclude that DTI changes are promising early biomarkers to help localize areas of GBM recurrence, but further larger prospective studies would need to be done to validate our findings before any clinical implementation could be considered.

5. Conclusions

The results from this retrospective longitudinal study suggest that the disruption of WM integrity near the site of recurrence in patients with GBM can precede the appearance of enhancing tumor on structural MRI. The FA values on images obtained before recurrence were different from those in the baseline images, and the microstructural feature NDI decreased significantly between 2–4 months before recurrence and baseline, suggesting that underlying progressive microstructural changes may precede the appearance of enhancing tumor. We further found that FA was more sensitive than other diffusion-derived features such as MD, AD, and RD for detecting subclinical tumor presence. FA may therefore be useful as an imaging biomarker to predict GBM recurrence, and DTI can provide important complementary information to conventional structural MRI to assist in the clinical diagnosis of recurrence. Our results also suggest that the underlying mechanism for FA reduction may be neurite loss rather than changes in neurite morphology. Future prospective studies of larger cohorts of patients with GBM using a more uniform imaging protocol and more detailed analysis are planned to evaluate the role of DTI in detecting subclinical GBM in a normal-appearing brain and, potentially, to refine the definition of clinical target volume for RT planning and for predicting GBM recurrence.

Author Contributions: Conceived and planned the work, Y.J., J.W.R., H.E., and C.C.; collected the data and performed the analysis, Y.J., J.W.R., and H.E.; took the lead in writing the manuscript, Y.J.; reviewed and edited the manuscript, A.M.E, K.A.A.F., L.L., and C.C.; provided critical feedback during the entire process, A.M.E., B.M.A., B.L.T., A.S.M., K.K.B., C.D.F., and C.C. All authors have read and agreed to the published version of the manuscript.

References

1. Thakkar, J.P.; Dolecek, T.A.; Horbinski, C.; Ostrom, Q.T.; Lightner, D.D.; Barnholtz-Sloan, J.S.; Villano, J.L. Epidemiologic and molecular prognostic review of glioblastoma. *Cancer Epidemiol Biomark. Prev.* **2014**, *23*, 1985–1996. [CrossRef] [PubMed]
2. Stupp, R.; Mason, W.P.; van den Bent, M.J.; Weller, M.; Fisher, B.; Taphoorn, M.J.; Belanger, K.; Brandes, A.A.; Marosi, C.; Bogdahn, U.; et al. Radiotherapy plus concomitant and adjuvant temozolomide for glioblastoma. *N. Engl. J. Med.* **2005**, *352*, 987–996. [CrossRef] [PubMed]
3. Ronning, P.A.; Helseth, E.; Meling, T.R.; Johannesen, T.B. A population-based study on the effect of temozolomide in the treatment of glioblastoma multiforme. *Neuro. Oncol.* **2012**, *14*, 1178–1184. [CrossRef] [PubMed]
4. Stupp, R.; Taillibert, S.; Kanner, A.A.; Kesari, S.; Steinberg, D.M.; Toms, S.A.; Taylor, L.P.; Lieberman, F.; Silvani, A.; Fink, K.L.; et al. Maintenance Therapy With Tumor-Treating Fields Plus Temozolomide vs Temozolomide Alone for Glioblastoma: A Randomized Clinical Trial. *JAMA* **2015**, *314*, 2535–2543. [CrossRef] [PubMed]

5. Belien, A.T.; Paganetti, P.A.; Schwab, M.E. Membrane-type 1 matrix metalloprotease (MT1-MMP) enables invasive migration of glioma cells in central nervous system white matter. *J. Cell Biol.* **1999**, *144*, 373–384. [CrossRef]
6. Pedersen, P.H.; Edvardsen, K.; Garcia-Cabrera, I.; Mahesparan, R.; Thorsen, J.; Mathisen, B.; Rosenblum, M.L.; Bjerkvig, R. Migratory patterns of lac-z transfected human glioma cells in the rat brain. *Int. J. Cancer* **1995**, *62*, 767–771. [CrossRef]
7. Lefranc, F.; Brotchi, J.; Kiss, R. Possible future issues in the treatment of glioblastomas: Special emphasis on cell migration and the resistance of migrating glioblastoma cells to apoptosis. *J. Clin. Oncol.* **2005**, *23*, 2411–2422. [CrossRef]
8. Basser, P.J.; Mattiello, J.; LeBihan, D. MR diffusion tensor spectroscopy and imaging. *Biophys. J.* **1994**, *66*, 259–267. [CrossRef]
9. Le Bihan, D.; Mangin, J.F.; Poupon, C.; Clark, C.A.; Pappata, S.; Molko, N.; Chabriat, H. Diffusion tensor imaging: concepts and applications. *J. Magn. Reson. Imaging.* **2001**, *13*, 534–546. [CrossRef]
10. Werring, D.J.; Clark, C.A.; Barker, G.J.; Thompson, A.J.; Miller, D.H. Diffusion tensor imaging of lesions and normal-appearing white matter in multiple sclerosis. *Neurology* **1999**, *52*, 1626–1632. [CrossRef]
11. Atkinson-Clement, C.; Pinto, S.; Eusebio, A.; Coulon, O. Diffusion tensor imaging in Parkinson's disease: Review and meta-analysis. *Neuroimage Clin.* **2017**, *16*, 98–110. [CrossRef] [PubMed]
12. Jin, Y.; Huang, C.; Daianu, M.; Zhan, L.; Dennis, E.L.; Reid, R.I.; Jack, C.R., Jr.; Zhu, H.; Thompson, P.M.; Alzheimer's Disease Neuroimaging, I. 3D tract-specific local and global analysis of white matter integrity in Alzheimer's disease. *Hum. Brain Mapp.* **2017**, *38*, 1191–1207. [CrossRef] [PubMed]
13. Svolos, P.; Kousi, E.; Kapsalaki, E.; Theodorou, K.; Fezoulidis, I.; Kappas, C.; Tsougos, I. The role of diffusion and perfusion weighted imaging in the differential diagnosis of cerebral tumors: a review and future perspectives. *Cancer Imaging* **2014**, *14*, 20. [CrossRef] [PubMed]
14. Darbar, A.; Waqas, M.; Enam, S.F.; Mahmood, S.D. Use of Preoperative Apparent Diffusion Coefficients to Predict Brain Tumor Grade. *Cureus* **2018**, *10*. [CrossRef]
15. Pauleit, D.; Langen, K.J.; Floeth, F.; Hautzel, H.; Riemenschneider, M.J.; Reifenberger, G.; Shah, N.J.; Muller, H.W. Can the apparent diffusion coefficient be used as a noninvasive parameter to distinguish tumor tissue from peritumoral tissue in cerebral gliomas? *J. Magn. Reson. Imaging* **2004**, *20*, 758–764. [CrossRef]
16. Price, S.J.; Jena, R.; Burnet, N.G.; Carpenter, T.A.; Pickard, J.D.; Gillard, J.H. Predicting patterns of glioma recurrence using diffusion tensor imaging. *Eur. Radiol.* **2007**, *17*, 1675–1684. [CrossRef]
17. Roberts, T.P.; Liu, F.; Kassner, A.; Mori, S.; Guha, A. Fiber density index correlates with reduced fractional anisotropy in white matter of patients with glioblastoma. *AJNR Am J. Neuroradiol.* **2005**, *26*, 2183–2186.
18. Zhang, H.; Schneider, T.; Wheeler-Kingshott, C.A.; Alexander, D.C. NODDI: practical in vivo neurite orientation dispersion and density imaging of the human brain. *Neuroimage* **2012**, *61*, 1000–1016. [CrossRef]
19. Shi, F.; Wang, L.; Dai, Y.; Gilmore, J.H.; Lin, W.; Shen, D. LABEL: pediatric brain extraction using learning-based meta-algorithm. *Neuroimage* **2012**, *62*, 1975–1986. [CrossRef]
20. Jenkinson, M.; Pechaud, M.; Smith, S. BET2: MR-based estimation of brain, skull and scalp surfaces. In Proceedings of the Eleventh Annual Meeting of the Organization for Human Brain Mapping, Toronto, ON, Canada, 12–16 June 2005.
21. Jenkinson, M.; Beckmann, C.F.; Behrens, T.E.; Woolrich, M.W.; Smith, S.M. FSL. *Neuroimage* **2012**, *62*, 782–790. [CrossRef]
22. Andersson, J.L.R.; Sotiropoulos, S.N. An integrated approach to correction for off-resonance effects and subject movement in diffusion MR imaging. *Neuroimage* **2016**, *125*, 1063–1078. [CrossRef] [PubMed]
23. Wen, J.H.; Zhang, H.; Alexander, D.C.; Durrleman, S.; Routier, A.; Rinaldi, D.; Houot, M.; Couratier, P.; Hannequin, D.; Pasquier, F.; et al. Neurite density is reduced in the presymptomatic phase of C9orf72 disease. *J. Neurol. Neurosurg. Psychiatry* **2019**, *90*, 387–394. [CrossRef] [PubMed]
24. Avants, B.B.; Tustison, N.J.; Song, G.; Cook, P.A.; Klein, A.; Gee, J.C. A reproducible evaluation of ANTs similarity metric performance in brain image registration. *Neuroimage* **2011**, *54*, 2033–2044. [CrossRef] [PubMed]
25. Connor, M.; Karunamuni, R.; McDonald, C.; White, N.; Pettersson, N.; Moiseenko, V.; Seibert, T.; Marshall, D.; Cervino, L.; Bartsch, H.; et al. Dose-dependent white matter damage after brain radiotherapy. *Radiother. Oncol.* **2016**, *121*, 209–216. [CrossRef] [PubMed]
26. Kassubek, R.; Gorges, M.; Westhoff, M.A.; Ludolph, A.C.; Kassubek, J.; Muller, H.P. Cerebral Microstructural

Alterations after Radiation Therapy in High-Grade Glioma: A Diffusion Tensor Imaging-Based Study. *Front. Neurol.* **2017**, *8*. [CrossRef]

27. Lundemann, M.; af Rosenschold, P.M.; Muhic, A.; Larsen, V.A.; Poulsen, H.S.; Engelholm, S.A.; Andersen, F.L.; Kjaer, A.; Larsson, H.B.W.; Law, I.; et al. Feasibility of multi-parametric PET and MRI for prediction of tumour recurrence in patients with glioblastoma. *Eur. J. Nucl. Med. Mol. Imaging* **2019**, *46*, 603–613. [CrossRef]
28. Zhang, J.F.; Liu, H.; Tong, H.P.; Wang, S.M.; Yang, Y.Z.; Liu, G.; Zhang, W.G. Clinical Applications of Contrast-Enhanced Perfusion MRI Techniques in Gliomas: Recent Advances and Current Challenges. *Contrast Media Mol. Imaging* **2017**. [CrossRef]
29. Chen, L.H.; Liu, M.; Bao, J.; Xia, Y.B.; Zhang, J.Q.; Zhang, L.; Huang, X.Q.; Wang, J. The Correlation between Apparent Diffusion Coefficient and Tumor Cellularity in Patients: A Meta-Analysis. *PLOS ONE* **2013**, 8. [CrossRef]
30. Jiang, R.S.; Ma, Z.J.; Dong, H.X.; Sun, S.H.; Zeng, X.M.; Li, X. Diffusion tensor imaging of breast lesions: evaluation of apparent diffusion coefficient and fractional anisotropy and tissue cellularity. *Brit. J. Radiol.* **2016**, *89*. [CrossRef]
31. Koh, D.M.; Collins, D.J.; Orton, M.R. Intravoxel incoherent motion in body diffusion-weighted MRI: Reality and challenges. *AJR Am. J. Roentgenol.* **2011**, *196*, 1351–1361. [CrossRef]
32. Park, M.J.; Kim, Y.K.; Choi, S.Y.; Rhim, H.; Lee, W.J.; Choi, D. Preoperative detection of small pancreatic carcinoma: value of adding diffusion-weighted imaging to conventional MR imaging for improving confidence level. *Radiology* **2014**, *273*, 433–443. [CrossRef] [PubMed]
33. Tang, L.; Zhang, X.P.; Sun, Y.S.; Shen, L.; Li, J.; Qi, L.P.; Cui, Y. Gastrointestinal stromal tumors treated with imatinib mesylate: apparent diffusion coefficient in the evaluation of therapy response in patients. *Radiology* **2011**, *258*, 729–738. [CrossRef] [PubMed]
34. Tang, L.; Zhou, X.J. Diffusion MRI of cancer: From low to high b-values. *J. Magn. Reson. Imaging* **2019**, *49*, 23–40. [CrossRef] [PubMed]
35. Chang, P.D.; Chow, D.S.; Yang, P.H.; Filippi, C.G.; Lignelli, A. Predicting Glioblastoma Recurrence by Early Changes in the Apparent Diffusion Coefficient Value and Signal Intensity on FLAIR Images. *AJR Am. J. Roentgenol.* **2017**, *208*, 57–65. [CrossRef] [PubMed]
36. Colman, H.; Berkey, B.A.; Maor, M.H.; Groves, M.D.; Schultz, C.J.; Vermeulen, S.; Nelson, D.F.; Mehta, M.P.; Yung, W.K.; Radiation Therapy Oncology, G. Phase II Radiation Therapy Oncology Group trial of conventional radiation therapy followed by treatment with recombinant interferon-beta for supratentorial glioblastoma: results of RTOG 9710. *Int. J. Radiat. Oncol. Biol. Phys.* **2006**, *66*, 818–824. [CrossRef] [PubMed]
37. Pilatus, U.; Shim, H.; Artemov, D.; Davis, D.; van Zijl, P.C.M.; Glickson, J.D. Intracellular volume and apparent diffusion constants of perfused cancer cell cultures, as measured by NMR. *Magn. Reson. Med.* **1997**, *37*, 825–832. [CrossRef]

3

Complications from Surgeries Related to Ovarian Cancer Screening

Lauren A. Baldwin, Edward J. Pavlik, Emma Ueland, Hannah E. Brown, Kelsey M. Ladd, Bin Huang, Christopher P. DeSimone, John R. van Nagell, Frederick R. Ueland and Rachel W. Miller *

Division of Gynecologic Oncology, Department of Obstetrics and Gynecology, The University of Kentucky Chandler Medical Center and the Markey Cancer Center, 800 Rose Street, Lexington, KY 40536-0293, USA; labald1@uky.edu (L.A.B.); Epaul1@uky.edu (E.J.P.); emmaueland_2017@depauw.edu (E.U.); hannah.e.brown@duke.edu (H.E.B.); Kelsey.ladd@uky.edu (K.M.L.); bhuang@kcr.uky.edu (B.H.); cpdesi00@uky.edu (C.P.D.); jrvann2@email.uky.edu (J.R.v.N.); fuela0@email.uky.edu (F.R.U.)

* Correspondence: raware00@uky.edu

Academic Editor: Andreas Kjaer

Abstract: The aim of this study was to evaluate complications of surgical intervention for participants in the Kentucky Ovarian Cancer Screening Program and compare results to those of the Prostate, Lung, Colorectal and Ovarian Cancer Screening trial. A retrospective database review included 657 patients who underwent surgery for a positive screen in the Kentucky Ovarian Cancer Screening Program from 1988–2014. Data were abstracted from operative reports, discharge summaries, and office notes for 406 patients. Another 142 patients with incomplete records were interviewed by phone. Complete information was available for 548 patients. Complications were graded using the Clavien–Dindo (C–D) Classification of Surgical Complications and considered minor if assigned Grade I (any deviation from normal course, minor medications) or Grade II (other pharmacological treatment, blood transfusion). C–D Grade III complications (those requiring surgical, endoscopic, or radiologic intervention) and C–D Grade IV complications (those which are life threatening) were considered "major". Statistical analysis was performed using SAS 9.4 software. Complications were documented in 54/548 (10%) subjects. For women with malignancy, 17/90 (19%) had complications compared to 37/458 (8%) with benign pathology ($p < 0.003$). For non-cancer surgery, obesity was associated with increased complications ($p = 0.0028$). Fifty patients had minor complications classified as C–D Grade II or less. Three of 4 patients with Grade IV complications had malignancy ($p < 0.0004$). In the Prostate, Lung, Colorectal and Ovarian Cancer Screening trial, 212 women had surgery for ovarian malignancy, and 95 had at least one complication (45%). Of the 1080 women with non-cancer surgery, 163 had at least one complication (15%). Compared to the Prostate, Lung, Colorectal and Ovarian Cancer Screening trial, the Kentucky Ovarian Cancer Screening Program had significantly fewer complications from both cancer and non-cancer surgery ($p < 0.0001$ and $p = 0.002$, respectively). Complications resulting from surgery performed as a result of the Kentucky Ovarian Cancer Screening Program were infrequent and significantly fewer than reported in the Prostate, Lung, Colorectal and Ovarian Cancer Screening trial. Complications were mostly minor (93%) and were more common in cancer versus non-cancer surgery.

Keywords: ovarian cancer screening; complications; ovary; cancer; screening

1. Introduction

Ovarian cancer is the most common cause of gynecologic cancer death in the United States with 22,280 new cases and 14,240 deaths from the disease in 2016 [1]. Despite the introduction of targeted therapies, refinements in novel chemotherapy regimens, and advances in surgical techniques, survival outcomes have remained essentially unchanged over time [2]. Most patients with ovarian cancer are diagnosed with advanced stage disease where survival outcomes are poor. Surgical stage at the time of diagnosis remains among the most important prognostic factors for patients with ovarian cancer. Women with Stage I disease, where cancer is confined to one or both ovaries have a 10-year survival rate of 74%, whereas those with Stages II, III, and IV disease have 10-year survival rates of 45%, 21%, and <5%, respectively [3]. Identifying women with early stage disease is difficult since early ovarian cancer does not reliably cause symptoms. A specific symptom profile has been described in patients with ovarian cancer; however, it is most often reported in those with advanced stage disease [4]. Early stage disease rarely demonstrates this symptom profile [5,6].

The key to a successful screening program is the increased detection of early stage disease and subsequent improved survival in the screen-detected cancers. Efforts in ovarian cancer screening have focused on the integration of transvaginal sonography and serum biomarkers, specifically CA 125 [7–10]. Improved survival from ovarian cancer screening has been reported [11–13], especially with regard to screen-detected incident ovarian cancers [9,14]. One large trial (the Prostate, Lung, Colorectal and Ovarian (PLCO) Randomized Controlled Screening Trial: *PLCO trial*) failed to observe improved survival in the intervention (screening) group [15] and reported a surprisingly high false positive rate with 19 women recommended for surgery for every malignancy that was identified [16]. This is in contrast to other screening studies that reported lower false positive rates [9,11,13]. In the PLCO trial, screen positive cases found to be non-malignant at surgery had an unexpectedly high complication rate (15%) [15] and led to announcements that ovarian cancer screening does more harm than good [17]. In comparison, the United Kingdom Controlled Trial on Ovarian Cancer Screening (UKCTOCS trial) reported a surgical complication rate of less than 1% [9].

The present study examines complications in women undergoing surgery as a result of an abnormality detected in the Kentucky Ovarian Cancer Screening Program, an ultrasound-based program that has screened over 40,000 women from 1988 to present. We objectively evaluated the number and type of complications observed in these women using the Clavien–Dindo (C–D) Classification of Surgical Complications [18,19] and compared findings to those reported in the PLCO trial.

2. Methods

The study was approved by the (University of Kentucky Institutional Review Board protocol 88-0021-9F with the most recent renewal on 11 August 2016. Women enrolled in the Kentucky Ovarian Cancer Screening Program from 26 May 1988 to 1 June 2014 were included in the study group (n = 41,529). The University of Kentucky Institutional Review Board approved this study. Women were recruited by physician referral, media announcements, and word of mouth. Eligibility criteria included asymptomatic women age 50 years or older without a family history of ovarian cancer, or those 25 years or older with a documented family history of ovarian cancer in at least one first or second-degree relative, and the ability to read and understand the informed consent presented in English. Women under clinical evaluation because of pelvic symptoms, a known ovarian tumor, or a personal history of ovarian cancer were excluded. Women enrolled in the Kentucky Ovarian Cancer Screening Program underwent annual screening with transvaginal sonography. Abnormalities were managed according to the study algorithm (Figure 1), which included increased frequency of screening with transvaginal sonography, assessment of morphology index score, and serum CA 125 (Figure 2). Diagnostic surgical intervention was recommended if results indicated at least moderate risk of malignancy according to the published protocol [20]. Minimally invasive surgical technique was preferred, unless medical issues prohibited this approach. Details of the study algorithm, threshold for intervention, and cancer outcomes have been previously published [12,20].

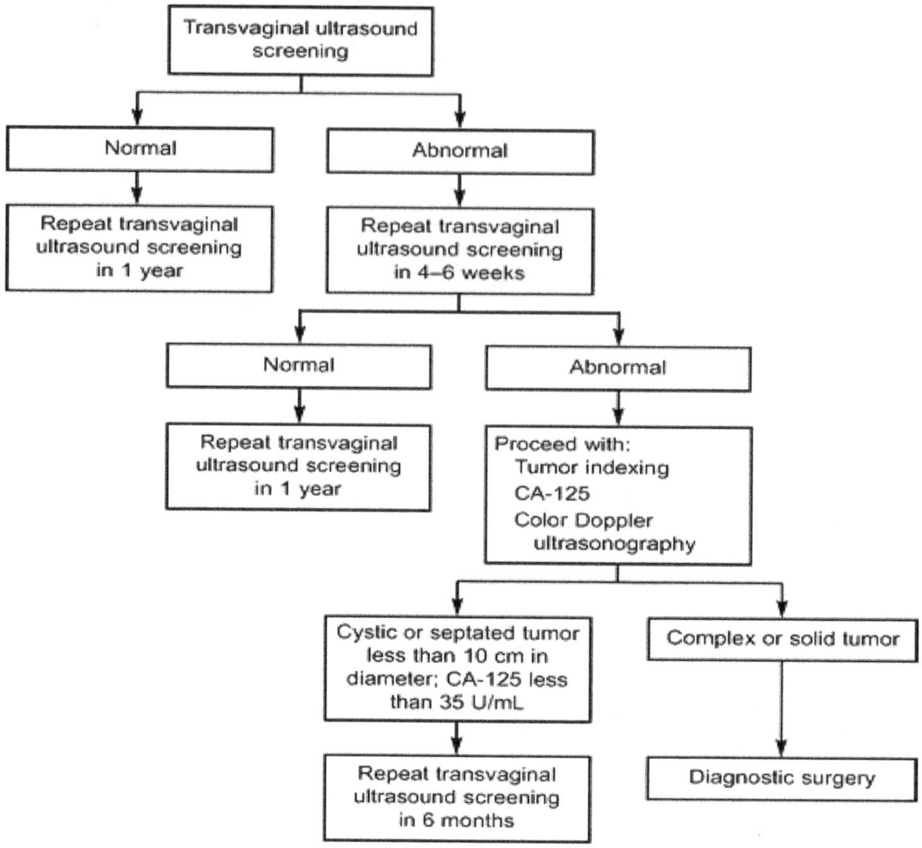

Figure 1. Study algorithm for the Kentucky Ovarian Cancer Screening Program. Reprinted from [12].

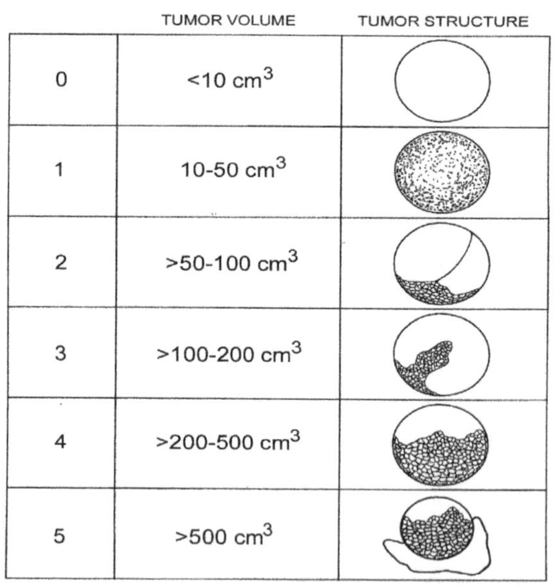

Figure 2. Morphology Index (numeric value 0–10). Reprinted from [12].

In the first 26 years of the Kentucky Ovarian Cancer Screening Program, 657 patients underwent surgical intervention for positive screens. Three investigators performed a thorough review of all available medical records including operative reports, discharge summaries, and office notes. Phone interviews were conducted when medical records were incomplete. A complication was defined as any deviation from the normal postoperative course within 60 days of surgery. Complete information was obtained for 548 patients. Physician investigators graded all surgical complications that were identified in these 548 patients according to the C–D Classification of Surgical Complications (Table 1) [18,19]. Complications were considered "minor" if they were C–D Grades I or II. Grade I complications included any minor deviations from a normal postoperative course without the need for pharmacologic intervention. Grade II complications consisted of complications treated pharmacologically. C–D Grade III complications (those requiring surgical, endoscopic, or radiologic intervention) and C–D Grade IV complications (those which are life threatening) were considered "major."

Table 1. Classification of Surgical Complications. Modified from [19].

C–D Grades	Definition
Grade I	Any deviation from normal postoperative course without the need for pharmacological treatment or surgical, endoscopic and radiological interventions. Acceptable therapeutic regimens are: drugs as antiemetics, antipyretics, analgetics, diuretics, and electrolytes and physiotherapy.
Grade II	Requiring pharmacological treatment with drugs other thanthan such allowed for Grade I complications.
Grade III	Requiring surgical, endoscopic or radiologic intervention.
Grade III-a	Intervention not under general anesthesia.
Grade III-b	Intervention under general anesthesia.
Grade IV	Life threatening complications (including CNS complications) ‡ requiring IC/ICU management.
Grade IV-a	Single organ dysfunction (including dialysis).
Grade IV-b	Multi organ dysfunction.
Grade V	Death of patient.
Suffix "d"	If the patient suffers from a complication at the time of discharge (see examples in Appendix B, http://Links.Lww.com/SLA/A3), the suffix "d" (for "disability") is added to the respective grade of complication. This label indicates the need for a follow-up to fully evaluate the complication.

‡ Brain hemorrhage, ischemic stroke, subarachnoid bleeding, but excluding transient ischemic attacks (TIA); IC: intermediate care; ICU: intensive care unit (www.surgicalcomplications.info).

Descriptive analysis for demographics and clinical factors was performed. We used χ^2 tests to examine associations between complication status (yes and no) and other factors such as age, race, body mass index (BMI), type of surgery, cancer status, and type of hospital where surgery was performed. Multivariate logistic regressions were fitted to evaluate the association between complication status and other factors. The final model included only covariates with a significance level of 0.05 or less. Model goodness of fit, multicollinearity, and interactions were also examined. All analyses were performed using SAS Statistical software version 9.4. All statistical tests were two-sided with a p-value ≤ 0.05 used to identify statistical significance.

3. Results

Complete clinical information was available on 548 of the 657 patients who underwent surgery for positive screens in the Kentucky Ovarian Cancer Screening Program between the years of 1988–2014. A summary of demographic information is presented in Table 2 and shows that women with and without complications were similar. Complications were documented in 54 of 548 (10%) subjects. Fifty patients (93%) had minor complications classified as C–D Grade II or less, while four had complications categorized as C–D Grade IV. Complication profiles for individuals are shown relative to age and BMI in Figure 3.

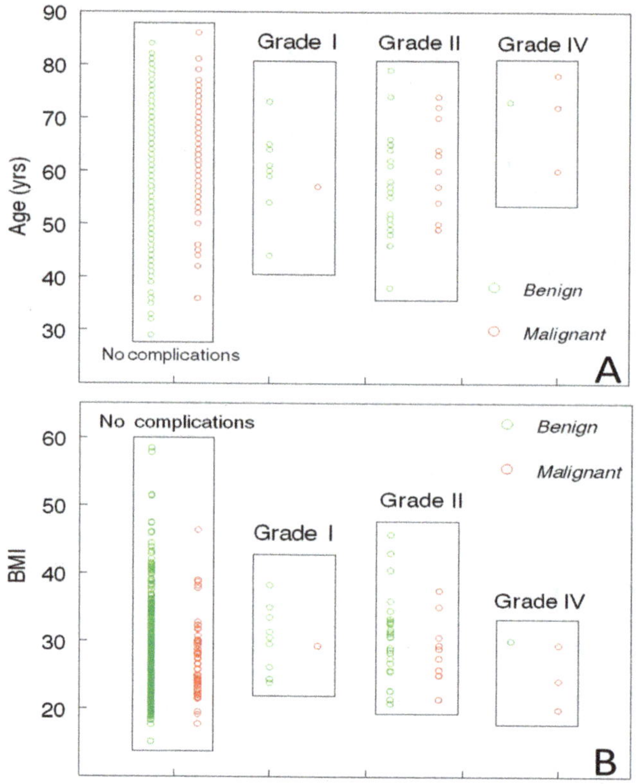

Figure 3. Clavien–Dindo classification of complication relative to age (**A**) and BMI (**B**) in women with benign (**green** circles) and malignant results (**red** circles) at surgery.

Table 2. Demographics of the group studied.

Variable	No Complications	Complications	Excluded
	N = 494	*N* = 54	*N* = 109
Age	59.7, 59 (29–86)	59.6, 59 (38–79)	59.6, 60 (36–84)
Weight	163.6, 158.5 (80–368)	173.7, 170 (121–274)	159.2, 150 (101–250)
Height	64.6, 64.5 (55–71)	64.4, 65 (60–70)	64.5, 64 (57–72)
BMI	27.6, 26.6 (15.1–58.4)	29.4, 29.2 (19.9–45.7)	26.9, 25.8 (18–43.9)
Family history of:			
Ovarian cancer	132 (26.7%)	15 (27.8%)	36 (33%)
Breast cancer	27 (50%)	217 (43.9%)	46 (42.2%)
Breast cancer personal history	8 (14.8%)	39 (7.9%)	8 (7.3%)
Colon cancer	128 (25.9%)	11 (20.3%)	46 (24.7%)
Colon cancer personal history	3 (0.6%)	0 (0%)	1 (0.9%)
No history of hormone replacement therapy	372 (75.3%)	43 (79.6%)	65 (59.6%)
History of hormone replacement therapy	122 (24.7%)	11 (20.4%)	38 (34.9%)
Menopausal Status			
Premenopausal	73 (14.8%)	6 (11.1%)	18 (16.5%)
Perimenopausal	18 (3.6%)	0	7 (6.4%)
Postmenopausal	403 (81.6%)	48 (88.9%)	84 (77.1%)
Any symptoms	254 (51%)	30 (55.5%)	51 (46.8%)
Ovarian cancer symptoms *	27 (14.8%)	4 (7.4%)	5 (4.6%)
Other symptoms **	248 (50.2%)	30 (55.6%	48 (44%)

Mean, median (range) * Women reporting pelvic or abdominal pain, being unable to eat normally, feeling full quickly, feeling abdominal bloating or increased abdominal size presenting for >12 days per month with an onset in less than the last 12 months. ** Women reporting back pain, indigestion, nausea, vomiting, weight loss, urinary urgency, frequent urination, constipation, menstrual irregularities, bleeding after menopause, pain during intercourse, fatigue, leg swelling, difficulty breathing. Any symptoms: any symptom included under ovarian cancer symptoms or other symptoms without regard to frequency of duration.

Complication rates were compared for surgeries that resulted in the diagnosis of malignancy versus surgery for false positive screens with benign pathology. For women with malignancy, 17 of 90 (19%) had complications compared to 37 of 458 (8%) with benign pathology ($p < 0.003$), Figure 4. Thus, a diagnosis of cancer increased the likelihood of complications with an odds ratio of 2.65. Three of four patients with C–D Grade IV complications had malignancy, while one Grade IV complications occurred in the benign conditions group ($p < 0.0004$). In the PLCO trial, 212 women in the intervention group had surgery for ovarian malignancy, and 95 had at least one complication (45%). Of the 1080 women with surgery with a benign outcome, 163 had at least one complication (15%), yielding an odds ratio of 3 for complications in surgical cancer cases over benign surgical cases. Complication rates from the Kentucky Ovarian Cancer Screening Program were compared with the PLCO trial results. Compared to the PLCO trial, the Kentucky Ovarian Cancer Screening Program had significantly fewer complications from both cancer ($p < 0.001$) and non-cancer surgery ($p = 0.002$) based on chi-square analysis (Figure 4).

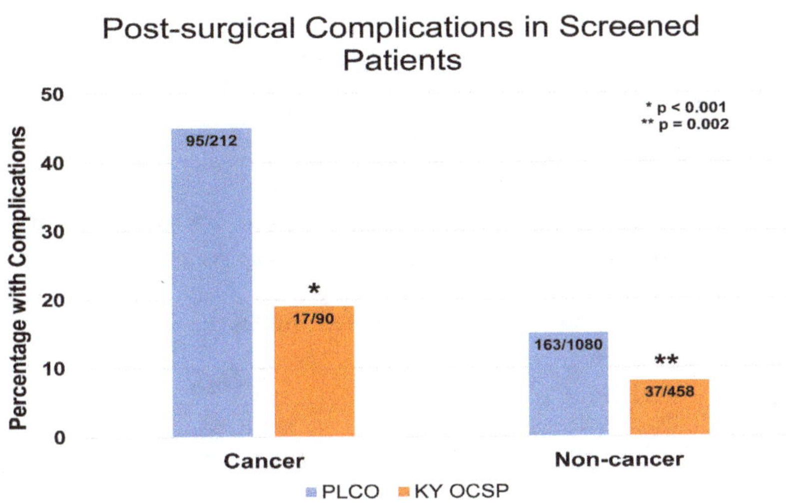

Figure 4. Complications associated with surgery.

Bivariate analysis of complication status versus other clinical variables was performed and obesity was associated with increased incidence of complication, $p = 0.049$ (Table 3). Evaluating clinical variables by cancer status, obesity was not associated with increased complications in surgeries performed for non-cancer pathology, $p = 0.458$ (Table 4). While patients with a cancer diagnosis were significantly older than those with a benign diagnosis, $p = 0.002$ (Table 4), age was not different for those who had complications when compared to those that did not, $p = 0.463$ (Table 3). Other factors evaluated in bivariate analysis did not show significant differences based on complication status.

Table 3. Associations between complications and other factors.

Variables	Complications		No Complications		*p*-Value
	N	%	*N*	%	
Age					0.463
<50	7	13.0	75	15.2	
50–64	32	59.3	257	52.0	
65–74	10	18.5	121	24.5	
75+	3	5.6	35	7.1	
Unknown	2	3.7	6	1.2	
Weight					0.049
Under-weight	0	0.0	5	1.0	
Normal	11	20.4	185	37.4	
Over-weight	20	37.0	175	35.4	
Obese	20	37.0	108	21.9	
Extreme obesity	3	5.6	21	4.3	

Table 4. Patient characteristics by cancer status.

Variables	Cancer		Non-Cancer		p-Value
	N	%	N	%	
Age					0.002
<50	6	6.7	76	16.6	
50–64	38	42.2	251	54.8	
65–74	33	36.7	98	21.4	
75+	11	12.2	27	5.9	
Unknown	2	2.2	6	1.3	
C–D Grade	N	%	N	%	<0.001
None	73	81.1	421	92.0	
Minor	14	15.6	36	7.9	
Severe	3	3.3	1	0.2	
Weight					0.458
Under-weight	1	1.1	4	0.9	
Normal	37	41.1	159	34.7	
Over-weight	31	34.4	164	35.8	
Obese	20	22.2	108	23.6	
Extreme obesity	1	1.1	23	5.0	

In multivariate analysis, obesity was determined to be associated with increased risk of complication versus normal weight (OR 3.17, 1.46–6.90). The location where the procedures were performed was also significantly associated with complication risk (OR 1.97, 1.07–3.65) (Table 5).

Table 5. Odds ratio estimates.

Effect	Odds Ratio	95% Confidence Limits
Age		
Unknown vs. 50–64	4.75	(0.86–26.19)
<50 vs. 50–64	0.76	(0.32–1.81)
75+ vs. 50–64	0.77	(0.22–2.71)
65–74 vs. 50–64	0.69	(0.33–1.48)
Weight		
Overweight vs. Underweight/Normal	2.06	(0.95–4.49)
Obese vs. Underweight/Normal	3.17	(1.46–6.90)
Location		
UK vs. Non-UK	1.97	(1.07–3.65)

4. Discussion

Ovarian cancer is the second most common gynecologic cancer, but the most common cause of gynecologic cancer death. Most women have advanced disease at the time of their diagnosis, with cancer spread throughout the peritoneal cavity and occasionally into the pleural cavity. Despite aggressive surgery and chemotherapy [21], the five-year overall survival for patients with advanced ovarian cancer is less than 30%. Unfortunately, only about 25% of women present with early stage ovarian cancer, where the five-year overall survival may exceed 80%–90% with appropriate surgical staging and adjuvant therapy.

Ovarian cancer screening with transvaginal sonography and serum biomarkers has been explored as a means for increasing the number of women diagnosed with early stage disease [7–13,20]. This shift in stage at diagnosis should result in an improved overall survival as a result of screening. There is a need for ovarian cancer screening because early stage disease rarely produces reliable symptoms. Goff and colleagues reported a symptom profile associated with ovarian cancer [4,22], which included abdominal pain or bloating, pelvic pain, and urinary symptoms present for more than two weeks out of the month and persisting for fewer than 12 months. The effectiveness of a symptom profile is limited as a screening tool because the profile is most useful for identifying advanced stage disease.

Ovarian cancer screening presents unique challenges that are inherent to the disease itself. First, ovarian cancer has a low incidence with only 22,280 new cases expected in 2016, compared to breast or colorectal cancer in women with 246,660 and 68,830 new cases, respectively [1]. The annual balance of deaths from disease to incident cases for ovarian cancer (0.639) is 3.9 times higher than for breast (0.164) and 1.8 times higher than for colorectal cancer (0.346), indicating that ovarian cancer is a much deadlier disease. This is reflected in the low prevalence of ovarian cancer with an estimated 195,767 women living with the disease in the United States in 2013, relative to colorectal (1,177,556) and breast cancers (3,053,450) [23].

A second challenge in ovarian cancer screening is the lack of a thorough understanding of the etiology and natural history of ovarian, primary peritoneal, and fallopian tube cancer. Historically, ovarian cancer was thought to arise from the surface epithelium of the ovary. However, this did not explain normal size ovaries as seen in primary peritoneal cancers. The similarities between serous ovarian and primary peritoneal cancers from the standpoint of genetic mutations, histology, behavior, and response to treatment suggest similar etiologic factors. More recently, investigators have hypothesized that ovarian, primary peritoneal, and fallopian tube cancers originate from serous intraepithelial carcinomas in the fallopian tube [24–33]. If this is the case, then screening for abnormalities of the ovary with transvaginal sonography will prove futile because the early abnormalities exist in the fallopian tube. This model is founded on the presence of microscopic disease that is below the resolution of biomarkers and ultrasonography, and consequently implies that these screening tools cannot be effective. However, the discovery of Stage I cancers in several screening studies indicates that biomarker and ultrasonography screening modalities are sufficiently effective in detecting ovarian cancer early enough to decrease mortality and increase survival [9–12]. Thus, cases that have progressed beyond microscopic disease in the distal fallopian tube can be detected by biomarker and ultrasonography screening often enough to achieve a favorable prognosis for extending survival.

In the present report, we evaluate the complications related to surgery for a positive ovarian cancer screen. In other cancers, such as breast, colon, and cervical, a diagnostic biopsy is performed to determine the presence or absence of malignancy. Percutaneous or transvaginal biopsy of ovarian abnormalities is not recommended because of concern for "seeding" the needle track in the case of malignancy, or for rupturing a malignant tumor, resulting in potentially worse outcomes. Given the aggressive nature of ovarian cancer, these two possibilities could impact the need for adjuvant treatment, or increase the risk of recurrence in early stage disease. As a result, patients with a positive screen indicating a moderate to high risk of malignancy are offered definitive surgery for diagnosis. In most cases, removal of an ovary or ovaries because of an abnormality detected on ovarian cancer screening can be accomplished using a minimally invasive technique, but there are situations when this is not medically recommended. Surgical exploration for a positive screen introduces the possibility of intervention for benign or false positive ovarian abnormalities. The combination of a high percentage of surgeries for women without a malignancy in the PLCO trial (1 malignancy for every 19 surgeries) coupled with a high complication rate [15] led to published statements that screening is harmful [17].

In conclusion, little has been published regarding the nature of the complications reported from surgeries resulting from ovarian cancer screening. In this investigation, we report a low complication rate, with 93% classified as minor. Similarly, the UKCTOCS trial reported a very low complication rate of less than one percent in both screening groups [9]. The procedures of the PLCO trial were to notify the referring physician that a screen was abnormal, but not to make recommendations on whether surgery should be performed or by whom. It is possible that the high complication rates reported in the PLCO trial [15] are related to the recent recognition that better outcomes are achieved when ovarian cancer is treated by specialists at high volume hospitals [34–39], and this benefit may particularly apply to early stage ovarian cancers [40]. Ultimately, the methods used to decide who went to surgery and who would perform the operation may best explain the high false positive rates and high complication rates observed in the PLCO trial.

Acknowledgments: This work was supported by grants from the Telford Foundation, and the Department of Health and Human Services, Commonwealth of Kentucky. Bin Huang received support from the NCI Cancer Center Support Grant (P30 CA177558). No support was received to publish in open access.

Author Contributions: Lauren A. Baldwin contributed to data collection, review and grading of complications, abstract composition and original manuscript composition; Edward J. Pavlik contributed to data collection and manuscript composition; Emma Ueland, Hannah E. Brown, Kelsey M. Ladd contributed to data collection; Bin Huang performed statistical analysis and contributed to manuscript preparation; Christopher P. DeSimone, John R. van Nagell, Frederick R. Ueland contributed to manuscript preparation; and Rachel W. Miller developed the project concept and contributed to data collection, review and grading of complications, and manuscript composition.

References

1. Siegel, R.L.; Miller, K.D.; Jemal, A. Cancer Statistics. *CA Cancer J. Clin.* **2016**, *66*, 7–30. [CrossRef] [PubMed]
2. Bookman, M.A. Optimal primary therapy of ovarian cancer. *Ann. Oncol.* **2016**, *27*, i58–i62. [CrossRef] [PubMed]
3. Jelovac, D.; Armstrong, D.K. Recent progress in the diagnosis and treatment of ovarian Cancer. *CA Cancer J. Clin.* **2011**, *61*, 183–203. [CrossRef] [PubMed]
4. Goff, B.A.; Mandel, L.S.; Drescher, C.W.; Urban, N.; Gough, S.; Schurman, K.M.; Patras, J.; Mahony, B.S.; Andersen, M.R. Development of an ovarian cancer symptom index. *Cancer* **2007**, *109*, 221–227. [CrossRef] [PubMed]
5. Pavlik, E.J.; Saunders, B.A.; Doran, S.; McHugh, K.W.; Ueland, F.R.; DeSimone, C.P.; DePriest, P.D.; Ware, R.A.; Kryscio, R.J.; van Nagell, J.R. The search for meaning-symptoms and transvaginal sonography screening for ovarian cancer: Predicting malignancy. *Cancer* **2009**, *115*, 3689–3698. [CrossRef] [PubMed]
6. Rossing, M.A.; Wicklund, K.G.; Cushing-Haugen, K.L.; Weiss, N.S. Predictive value of symptoms for early detection of ovarian cancer. *J. Natl. Cancer Inst.* **2010**, *102*, 222–229. [CrossRef] [PubMed]
7. Van Nagell, J.R., Jr.; Pavlik, E.J. Ovarian cancer screening. *Clin. Obstet. Gynecol.* **2012**, *55*, 43–51. [CrossRef] [PubMed]
8. Pavlik, E.J.; Nagell, J.R., Jr. Early detection of ovarian tumors using ultrasound. *Women's Health* **2013**, *9*, 39–55. [CrossRef] [PubMed]
9. Jacobs, I.J.; Menon, U.; Ryan, A.; Gentry-Maharaj, A.; Burnell, M.; Kalsi, J.K.; Amso, N.N.; Apostolidou, S.; Benjamin, E.; Cruickshank, D.; et al. Ovarian cancer screening and mortality in the UK collaborative trial of ovarian cancer screening (UKCTOCS): A randomized controlled trial. *Lancet* **2016**, *387*, 945–956. [CrossRef]
10. Pavlik, E. Ovarian cancer screening effectiveness: A realization from the UKCTOCS. *Women's Health* **2016**, *12*, 475–479. [PubMed]
11. Kobayashi, H.; Yamada, Y.; Sado, T.; Sakata, M.; Yoshida, S.; Kawaguchi, R.; Kanayama, S.; Shigetomi, H.; Haruta, S.; Tsuji, Y.; et al. A randomized study of screening for ovarian cancer: A multicenter study in Japan. *Int. J. Gynecol. Cancer* **2008**, *18*, 414–420. [CrossRef] [PubMed]
12. Van Nagell, J.R., Jr.; Miller, R.W.; DeSimone, C.P.; Ueland, F.R.; Podzielinski, I.; Goodrich, S.T.; Elder, J.W.; Huang, B.; Kryscio, R.J.; Pavlik, E.J. Long-term survival of women with epithelial ovarian cancer detected by ultrasonographic screening. *Obstet. Gynecol.* **2011**, *118*, 1212–1221. [CrossRef] [PubMed]
13. Pavlik, E.J.; Ueland, F.R.; Miller, R.W.; Ubellacker, J.M.; Desimone, C.P.; Elder, J.; Hoff, J.; Baldwin, L.; Kryscio, R.J.; Nagell, J.R., Jr. Frequency and disposition of ovarian abnormalities followed with serial transvaginal ultrasonography. *Obstet. Gynecol.* **2013**, *122*, 210–217. [CrossRef] [PubMed]
14. Jacobs, I.J.; Parmar, M.; Skates, S.J.; Menon, U. Ovarian cancer screening: UKCTOCS trial—Authors' reply. *Lancet* **2016**, *387*, 2603–2604. [CrossRef]
15. Buys, S.S.; Partridge, E.; Black, A.; Johnson, C.C.; Lamerato, L.; Isaacs, C.; Reding, D.J.; Greenlee, R.T.; Yokochi, L.A.; Kessel, B.; et al. Effect of screening on ovarian cancer mortality—The Prostate, Lung, Colorectal and Ovarian (PLCO) Cancer Screening Randomized Controlled Trial. *JAMA* **2011**, *305*, 2295–2303. [CrossRef] [PubMed]
16. Partridge, E.; Greenlee, R.T.; Xu, J.L.; Kreimer, A.R.; Williams, C.; Riley, T.; Reding, D.J.; Church, T.R.; Kessel, B.; Johnson, C.C.; et al. Results from four rounds of ovarian cancer screening in a randomized trial. *Obstet. Gynecol.* **2009**, *113*, 775–782. [CrossRef] [PubMed]

17. Slomski, A. Screening women for ovarian cancer still does more harm than good. *JAMA* **2012**, *307*, 2474–2475. [CrossRef] [PubMed]
18. Clavien, P.A.; Barkun, J.; de Oliveira, M.L.; Vauthey, J.N.; Dindo, D.; Schulick, R.D.; de Santibañes, E.; Pekolj, J.; Slankamenac, K.; Bassi, C.; et al. The Clavien–Dindo classification of surgical complications: Five-year experience. *Ann. Surg.* **2009**, *250*, 187–196. [CrossRef] [PubMed]
19. Dindo, D.; Demartines, N.; Clavien, P.A. Classification of surgical complications: A new proposal with evaluation in a cohort of 6336 patients and results of a survey. *Ann. Surg.* **2004**, *240*, 205–213. [CrossRef] [PubMed]
20. Nagell, J.R., Jr.; Miller, R.W. Evaluation and management of ultrasonographically detected ovarian tumors in asymptomatic women. *Obstet. Gynecol.* **2016**, *127*, 848–858. [CrossRef] [PubMed]
21. National Comprehensive Cancer Network. Epithelial Ovarian Cancer/Fallopian Tube Cancer/Primary Peritoneal Cancer (Version 1.2106). Available online: https://www.nccn.org/professionals/physician_gls/pdf/ovarian.pdf (accessed on 15 November 2016).
22. Goff, B. Symptoms associated with ovarian cancer. *Clin. Obstet. Gynecol.* **2012**, *55*, 36–42. [CrossRef] [PubMed]
23. National Cancer Institute. Surveillance, Epidemiology, and End results Program, Cancer Statistics. Available online: http://seer.cancer.gov/statfacts/ (accessed on 15 November 2016).
24. Alvarado-Cabrero, I.; Navani, S.S.; Young, R.H.; Scully, R.E. Tumors of the fimbriated end of the fallopian tube: A clinicopathologic analysis of 20 cases, including nine carcinomas. *Int. J. Gynecol. Pathol.* **1997**, *16*, 189–196. [CrossRef] [PubMed]
25. Colgan, T.J.; Murphy, J.; Cole, D.E.; Narod, S.; Rosen, B. Occult carcinoma in prophylactic oophorectomy specimens: Prevalence and association with BRCA germline mutation status. *Am. J. Surg. Pathol.* **2001**, *25*, 1283–1289. [CrossRef] [PubMed]
26. Cass, I.; Holschneider, C.; Datta, N.; Barbuto, D.; Walts, A.E.; Karlan, B.Y. BRCA-mutation-associated fallopian tube carcinoma: A distinct clinical phenotype? *Obstet. Gynecol.* **2005**, *106*, 1327–1334. [CrossRef] [PubMed]
27. Medeiros, F.; Muto, M.G.; Lee, Y.; Elvin, J.A.; Callahan, M.J.; Feltmate, C.; Garber, J.E.; Cramer, D.W.; Crum, C.P. The tubal fimbria is a preferred site for early adenocarcinoma in women with familial ovarian cancer syndrome. *Am. J. Surg. Pathol.* **2006**, *30*, 230–236. [CrossRef] [PubMed]
28. Kindelberger, D.W.; Lee, Y.; Miron, A.; Hirsch, M.S.; Feltmate, C.; Medeiros, F.; Callahan, M.J.; Garner, E.O.; Gordon, R.W.; Birch, C.; et al. Intraepithelial carcinoma of the fimbriae and pelvic serous carcinoma: Evidence for a causal relationship. *Am. J. Surg. Pathol.* **2007**, *31*, 161–169. [CrossRef] [PubMed]
29. Crum, C.P.; Drapkin, R.; Miron, A.; Ince, T.A.; Muto, M.; Kindelberger, D.W.; Lee, Y. The distal fallopian tube: A new model for pelvic serous carcinogenesis. *Curr. Opin. Obstet. Gynecol.* **2007**, *19*, 3–9. [CrossRef] [PubMed]
30. Landen, C.N.; Birrer, M.J.; Sood, A.K. Early events in the pathogenesis of epithelial ovarian cancer. *J. Clin. Oncol.* **2008**, *26*, 995–1005. [CrossRef] [PubMed]
31. Lengyel, E. Ovarian cancer development and metastasis. *Am. J. Pathol.* **2010**, *177*, 1053–1064. [CrossRef] [PubMed]
32. Kurman, R.J.; Shih, L.M. The origin and pathogenesis of epithelial ovarian cancer: A proposed unifying theory. *Am. J. Surg. Pathol.* **2010**, *34*, 433–4439. [CrossRef] [PubMed]
33. Crum, C.P.; Mckeon, F.D.; Xian, X. The oviduct and ovarian cancer: Causality, clinical implications, and "Targeted Prevention". *Clin. Obstet. Gynecol.* **2012**, *55*, 24–35. [CrossRef] [PubMed]
34. Cliby, W.A.; Powell, M.A.; Al-Hammadi, N.; Chen, L.; Philip, M.J.; Roland, P.Y.; Mutch, D.G.; Bristow, R.E. Ovarian cancer in the United States: Contemporary patterns of care associated with improved survival. *Gynecol. Oncol.* **2015**, *136*, 11–17. [CrossRef] [PubMed]
35. Bristow, R.E.; Chang, J.; Ziogas, A.; Campos, B.; Chavez, L.R.; Anton-Culver, H. Impact of National Cancer Institute Comprehensive Cancer Centers on ovarian cancer treatment and survival. *J. Am. Coll. Surg.* **2015**, *220*, 940–950. [CrossRef] [PubMed]
36. Bristow, R.E.; Chang, J.; Ziogas, A.; Anton-Culver, H. Adherence to treatment guidelines for ovarian cancer as a measure of quality care. *Obstet. Gynecol.* **2013**, *121*, 1226–1234. [CrossRef] [PubMed]

37. Bristow, R.E.; Palis, B.E.; Chi, D.S.; Cliby, W.A. The National Cancer Database report on advanced-stage epithelial ovarian cancer: Impact of hospital surgical case volume on overall survival and surgical treatment paradigm. *Gynecol. Oncol.* **2010**, *118*, 262–267. [CrossRef] [PubMed]
38. Bristow, R.E.; Chang, J.; Ziogas, A.; Randall, L.M.; Anton-Culver, H. High-volume ovarian cancer care: Survival impact and disparities in access for advanced-stage disease. *Gynecol. Oncol.* **2014**, *132*, 403–410. [CrossRef] [PubMed]
39. Lee, J.Y.; Kim, T.H.; Suh, D.H.; Kim, J.W.; Kim, H.S.; Chung, H.H.; Park, N.H.; Song, Y.S.; Kang, S.B. Impact of guideline adherence on patient outcomes in early-stage epithelial ovarian cancer. *Eur. J. Surg. Oncol.* **2015**, *41*, 585–591. [CrossRef] [PubMed]
40. Vernooij, F.; Heintz, A.P.; Witteveen, P.O.; Coebergh, J.W.; van der Graaf, Y. Specialized care and survival of ovarian cancer patients in The Netherlands: Nationwide cohort study. *J. Natl. Cancer Inst.* **2008**, *100*, 399–406. [CrossRef] [PubMed]

4

^{18}F-FDG Pet Parameters and Radiomics Features Analysis in Advanced NSCLC Treated with Immunotherapy as Predictors of Therapy Response and Survival

Giulia Polverari [1,2,†], Francesco Ceci [1,*,†], Valentina Bertaglia [3], Maria Lucia Reale [3], Osvaldo Rampado [4], Elena Gallio [4], Roberto Passera [1], Virginia Liberini [1], Paola Scapoli [5], Vincenzo Arena [2], Manuela Racca [5], Andrea Veltri [6], Silvia Novello [3] and Désirée Deandreis [1]

1 Division of Nuclear Medicine, Department of Medical Sciences, University of Turin, AOU Città della Salute e della Scienza, 10126 Turin, Italy; giuliapolverari@yahoo.com (G.P.); passera.roberto@gmail.com (R.P.); v.liberini@gmail.com (V.L.); desiree.deandreis@unito.it (D.D.)
2 PET/CT Center, Affidea IRMET, 10135 Turin, Italy; vincenzo.arena@affidea.it
3 Department of Oncology, University of Turin, San Luigi Gonzaga Hospital, Orbassano, 10043 Torino, Italy; valentina.bertaglia@gmail.com (V.B.); realemarialucia@gmail.com (M.L.R.); silvia.novello@unito.it (S.N.)
4 Medical Physics Unit, S.C. Fisica Sanitaria, A.O.U. Città della Salute e della Scienza, 10135 Turin, Italy; orampado@cittadellasalute.to.it (O.R.); gallio.elena@gmail.com (E.G.)
5 Nuclear Medicine, Istituto per la Ricerca e la Cura del Cancro (IRCC), 10060 Candiolo, Italy; paola.scapoli@ircc.it (P.S.); manuela.racca@ircc.it (M.R.)
6 Radiology Unit, Department of Oncology, University of Turin, San Luigi Gonzaga Hospital, Orbassano, 10043 Torino, Italy; andrea.veltri@unito.it
* Correspondence: francesco.ceci@unito.it
† These authors contributed equally to this work.

Abstract: Objectives: (1.1) to evaluate the association between baseline 18F-FDG PET/CT semi-quantitative parameters of the primary lesion with progression free survival (PFS), overall survival (OS) and response to immunotherapy, in advanced non-small cell lung carcinoma (NSCLC) patients eligible for immunotherapy; (1.2) to evaluate the application of radiomics analysis of the primary lesion to identify features predictive of response to immunotherapy; (1.3) to evaluate if tumor burden assessed by 18F-FDG PET/CT (N and M factors) is associated with PFS and OS. Materials and Methods: we retrospectively analyzed clinical records of advanced NCSLC patients (stage IIIb/c or stage IV) candidate to immunotherapy who performed 18F-FDG PET/CT before treatment to stage the disease. Fifty-seven (57) patients were included in the analysis (F:M 17:40; median age = 69 years old). Notably, 38/57 of patients had adenocarcinoma (AC), 10/57 squamous cell carcinoma (SCC) and 9/57 were not otherwise specified (NOS). Overall, 47.4% patients were stage IVA, 42.1% IVB and 8.8% IIIB. Immunotherapy was performed as front-line therapy in 42/57 patients and as second line therapy after chemotherapy platinum-based in 15/57. The median follow up after starting immunotherapy was 10 months (range: 1.5–68.6). Therapy response was assessed by RECIST 1.1 criteria (CT evaluation every 4 cycles of therapy) in 48/57 patients or when not feasible by clinical and laboratory data (fast disease progression or worsening of patient clinical condition in nine patients). Radiomics analysis was performed by applying regions of interest (ROIs) of the primary tumor delineated manually by two operators and semi-automatically applying a threshold at 40% of SUVmax. Results: (1.1) metabolic tumor volume (MTV) ($p = 0.028$) and total lesion glycolysis (TLG) ($p = 0.035$) were significantly associated with progressive vs. non-progressive disease status. Patients with higher values of MTV and TLG had higher probability of disease progression, compared to those patients presenting with lower values. SUVmax did not show correlation with PD status, PFS and OS. MTV ($p = 0.027$) and TLG ($p = 0.022$) also resulted in being significantly different among PR, SD and PD groups, while SUVmax was confirmed to not be associated with response to therapy ($p = 0.427$). (1.2) We observed the association of several radiomics features with PD status. Namely, patients with high tumor volume, TLG and heterogeneity expressed by "skewness" and "kurtosis" had a higher probability of failing immunotherapy. (1.3) M status at 18F-FDG PET/CT was significantly associated with PFS ($p = 0.002$) and OS ($p = 0.049$). No significant associations were observed for N status. Conclusions: 18F-FDG PET/CT performed before the start of immunotherapy might be an important prognostic tool able to predict the disease progression and response to immunotherapy in patients with advanced NSCLC, since MTV, TLG and radiomics features (volume and heterogeneity) are associated with disease progression.

Keywords: PET/CT; immunotherapy; PD-1; PD-L1; response to therapy; NSCLC

1. Introduction

Lung cancer remains the leading cause of cancer-related death, despite continuous progresses in diagnosis and therapy [1]. Non-small cell lung carcinoma (NSCLC) accounts for 80–85% of all cases of lung cancer [1]. In almost half of the patients, the diagnosis of NSCLC is performed when the disease is already in advanced stages (stage III or stage IV), having an estimated overall 5-year survival rate of 18% [2]. In more than half of patients, the diagnosis of NSCLC is performed when the disease is already in advanced stage with an estimated overall 5-year survival rate of 18% [2,3]. Platinum-based chemotherapy can improve outcome, but the rise of immunotherapy has changed this scenario. Multiple molecules targeting the programmed cell death-1 (PD-1) and the programmed death ligand-1 (PD-L1) axis have been proposed [3]. Different immune checkpoint inhibitors have been approved in the second line setting on the basis of an improving in overall survival (OS) compared to chemotherapy, irrespective to PDL1 expression or with a PD-L1 expression ≥1% for pembrolizumab. Pembrolizumab has also been approved as first-line treatment for advanced NSCLC with PD-L1 higher than 50%, given the significant increase in both progression free survival (PFS) (10.3 versus 6 months) and OS (30 vs. 14.2 months) compared to chemotherapy [3,4]. Moreover, combination strategies of chemo-immunotherapy have recently enriched the upfront therapy approach. However, the benefit with immunotherapy is not seen for the entire population, making the identification of biomarkers and predicting tools a critical step in selecting the ideal candidate population. In NSCLC adenocarcinoma, platinum chemotherapy, plus pemetexered and pembrolizumab, reached a disease control rate of 84.6%, while it was 70.4% for chemotherapy only [5]. However, approximately 15% of positive PD-L1 patients will have disease progression within two months and a median survival of only three months [4]. The inter-patient, inter-tumour and even intra-tumour heterogeneity seem to be the major reasons of such a large prognosis variability, representing a key challenge for the scientific community. In this scenario, the application of new generation image analysis, such as radiomics, might provide further and useful information [6].

Radiomics is an emerging field, defined as the high-throughput extraction of quantitative features from medical images [6,7]. This approach provides high-dimensional data describing the properties of shape and texture of tumors captured in different diagnostic procedures, including PET imaging. The radiomics features are believed to contain information that reflects underlying tumor pathophysiology and allow evaluation of tumor heterogeneity [6,7]. The primary goal of radiomics is to build a clinically relevant predictive, descriptive, or prognostic model using these parameters. Focusing on the relationship between quantitative biological features and cancer prognosis by non-invasive method and aiding clinicians in selecting the appropriate treatments, radiomics is considered a step toward the application of personalized medicine in routine practice. In this respect, NSCLC is a key example to show the advantages of a tailored approach [8,9].

2. Materials and Methods

2.1. Objectives

The objectives of this study were:

(1.1) to evaluate the association between 18F-FDG PET/CT baseline semi-quantitative parameters of the primary lesion in advanced NSCLC patients eligible for immunotherapy with patient's outcome (PFS and OS) and response to immunotherapy,

(1.2) to evaluate the application of radiomics analysis of the primary lesion for texture analysis to extract characteristics (quantitative biomarkers) from PET/CT images to represent tumor pathology or heterogeneity (phenotype),

(1.3) to evaluate if tumor burden assessed by 18F-FDG PET/CT, as nodal (N) and metastatic (M) status, is associated with PFS and OS.

2.2. Study Design and Inclusion Criteria

This is a retrospective, observational study approved by the ethical committee A.O.U. Città della Salute e della Scienza di Torino (IRB number: 0011604; code: IMMUNO PET-19). We analyzed the records and clinical/pathological characteristics of patients referred to Pulmonary Oncology Department, San Luigi Gonzaga Hospital, University of Turin. Eligible patients matched all the following inclusion criteria: (a) biopsy proven advanced NSCLC (stage IIIb/c or stage IV); (b) candidate to immunotherapy targeting the PD-1 or PD-L1; (c) 18F-FDG PET/CT performed at baseline, during the diagnostic work-up, within the start of immunotherapy. Patients with missing data and lost follow-up were excluded from the analysis. Compliance with ethical standards: Ethical approval for all procedures performed in studies involving human participants was in accordance with the ethical standards of the institutional and/or national research committee and with the principles of the 1964 Declaration of Helsinki and its later amendments or comparable ethical standards. Informed consent and local ethical committee approval: informed consent form (ICF) was obtained from all individual participants enrolled in this retrospective analysis. ICF has been provided.

2.3. ^{18}F-FDG PET/CT Image Acquisition and Interpretation

Here, 18F-FDG PET/CT were performed with a standard protocol. Patients were instructed to fast for at least 6 h before the scan, and blood glucose levels were measured before the injection of 18F-FDG. Patients were excluded if their blood glucose levels at the time of the scans exceeded 150 mg/dL. Patient protocol included the intravenous injection of 2.5–3 MBq/kg of 18F-FDG, up to a maximum of 370 MBq (10 mCi), followed by a 60-min uptake period. All patients underwent PET/CT scan in a dedicated tomograph: AOU Città della Salute e della Scienza and IRCSS Istituto di Candiolo (Philips Gemini Dual-slice EXP, Philips Medical Systems, Cleveland, OH, USA)); Affidea-IRMET (Discovery 610, GE Healthcare, Chicago, IL, USA). An attenuation-corrected whole-body scan (base of the skull to mid thighs), 2 to 2.5 min per bed position (with an axial field-of-view of 18 cm per bed position), starting 60 min after tracer injection, was acquired. All patients performed a low-dose CT for attenuation correction and anatomical correlation of PET findings. The tomographs results were validated for a proper quantification and quality of the images recorded. The PET scans were reconstructed by ordered subset expectation maximization (OSEM)-based algorithms. All PET/CT images were analyzed with dedicated workstation (Advantage; GE Healthcare) and were independently interpreted with central reading by two nuclear medicine physicians, aware of clinical data.

2.4. PET Semi-Quantitative Parameters and Radiomics Analysis

Semi-quantitative PET parameters and radiomics features of the primary lesion were extracted using the open-access LIFEx platform v5.1 (IMIV/CEA, Orsay, France) [10]. For each primary lesion were evaluated PET semi-quantitative parameters, including maximum standardized uptake value

(SUVmax), metabolic tumor volume (MTV) and total lesion glycolysis (TLG). The delineation of each primary lung lesion was performed manually, slice-by-slice, independently by two expert operators. Region of interest (ROI) with a threshold at 40% of SUVmax was also applied. MTV represents the volume of the above given ROIs. 3D ROIs based on percentage of SUVmax were applied (3D isocontour at 41% of the maximum pixel value [VOI41]). TLG was calculated as the product of the ROI average SUVmean multiplied by the corresponding MTV. In the longitudinal setting, the quantitative metrics described above were derived using the same approach for all PET/CT examinations in the same patient. Radiomics features were extracted from each of the two ROIs. The following radiomics features were analyzed: size and shape based–features such as volume, maximum diameter along different orthogonal directions, maximum surface, tumor compactness, and sphericity; first-order statistics features reporting the mean, median, maximum, minimum values of the voxel intensities on the image, as well as their skewness (asymmetry), kurtosis (flatness), uniformity, and randomness (entropy) and second-order statistics features include the so-called textural features. Lymph node and systemic metastasis were evaluated and grouped as N and M status.

2.5. *Evaluation of the Response to Immunotherapy*

Therapy response was routinely assessed by CT evaluation every 4 cycles of therapy and by clinical/laboratory evaluation. The diagnostic assessment of response to immunotherapy was performed with response evaluation criteria in solid tumors (RECIST) 1.1 criteria. Complete response (CR) was the disappearance of the primary tumor, partial response (PR) was a decrease of 30% or more in the longest diameter of the primary tumor, progressive disease (PD) was an increase of 20% or more in the longest diameter of the primary tumor, and stable disease (SD) was noted in patients whose tumors did not show either sufficient shrinkage to qualify for PR or a sufficient increase to qualify for PD [11,12]. When CT evaluation was not feasible for fast disease progression or the worsening of patient clinical condition, the response to immunotherapy was performed by clinical and laboratory evaluation only.

2.6. *Outcome Measurements and Statistical Analysis*

Demographic and baseline disease characteristics were recorded, censoring the times of observation on July 2019, at a median follow-up of 10 months (IQR 6–14 months). The primary endpoint was PFS, while the secondary one was OS. PFS was defined as the time from the start of immunotherapy to progression/death for any cause. OS was defined as the time from the start of immunotherapy to death as a result of any cause; patients still alive were censored at the date of last contact. The response to immunotherapy was assessed considering both clinical follow-up and RECIST 1.1 criteria.

Patient characteristics were compared using the Fisher's exact test for categorical variables and the Mann–Whitney test for continuous ones. PFS and OS curves were estimated by the Kaplan–Meier method, comparing the two arms by the log-rank test and calculating 95% CIs. All p-values were obtained by 2-sided exact method at the conventional 5% significance level. All statistical analyses were performed in R 3.6.1.

Considering the radiomics analysis, univariate analysis with Kruskal–Wallis test was performed for each variable (histology, PDL-1 expression, disease stage, progression and response to therapy). The intraclass correlation coefficient (ICC) was used to assess intra- (by observer 1) and inter-observer (by observers 1 and 2) differences in texture and evaluate the reproducibility of textural parameters. The ICC was also used to assess differences in texture between manual and semi-automatic segmentation.

3. Results

3.1. Population Characteristics

Fifty-seven patients have been retrospectively enrolled: 17 females and 40 males, with a median age of 69 years old (range 39–84 years old). Three out of 57 patients were non-smokers, 33/57 were former smokers, while 21/57 were current smokers. Sixty-six percent (38/57) of patients had adenocarcinoma (AC), 17.5% (10/57) squamous cell carcinoma (SCC) and 15.7% (9/57) were not otherwise specified (NOS). According to the 8th Edition of TNM in Lung Cancer (8), about half of the patients (47.4%) were stage IVa, 42.1% were IVb and 8.8% of patients were IIIb. The Eastern Cooperative Oncology Group, performance status (ECOG PS) was 0 in 20/57 patients, 1 in 35/57 and two patients had an ECOG PS of 2. All patients were wildtype (no EGFR mutations, no ALK rearrangements detected). The PD-L1 expression on the bioptic specimen was evaluated in 51/57 patients. Notably, 80.4% of patients (41/51) presented a PD-L1 expression higher than 50%, 7.8% (4/51) between 1 and 49% and 11.8% (6/51) patients lower than 1%. All patients' characteristics are listed in Table 1.

Table 1. Overall population ($n = 57$) characteristics.

Characteristics	Value
Age	Median 69 years old (range 39–84)
Sex	
Male	40/57 (70.2%)
Female	17/57 (29.8%)
Smoking Status	
Non-smoker	3/57 (5.3%)
Ex-smoker	33/57 (57.9%)
Current smoker	21/57 (36.8%)
Histological Variant	
Adenocarcinoma	38/57 (66.6%)
Squamous cell carcinoma	10/57 (17.5%)
NOS	9/57 (15.7%)
ECOG PS	
0	20/57 (35.1%)
1	35/57 (61.4%)
2	2/57 (3.5%)
Stage at Diagnosis	
IB	1/57 (1.75%)
IIB	1/57 (1.75%)
IIIA	5/57 (8.8%)
IIIB	7/57 (12.3%)
IIIC	1/57 (1.7%)
IVA	26/57 (45.6%)
IVB	16/57 (28.1%)
Stage before IO	
IIIB	6/57 (8.8%)
IVA	27/57 (47.4%)
IVB	24/57 (42.1%)
PD-L1 expression analysis	
Not Performed	6/57 (10.5%)
<1%	6/57 (10.5%)
1–49%	4/57 (7.0%)
>50%	41/57 (72.0%)
Immunotherapy	
First line IO	42/57 (73.7%)
Second line IO	15/57 (26.3%)

NOS: Not Otherwise Specified; ECOG PS: Eastern Cooperative Oncology Group Performance Status; IO: Immuno-Oncology therapy.

3.2. Immunotherapy Scheme

Treatment was decided by referent physicians considering tumor histology, PD-L1 expression and patients' risk factors. Immunotherapy was performed as a frontline therapy in 42/57 (73.7%) patients and as a second line therapy after chemotherapy in 15/57 (26.3%) patients. The formers were all treated with Pembrolizumab after the assessment of PD-L1 expression higher than 50%. The latter were treated with Pembrolizumab in 5 cases, Nivolumab in 5 cases and Atezolizumab in 5 cases as well. Of these 15 cases treated with immunotherapy as second line, 8 patients received platinum + pemetrexed, 5 patients platinum + gemcitabine and 2 patients platinum + docetaxel. Six out of fifteen patients underwent surgery on the primary lesion before starting immunotherapy. Pembrolizumab, nivolumab and atezolizumab were administered intravenously at the standard dose.

3.3. Follow-Up and Therapy Response to Immunotherapy

The median follow-up was 10 months (range 1.5–68.6; IQR 6–14 months). Forty percent (23/57) of patients died from cancer-related causes, while 59.6% (34/57) were alive with evidence of disease. At the last follow-up, 30 patients were PD, 19 were SD and 8 were PR. No CR was observed. Thirty patients (52.6%) experienced disease progression during therapy. Among patients with progressive disease, 21 had the appearance of new lesions on CT performed as part of monitoring therapy response (RECIST 1.1). In 9 cases, CT evaluation was not feasible (fast disease progression or worsening of patient clinical condition) and disease progression was observed by clinical and laboratory evaluation.

Four patients experienced immunotherapy-induced toxicity (skin reaction, cough and rising liver enzymes) and four patients experienced acute events (transient ischemic attack, pneumonia and acute respiratory failure).

Immunotherapy was suspended in 30/57 patients. The causes of suspension were: progression (clinical and/or radiological) of disease in 27 cases assessed through CT and/or clinical evaluation, severe toxicity in 2 cases and death in 1 case. In 25/57 patients, immunotherapy was ongoing at the time of the last follow-up. The median number of cycles of therapy was 7 (mean = 11; range 1–69).

3.4. ^{18}F-FDG PET/CT Findings

First, 18F-FDG PET/CT was performed as routine diagnostic procedure to stage the disease before the start of immunotherapy. The median time from PET/CT and the start of immunotherapy was 37 days (mean = 45; range 4–133 days). All primary tumors, observed in the 51/57 patients who did not receive surgery and/or radiation therapy with radical intent, exhibited increased FDG uptake.

Twenty-two patients were N0, while 35/57 had positive lymph nodes (N+). In details, 10 were N1 (ipsilateral peribronchial and/or hilar and intrapulmonary), 12 patients were N2 (ipsilateral mediastinal and/or subcarinal nodes), and 13 patients were N3 (contralateral mediastinal or hilar nodes or supraclavicular nodes). Systemic metastases were seen in 34/57 patients, while 23 patients were staged as M0. 18F-FDG PET/CT observed adrenal metastases in 10 cases, contralateral lung nodules in 9, bone metastases in 9, liver lesions in 6, pleural involvement or malignant effusion in 5, extra-pulmonary lymph nodes in 2, soft tissue localization in 2 cases and 1 mesenterial nodule. Eleven patients were classified as M1a (contralateral lung or pleural/pericardial nodule or effusion), six were M1b (single extra-thoracic metastasis) and seventeen were M1c (multiple extra-thoracic metastases).

3.5. PET Semi-Quantitative Parameters Analysis (Objective 1.1)

The values of baseline 18F-FDG PET/CT semi-quantitative parameters of the primary lesion are listed in Table 2. At the Mann–Whitney test, MTV (p = 0.028) and TLG (p = 0.035) were significantly associated with progressive vs. non-progressive disease status (Table 3). Patients with higher values of MTV and TLG of the primary lesion at the baseline PET/CT had higher probability of disease progression, compared to those patients presenting with lower values. SUVmax values did not show significant association between the two groups (PD vs. non-PD patients) ($p = 0.55$). In the Kaplan–Meier plot analysis, the variables resulted associated with PD vs. non-PD status (MTV and TLG) were compared with PFS and OS (Figure 1). MTV and TLG were stratified according to the median value: upper and lower median value (MTV = 74.1 ml3; TLG = 310.8). Kaplan–Meier curves showed a trend to predict disease progression among patients with MTV and TLG lower or higher the median values. However, the log rank test of the two curves showed them not to be significantly different (Figure 1). In patients with MTV and TLG upper median values, PFS was 5 months, while OS was 15 months. In patients with MTV and TLG lower median values, PFS and OS were not reached (minimum 50% of events at last follow-up not reached).

Table 2. In this table; 18F-FDG PET/CT semi-quantitative parameters: SUVmax, metabolic tumor volume (MTV) and total lesion glycolysis (TLG) values.

PET Parameters	Minimum	Percentile 25	Median	Percentile 75	Maximum
SUVmax (g/mL)	1.4	5.8	9.5	13.5	30.5
MTV (mL^3)	3.1	36.7	74.1	163.3	695.2
TLG	2.8	87.3	310.8	852.9	4639.8

Table 3. SUVmax, MTV and TLG values among patients with progressive (PD) and non-progressive (non-PD) disease.

Associations Between Baseline PET Parameters and PD vs. non-PD							
PET Parameters	Status	Minimum	Percentile 25	Median	Percentile 75	Maximum	*p* Value
SUVmax (g/mL)	PD	2.5	5.8	11.5	13.6	30.5	0.55
	non-PD	1.4	5.9	9.3	13.4	28.9	
MTV (mL^3)	PD	3.1	47.0	124.4	203.1	695.2	0.028
	non-PD	3.1	19.7	57.4	86.6	548.5	
TLG	PD	4.5	165.9	536.1	988.1	2820.3	0.035
	non-PD	2.8	55.0	205.8	417.8	4639.8	

In the Kruskal–Wallis test, MTV ($p = 0.027$) and TLG ($p = 0.022$) resulted in being significantly different among PR, SD and PD groups (Table 4). SUVmax was confirmed to not be associated with response to therapy criteria ($p = 0.427$) (Table 4).

Table 4. Association of MTV and TLG with response to immunotherapy, as assessed by response evaluation criteria in solid tumors (RECIST) 1.1 criteria and clinical follow-up.

PET Parameters	Associations Between Baseline PET Parameters and Response to Immunotherapy						
	Status	Minimum	Percentile 25	Median	Percentile 75	Maximum	*p* Value
SUVmax (g/mL)	PR	1.4	5.8	8.8	13.2	15.3	0.427
	SD	5.7	9.2	11.9	15.0	28.9	
	PD	2.5	6.4	10.7	13.5	30.5	
MTV (mL^3)	PR	3.1	15.3	49.5	79.6	173.9	0.027
	SD	26.9	72.2	75.0	375.9	548.5	
	PD	3.1	44.3	124.3	202.6	695.2	
TLG	PR	2.8	30.4	139.3	251.3	865.6	0.022
	SD	83.4	310.8	417.8	852.9	4639.8	
	PD	4.5	151.3	440.8	979.9	2820.3	

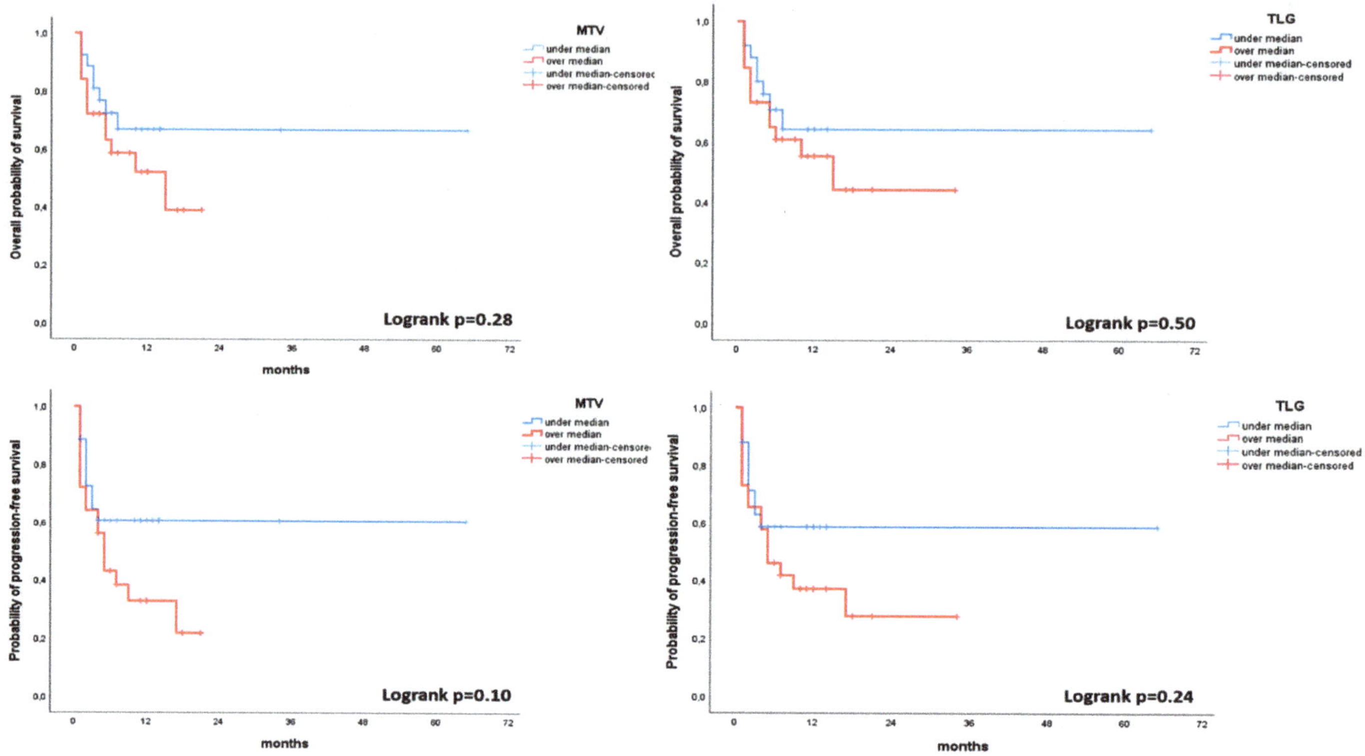

Figure 1. Kaplan–Meier plot analysis for MTV and TLG with both progression free survival (PFS) and overall survival (OS). Population was grouped by the median value of MTV (74.1) and TLG (310.8).

3.6. Radiomics Analysis (Objective 1.2)

The intraclass correlation coefficient (ICC) analysis of the texture parameters of the primary lesion, based on two different delineations generated by two observers, showed that all parameters presented good reproducibility (ICC > 0.95), except for GLZLM_SZLGE (ICC = 0.37). However, when applying a semi-automatic segmentation (threshold = 40% of the SUVmax), only 8 features showed good reproducibility (SUVmax, sphericity, two first-order statistics features and 4 textural features. ICC > 0.95). The univariate analysis with the Kruskal–Wallis test was performed for the following variables: histology, PDL-1 expression, disease stage, progression and response to therapy.

Histological variants: the only feature associated with different histological subtypes was SUVmax (Figure 2). Namely, SCC showed higher SUVmax values than AC and NOS subtype.

PD-L1 expression: several features (including SUVmax, volume, busyness, coarseness, GLZML_ZLNU and GLZML_GLNU) resulted in being significantly different between patients with PD-L1 expression lower than 1%, between 1% and 49% and higher than 50%. Considering the semi-automatic ROIs, only two features (coarseness and GLZLM_ZLNU) maintained the statistical correlation (Figure 3).

Disease stage: radiomics features did not show significant difference between IIIb, IVa and IVb patients at both manual and semi-automatic segmentation.

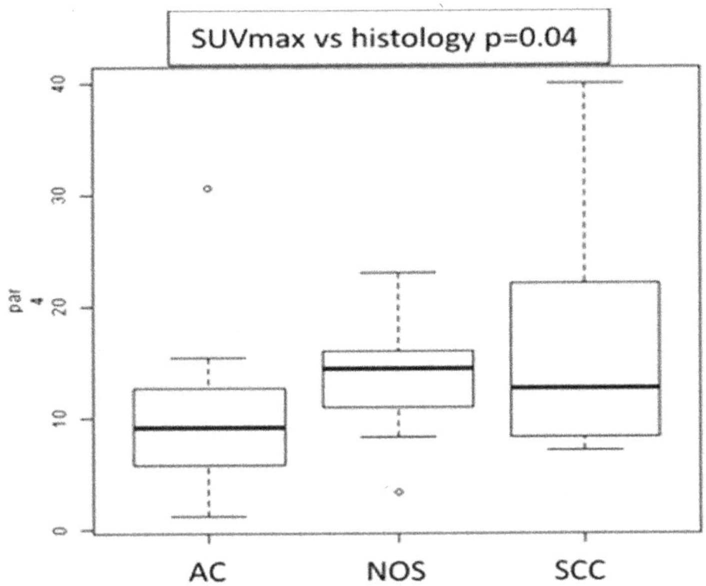

Figure 2. Box plot of SUVmax values showing differences between histological subtypes.

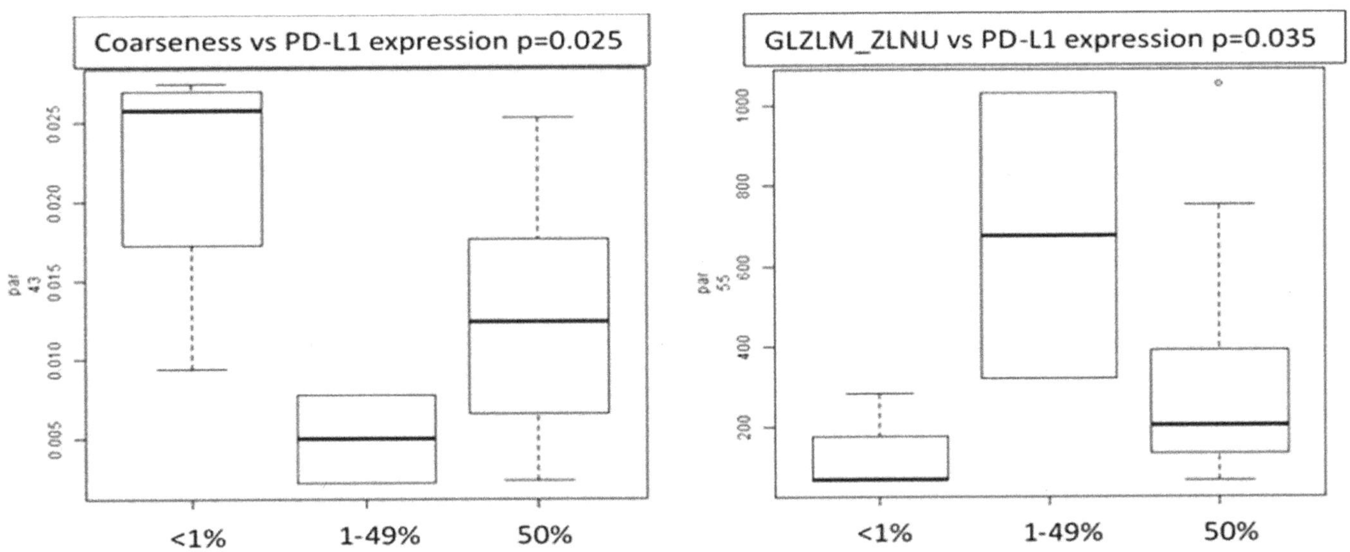

Figure 3. Box plots of radiomics features (coarseness and GLZLM_ZLNU) showing correlation with PD-L1 expression.

Progression status: several features showed differences between PD vs. non-PD patients, such as volume ($p = 0.035$), TLG ($p = 0.037$), three first-order histograms-based features (kurtosis, excess-kurtosis and skewness) and six textural features (GLZLM_LZE, GLRLM_RP, GLRLM_SRE, GLRLM_HGRE, GLRLM_SRHGE and GLCM Homogeneity) (Figure 4). GLZLM represents the grey-level zone length matrix and provides information on the size of homogeneous zones for each grey-level in 3 dimensions. GLZLM_LZE is the distribution of long homogeneous zones in an image. GLRLM represents the size of homogeneous runs for each grey level. "Run" means the presence of elements in the image with the same gray-level on in a row/line. GLCM_homogeneity considers the arrangements of pairs of voxels to calculate textural indices and represents the homogeneity of grey-level voxel pairs.

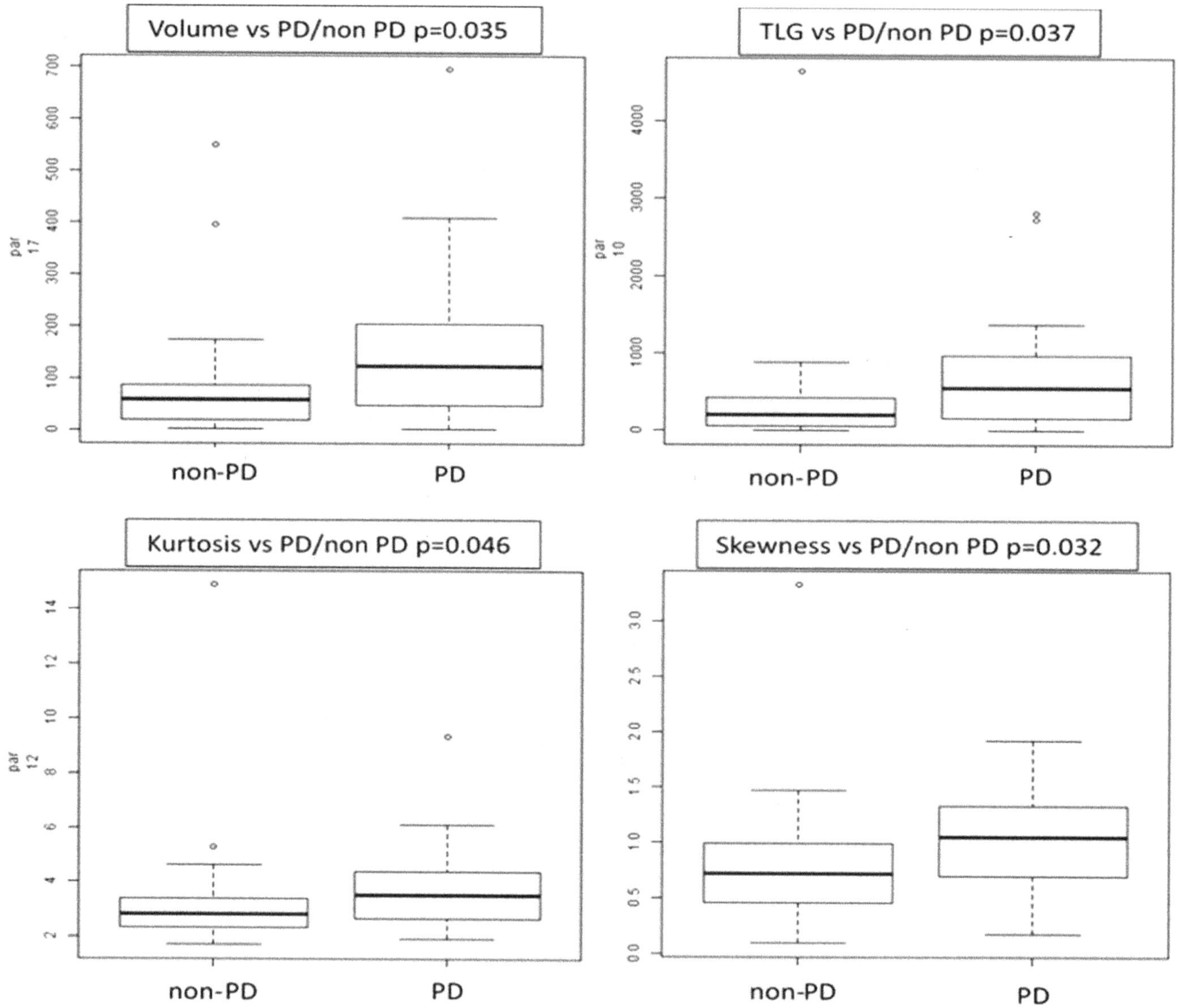

Figure 4. Box plots of radiomics features correlated with progressive (PD) vs. non-progressive disease status (non-PD).

Accordingly, patients with primary lung tumor presenting with higher TLG value, higher volume, higher asymmetry and kurtosis had higher probability to progress.

Response to therapy: TLG, volume and two textural features showed a significant difference between PR, SD and PD patients at both manual and semiautomatic evaluation.

3.7. Tumor Burden Analysis (Objective 1.3)

In the Kaplan–Meier plot analysis, M status (M0, M1a, M1b, M1c) as assessed by 18F-FDG PET/CT was significantly associated with PFS ($p = 0.002$) and OS ($p = 0.049$). Namely, patients with no visible metastases at PET/CT had significantly better outcome compared with those patients presenting with FDG avid metastases. No significant associations were observed for N status (N0, N1, N2, N3) as assessed by 18F-FDG PET/CT and PFS or OS. (Figure 5).

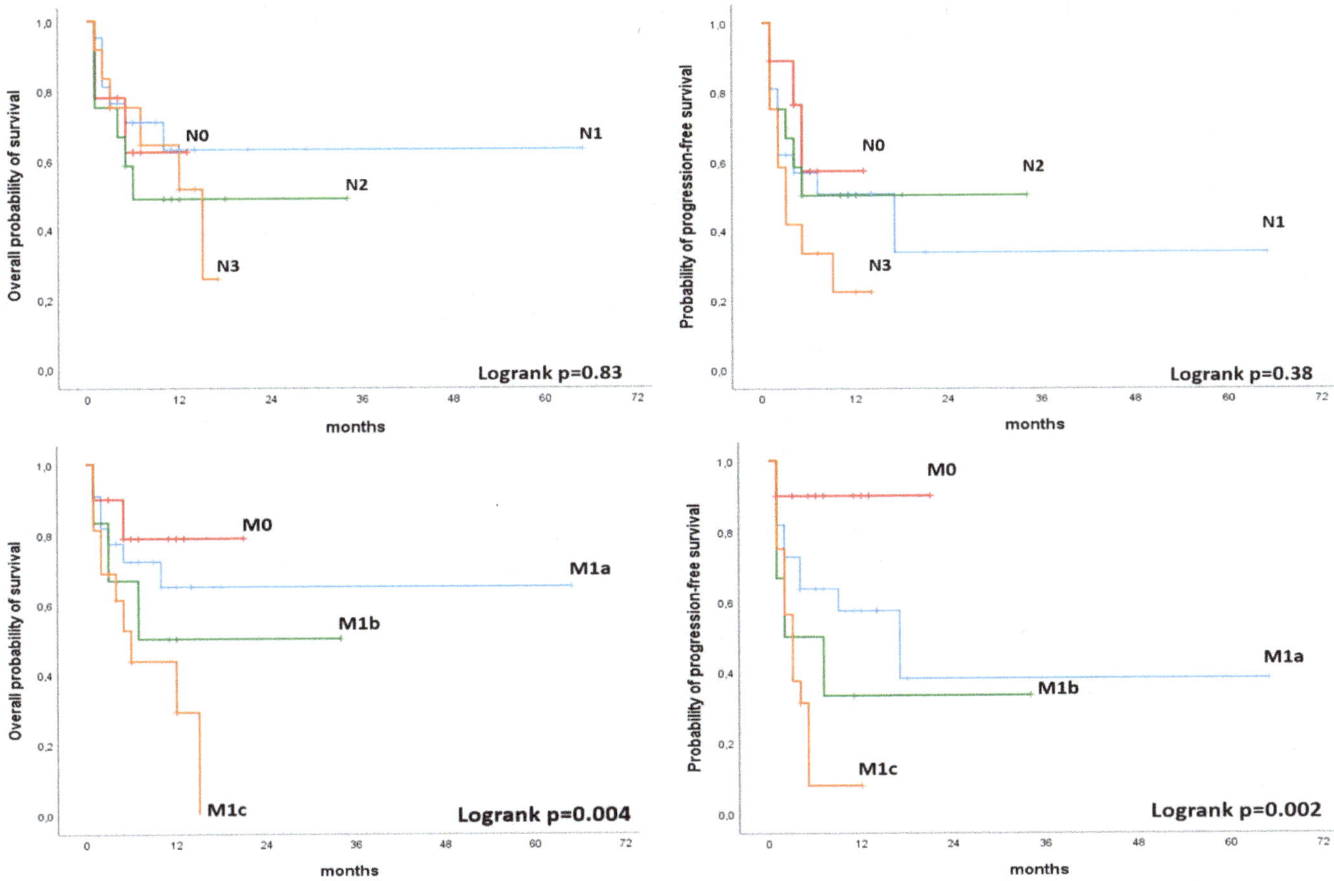

Figure 5. Kaplan–Meier plot analysis for N status (N0, N1, N2, N3) and M status (M0, M1a, M1b, M1c) with PFS and OS.

4. Discussion

Over the past decade 18F-FDG PET/CT demonstrated to be a powerful tool for staging and assessing treatment response in patients suffering from NSCLC [13,14]. Even if PET/CT is widely used in this clinical scenario, limited data are currently available regarding the role of PET/CT semi-quantitative parameters as predictors of patient outcome [15,16]. Findings are generally heterogeneous and this variability might be probably related to the heterogeneity of the population enrolled. Furthermore, the association of semi-quantitative parameters with patients' outcome can be related to the clinical stage of the disease (locally vs. advanced disease) and to the therapy investigated (chemo-radiotherapy vs. biological therapy) [15–18]. At present, SUV values, MTV and TLG are the PET-derived parameters used to assess the tumor metabolic activity in NSCLC [18]. MTV and TLG can easily be calculated in the primary tumor by means of a segmentation technique. The manual or semi-automatic measurement of the pre-treatment MTV has been shown to be better than SUVmax for predicting patients' prognosis in different solid neoplasms such as head and neck cancer, with or without metastases [19,20].

Our study aimed to investigate the relationship between the functional tumor parameters at baseline (SUVmax, MTV, and TLG) and PFS and OS in patients with advanced NSCLC, presenting with stage IIIB, IIIC, IVa and IVb, for whom immunotherapy was shortly planned. A significant association of MTV and TLG of the primary lesions with PD was observed, since lower MTV and TLG values were associated with non-PD status; while, on the contrary, primary lesions presenting with higher values were more likely associated with the progression of the disease during immunotherapy. On the contrary, SUVmax did not show significant association with both PFS and OS. These results are in accordance with recent studies, suggesting a superior correlation of volumetric 18F-FDG PET/CT parameters, rather than SUVmax only [7,9,21,22]. However, despite the fact that in the Kaplan–Meier analysis, MTV and TLG showed a trend in predicting disease progression, the curves associated with PFS and OS were not statistically significant. This is probably due to the relatively small sample size and the limited number of events that occurred.

Grizzi et al., in a preliminary analysis on 27 patients with NSCLC, found an antithetical correlation between 18F-FDG PET/CT pre-treatment parameters and the response to immunotherapy. Authors observed a rapid progression of disease after 8 weeks from the start of immunotherapy in patients with a SUVmax up to 17.1 and a SUVmean up to 8.3, with a sensitivity of 88.9% and 100%, respectively [23]. Similarly, Evangelista et al. investigated the role of semi-quantitative 18F-FDG PET/CT parameters in NSCLC treated with Nivolumab. Authors observed an association between the sum of metabolic parameters of all lesions and PD status, with SUVmax having the strongest association [24]. Their data seem to be in contrast with our analysis. However, authors considered all the lesions together as the cumulative sum of all FDG deposits detected by PET/CT, while we specifically designed our study to analyze semi-quantitative parameters of the primary lesion only, and we analyzed the correlation of the tumor burden (N and M status assessed by 18F-FDG PET/CT) separately, with a dedicated objective (objective 1.3). In our study, MTV and TLG were also significantly associated with immunotherapy response. Patients with SD or PR had lower values of MTV and TLG compared to patients with PD. No correlation was observed again between SUVmax values and response to therapy. Accordingly, since MTV and TLG are parameters that accurately reflect the glycolytic metabolic status of a lesion and thus the disease aggressiveness, 18F-FDG PET/CT might be considered as a prognostic tool to stratify patients presenting with higher metabolic primary tumors that, most likely, will fail immunotherapy. In our study, we also observed a significant association between the M status at 18F-FDG PET/CT and PFS and OS. It is worth noting that 18F-FDG PET/CT offers the possibility of having a single-step whole body examination that can clearly identify distant metastases and select NSCLC patients treated with immunotherapy with a higher probability of experiencing rapid disease progression and poor survival outcomes.

Immunotherapy has completely changed the prognosis and the care of patients with NSCLC. However, the benefit with immunotherapy is not seen for the entire population, making the identification of biomarkers a critical step in selecting the candidate population. Therefore, radiomics aims to identify biomarkers that better predict patient response [25,26]. Radiomics has been investigated in various studies to identify clinical and computational image-based predictors of rapid disease progression phenotypes in NSCLC patients [7,27,28]. However, there are only few studies investigating the application of this new field in patients with NSCLC treated with checkpoint-based immunotherapy and most of them based radiomics analysis on CT images and enrolled heterogeneous population with different primaries (e.g., lung and melanoma) [29,30]. Recently, Mu et al. presented promising data and a novel methodological approach on the application of radiomics analysis in NSCLC treated with immune checkpoint blockades. In their study, authors tested the hypothesis that radiomics features from baseline pretreatment 18F-FDG PET/CT scans can predict the clinical outcomes of NSCLC patients treated with checkpoint blockade immunotherapy. Among other findings, authors reported that when investigating the informative components of multi-parametric radiomics signature (mp-RS) formula, they found that multiple texture features (PET_SRLGE, KLD_SZE) positively correlated, suggesting that the more heterogeneous tumors had a larger probability to have a durable clinical benefit (DCB). These results are slightly in contrast with prior studies, which showed that more heterogeneous tumors with CT textures had worse response to radiation or chemotherapy [31]. Our results were slightly in contrast with Mu et al. [7] as well. In our study, the most interesting difference of features was seen between patients with PD and patients with non-PD. Namely, patients with primary lung tumor presenting with high TLG value, high volume and tumor heterogeneity represented by asymmetry (skewness feature) and kurtosis (how heavily the tails of a distribution differ from the tails of a normal distribution) had a higher probability of progression and were associated with non-response to immunotherapy. However, differences in features extraction methodology and different endpoints (DCB vs. PD) make these findings not completely comparable. Finally, segmentation is currently the rate-limiting step in radiomics analysis. To overcome this issue, in our study, the segmentation of the ROIs was performed manually by two independent operators and semi-automatically, applying a threshold of 40% of the SUVmax.

Limitation

This work is not exempt from limitations. The retrospective design of this analysis might have probably affected population selection. A prospective design would probably offer the chance to recruit a more homogenous population (e.g., same immunotherapy scheme, shorter range for PET scan before immunotherapy, immunotherapy administrated as first-line). Namely, in our cohort, 26.3% of patients received immunotherapy after platinum-based chemotherapy. However, the population enrolled represents the typical cohort of patients generally referred to 18F-FDG PET/CT before immunotherapy in daily clinical practice.

This analysis was performed in a relatively small sample size. A larger cohort would be preferable. In our study, we observed an association of MTV and TLG with PD vs. non-PD status. Nevertheless, this association was not maintained in the Kaplan–Meier analysis and, despite a non-negligible trend, MTV and TLG were not statistically significantly associated with PFS. The limited number of events at the end of follow-up, namely for patients with lower than median values for MTV and TLG, influenced the correlation between these metabolic parameters and PFS and OS. It is probable that our statistical model might rich significance in a larger cohort.

Another limitation is related to the lack of "early intermediate" PET performed while immunotherapy was still on-going, in order to evaluate PET response to therapy. However, since the role of PET imaging during immunotherapy is not yet established, 18F-FDG PET/CT is generally performed in clinical practice at baseline only. Thus, none of the patients enrolled in our study performed a second PET scan.

Considering radiomics analysis, the ideal setting would require a robust validation regarding reconstruction and segmentation on different tomographs. In our analysis, despite similar 18F-FDG PET/CT protocols and using the same reconstruction algorithm, the texture analysis was performed on images derived by three different tomographs. A common issue with radiomics analysis is represented by segmentation process (manual vs. automatic) and a comparison between the two approaches would be preferable. However, to strengthen our analysis, we included two operators who independently perform the segmentation. Furthermore, a threshold of 40% of SUVmax was also applied to both operators' ROI. Finally, in our study, segmentation was performed on PET images only, while low-dose CT images were not segmented, and so not considered in our radiomics analysis.

5. Conclusions

According to our results, baseline 18F-FDG PET/CT performed before the start of immunotherapy might be important, since it offers the chance to evaluate different quantitative parameters potentially associated with different response to therapy in patients with advanced NSCLC. In our study, and considering the limitations exposed above, MTV, TLG and radiomics features (volume and heterogeneity) were associated with disease progression, while metastatic tumor stages assessed with PET/CT were associated with different patients' outcome.

These results, while far from definitive evidence, encouraged us to initiate a prospective trial to investigate the role of radiomics features extracted from 18F-FDG PET/CT in NSCLC eligible to immunotherapy.

Author Contributions: Conceptualization, G.P., F.C., V.B., S.N. and D.D.; methodology, F.C. and R.P.; software, O.R., E.G. and V.L., validation; F.C., D.D.; formal analysis, R.P., F.C., G.P. and O.R.; investigation, F.C. and G.P.; resources, D.D., S.N. and A.V.; data curation, G.P., V.A., P.S., M.R., V.B., and M.L.R.; writing—original draft preparation, G.P. and F.C.; writing—review and editing, F.C., G.P., D.D., V.B. and S.N.; visualization, F.C., G.P., V.A., M.R. and P.S.; supervision, F.C., A.V., S.N. and D.D.; project administration, G.P. and F.C. All authors have read and agreed to the published version of the manuscript.

References

1. Siegel, R.L.; Miller, K.D.; Jemal, A. Cancer statistics, 2018. *CA Cancer J. Clin.* **2018**, *68*, 7–30. [CrossRef] [PubMed]
2. Cancer statistics. *JAMA* **2013**, *310*, 982. [CrossRef] [PubMed]
3. Reck, M.; Rodríguez-Abreu, D.; Robinson, A.G.; Hui, R.; Csőszi, T.; Fülöp, A.; Gottfried, M.; Peled, N.; Tafreshi, A.; Cuffe, S.; et al. Pembrolizumab versus Chemotherapy for PD-L1-Positive Non-Small-Cell Lung Cancer. *N. Engl. J. Med.* **2016**, *375*, 1823–1833. [CrossRef] [PubMed]
4. Mezquita, L.; Auclin, E.; Ferrara, R.; Charrier, M.; Remon, J.; Planchard, D.; Ponce, S.; Ares, L.P.; Leroy, L.; Audigier-Valette, C.; et al. Association of the Lung Immune Prognostic Index with Immune Checkpoint Inhibitor Outcomes in Patients with Advanced Non–Small Cell Lung Cancer. *JAMA Oncol.* **2018**, *4*, 351–357. [CrossRef]
5. Paz-Ares, L.; Luft, A.; Vicente, D.; Tafreshi, A.; Gümüş, M.; Mazières, J.; Hermes, B.; Çay Şenler, F.; Csőszi, T.; Fülöp, A.; et al. Pembrolizumab plus Chemotherapy for Squamous Non-Small-Cell Lung Cancer. *N. Engl. J. Med.* **2018**, *379*, 2040–2051. [CrossRef]
6. Scrivener, M.; de Jong, E.E.; van Timmeren, J.E.; Pieters, T.; Ghaye, B.; Geets, X. Radiomics applied to lung cancer: A review. *Transl. Cancer Res.* **2016**, *5*, 398–409. [CrossRef]
7. Mu, W.; Tunali, I.; Gray, J.E.; Qi, J.; Schabath, M.B.; Gillies, R.J. Radiomics of 18F-FDG PET/CT images predicts clinical benefit of advanced NSCLC patients to checkpoint blockade immunotherapy [published online ahead of print, 2019 Dec 5]. *Eur. J. Nucl. Med. Mol. Imaging* **2019**. [CrossRef]
8. Sollini, M.; Cozzi, L.; Antunovic, L.; Chiti, A.; Kirienko, M. PET Radiomics in NSCLC: State of the art and a proposal for harmonization of methodology. *Sci. Rep.* **2017**, *7*, 358. [CrossRef]
9. Grizzi, F.; Castello, A.; Qehajaj, D.; Toschi, L.; Rossi, S.; Pistillo, D.; Paleari, V.; Veronesi, G.; Novellis, P.; Monterisi, S.; et al. Independent expression of circulating and tissue levels of PD-L1: Correlation of clusters with tumor metabolism and outcome in patients with non-small cell lung cancer. *Cancer Immunol. Immunother.* **2019**, *68*, 1537–1545. [CrossRef]
10. Nioche, C.; Orlhac, F.; Boughdad, S.; Reuzé, S.; Goya-Outi, J.; Robert, C.; Pellot-Barakat, C.; Soussan, M.; Frouin, F.; Buvat, I. LIFEx: A freeware for radiomic feature calculation in multimodality imaging to accelerate advances in the characterization of tumor heterogeneity. *Cancer Res.* **2018**, *78*, 4786–4789. [CrossRef]
11. Eisenhauer, E.A.; Therasse, P.; Bogaerts, J.; Schwartz, L.H.; Sargent, D.; Ford, R.; Dancey, J.; Arbuck, S.; Gwyther, S.; Mooney, M.; et al. New response evaluation criteria in solid tumours: Revised RECIST guideline (version 1.1). *Eur. J. Cancer* **2009**, *45*, 228–247. [CrossRef]
12. Detterbeck, F.C.; Boffa, D.J.; Kim, A.W.; Tanoue, L.T. The Eighth Edition Lung Cancer Stage Classification. *Chest* **2017**, *151*, 193–203. [CrossRef] [PubMed]
13. Huang, W.; Zhou, T.; Ma, L.; Sun, H.; Gong, H.; Wang, J.; Yu, J.; Li, B. Standard uptake value and metabolic tumor volume of 18F-FDG PET/CT predict short-term outcome early in the course of chemoradiotherapy in advanced non-small cell lung cancer. *Eur. J. Nucl. Med. Mol. Imaging* **2011**, *38*, 1628–1635. [CrossRef] [PubMed]
14. Banna, G.L.; Anile, G.; Russo, G.; Vigneri, P.; Castaing, M.; Nicolosi, M.; Strano, S.; Gieri, S.; Spina, R.; Patanè, D.; et al. Predictive and Prognostic Value of Early Disease Progression by PET Evaluation in Advanced Non-Small Cell Lung Cancer. *Oncology* **2017**, *92*, 39–47. [CrossRef] [PubMed]
15. Van de Wiele, C.; Kruse, V.; Smeets, P.; Sathekge, M.; Maes, A. Predictive and prognostic value of metabolic tumour volume and total lesion glycolysis in solid tumours. *Eur. J. Nucl. Med. Mol. Imaging* **2013**, *40*, 290–301. [CrossRef]
16. Visser, E.P.; Philippens, M.E.; Kienhorst, L.; Kaanders, J.H.; Corstens, F.H.; de Geus-Oei, L.F.; Oyen, W.J. Comparison of tumor volumes derived from glucose metabolic rate maps and SUV maps in dynamic 18F-FDG PET. *J. Nucl. Med.* **2008**, *49*, 892–898. [CrossRef]
17. Hofheinz, F.; Van den Hoff, J.; Steffen, I.G.; Lougovski, A.; Ego, K.; Amthauer, H.; Apostolova, I. Comparative evaluation of SUV, tumor-to-blood standard uptake ratio (SUR), and dual time point measurements for assessment of the metabolic uptake rate in FDG PET. *EJNMMI Res.* **2016**, *6*, 53. [CrossRef]
18. Dosani, M.; Yang, R.; McLay, M.; Wilson, D.; Liu, M.; Yong-Hing, C.J.; Hamm, J.; Lund, C.R.; Olson, R.; Schellenberg, D. Metabolic tumour volume is prognostic in patients with non-small-cell lung cancer treated with stereotactic ablative radiotherapy. *Curr. Oncol.* **2019**, *26*, e57–e63. [CrossRef]

19. Sharma, A.; Mohan, A.; Bhalla, A.S.; Sharma, M.C.; Vishnubhatla, S.; Das, C.J.; Pandey, A.K.; Sekhar Bal, C.; Patel, C.D.; Sharma, P.; et al. Role of Various Metabolic Parameters Derived From Baseline 18F-FDG PET/CT as Prognostic Markers in Non-Small Cell Lung Cancer Patients Undergoing Platinum-Based Chemotherapy. *Clin. Nucl. Med.* **2018**, *43*, e8–e17. [CrossRef]
20. Salavati, A.; Duan, F.; Snyder, B.S.; Wei, B.; Houshmand, S.; Khiewvan, B.; Opanowski, A.; Simone, C.B., 2nd; Siegel, B.A.; Machtay, M.; et al. Optimal FDG PET/CT volumetric parameters for risk stratification in patients with locally advanced non-small cell lung cancer: Results from the ACRIN 6668/RTOG 0235 trial. *Eur. J. Nucl. Med. Mol. Imaging* **2017**, *44*, 1969–1983. [CrossRef]
21. Chen, H.H.; Chiu, N.T.; Su, W.C.; Guo, H.R.; Lee, B.F. Prognostic value of whole-body total lesion glycolysis at pretreatment FDG PET/CT in non-small cell lung cancer. *Radiology* **2012**, *264*, 559–566. [CrossRef]
22. Liao, S.; Penney, B.C.; Wroblewski, K.; Zhang, H.; Simon, C.A.; Kampalath, R.; Shih, M.C.; Shimada, N.; Chen, S.; Salgia, R.; et al. Prognostic value of metabolic tumor burden on 18F-FDG PET in nonsurgical patients with non-small cell lung cancer. *Eur. J. Nucl. Med. Mol. Imaging* **2012**, *39*, 27–38. [CrossRef]
23. Grizzi, F.; Castello, A.; Lopci, E. Is it time to change our vision of tumor metabolism prior to immunotherapy? *Eur. J. Nucl. Med. Mol. Imaging* **2018**, *45*, 1072–1075. [CrossRef] [PubMed]
24. Evangelista, L.; Cuppari, L.; Menis, J.; Bonanno, L.; Reccia, P.; Frega, S.; Pasello, G. 18F-FDG PET/CT in non-small-cell lung cancer patients: A potential predictive biomarker of response to immunotherapy. *Nucl. Med. Commun.* **2019**, *40*, 802–807. [CrossRef] [PubMed]
25. Dennie, C.; Thornhill, R.; Sethi-Virmani, V.; Souza, C.A.; Bayanati, H.; Gupta, A.; Maziak, D. Role of quantitative computed tomography texture analysis in the differentiation of primary lung cancer and granulomatous nodules. *Quant Imaging Med. Surg.* **2016**, *6*, 6. [PubMed]
26. Kirienko, M.; Cozzi, L.; Rossi, A.; Voulaz, E.; Antunovic, L.; Fogliata, A.; Chiti, A.; Sollini, M. Ability of FDG PET and CT radiomics features to differentiate between primary and metastatic lung lesions. *Eur. J. Nucl. Med. Mol. Imaging* **2018**, *45*, 1649–1660. [CrossRef]
27. Nappi, A.; Gallicchio, R.; Simeon, V.; Nardelli, A.; Pelagalli, A.; Zupa, A.; Vita, G.; Venetucci, A.; di Cosola, M.; Barbato, F.; et al. FDG-PET/CT parameters as predictors of outcome in inoperable NSCLC patients. *Radiol. Oncol.* **2015**, *49*, 320–326. [CrossRef]
28. Pyka, T.; Bundschuh, R.A.; Andratschke, N.; Mayer, B.; Specht, H.M.; Papp, L.; Zsótér, N.; Essler, M. Textural features in pre-treatment [F18]-FDG-PET/CT are correlated with risk of local recurrence and diseasespecific survival in early stage NSCLC patients receiving primary stereotactic radiation therapy. *Radiat. Oncol.* **2015**, *10*, 100. [CrossRef]
29. Deutsch, E.; Paragios, N. Radiomics to predict response to immunotherapy, bridging the gap from proof of concept to clinical applicability? *Ann. Oncol.* **2019**, *30*, 879–881. [CrossRef]
30. Trebeschi, S.; Drago, S.G.; Birkbak, N.J.; Kurilova, I.; Călin, A.M.; Pizzi, A.D.; Lalezari, F.; Lambregts, D.M.J.; Rohaan, M.W.; Parmar, C.; et al. Predicting Response to Cancer Immunotherapy using Non-invasive Radiomic Biomarkers. *Ann. Oncol.* **2019**, *30*, 998–1004. [CrossRef]
31. Aerts, H.J.; Velazquez, E.R.; Leijenaar, R.T.; Parmar, C.; Grossmann, P.; Carvalho, S.; Bussink, J.; Monshouwer, R.; Haibe-Kains, B.; Rietveld, D.; et al. Decoding tumour phenotype by noninvasive imaging using a quantitative radiomics approach. *Nat. Commun.* **2014**, *5*, 4006. [CrossRef]

5

Usefulness of Hybrid PET/MRI in Clinical Evaluation of Head and Neck Cancer Patients

Natalia Samolyk-Kogaczewska [1], Ewa Sierko [1,2,*], Dorota Dziemianczyk-Pakiela [3], Klaudia Beata Nowaszewska [4], Malgorzata Lukasik [5] and Joanna Reszec [5]

1 Department of Radiotherapy, Comprehensive Cancer Center, 15-027 Bialystok, Poland; natalia.samolyk@gmail.com
2 Department of Oncology, Medical University of Bialystok, 15-027 Bialystok, Poland
3 Department of Otolaryngology and Maxillofacial Surgery, Jedrzej Sniadecki Memorial Regional Hospital, 15-950 Bialystok, Poland; dyrka2@wp.pl
4 Department of Maxillofacial and Plastic Surgery, Medical University of Bialystok, 15-276 Bialystok, Poland; beata.nowaszewska@wp.pl
5 Department of Medical Pathology, Medical University of Bialystok, 15-089 Bialystok, Poland; mblukasik@gmail.com (M.L.); joannareszec@gmail.com (J.R.)
* Correspondence: ewa.sierko@iq.pl

Abstract: (1) Background: The novel hybrid of positron emission tomography/magnetic resonance (PET/MR) examination has been introduced to clinical practice. The aim of our study was to evaluate PET/MR usefulness in preoperative staging of head and neck cancer (HNC) patients (pts); (2) Methods: Thirty eight pts underwent both computed tomography (CT) and PET/MR examination, of whom 21 pts underwent surgical treatment as first-line therapy and were further included in the present study. Postsurgical tissue material was subjected to routine histopathological (HP) examination with additional evaluation of p16, human papillomavirus (HPV), Epstein-Barr virus (EBV) and Ki67 status. Agreement of clinical and pathological T staging, sensitivity, specificity, positive predictive value (PPV), negative predictive value (NPV) of CT and PET/MR in metastatic lymph nodes detection were defined. The verification of dependences between standardized uptake value (SUV value), tumor geometrical parameters, number of metastatic lymph nodes in PET/MR and CT, biochemical parameters, Ki67 index, p16, HPV and EBV status was made with statistical analysis of obtained results; (3) Results: PET/MR is characterized by better agreement in T staging, higher specificity, sensitivity, PPV and NPV of lymph nodes evaluation than CT imaging. Significant correlations were observed between SUVmax and maximal tumor diameter from PET/MR, between SUVmean and CT tumor volume, PET/MR tumor volume, maximal tumor diameter assessed in PET/MR. Other correlations were weak and insignificant; (4) Conclusions: Hybrid PET/MR imaging is useful in preoperative staging of HNC. Further studies are needed.

Keywords: PET/MRI; head and neck cancer; HPV; EBV; p16

---

1. Introduction

Head and neck cancers (HNC) are the sixth most common cancers worldwide. The vast majority (more than 90%) are squamous cell carcinomas, so that the term HNC is often used to describe all carcinomas arising from the epithelium lining the sinonasal tract, oral cavity, pharynx and larynx and showing microscopic evidence of squamous differentiation. Approximately two-thirds of patients with HNC present with locally advanced disease at the primary site and/or spread to regional lymph nodes. The 5-year survival rate of HNC patients ranges between 40% and 70%, depending on the primary site and stage [1,2]. Positron emission tomography (PET) with fluorine-18 labelled fluorodeoxyglucose

(18F-FDG) as a radiotracer is an established procedure in head and neck squamous cell carcinoma (HNSCC) diagnosis [2]. It is vitally important to the characterization of local, regional and distant disease [3]. PET supports the initial staging of difficult cases, where other imaging methods produce equivocal results. It is useful in the detection of occult primary tumors and synchronous primary cancers. Furthermore, PET aids in assessing tumor response to therapy and helps in detecting cancer recurrence and metastasis during the follow-up period [3–5].

Contrary to anatomical imaging, 18F-FDG-PET takes into account biological differences in metabolism and the radiopharmacological uptake between the tumor and the surrounding normal tissue [6]. PET images are characterized by high contrast but low spatial resolution, which creates a need for combining PET with morphological imaging methods such as cone beam computed tomography (CBCT). A novel hybrid imaging technology, Positron Emission Tomography-Magnetic Resonance Imaging (PET/MRI), has been introduced to clinical practice [7]. The integrated PET/MRI technique combines the benefits of both methods such as superior soft tissue contrast, multiplanar image acquisition and functional imaging capability [8].

A suspicion of head and neck cancer (HNC) is predominantly based on the identification of a primary tumor or the presence of palpable metastatic lymph nodes in the head and neck region during a clinical examination [9]. Accurate, pre-treatment staging is crucial in newly diagnosed HNSCC patients since it enables clinicians to determine patient prognosis and develop an optimal treatment strategy [5]. Precision imaging methods play an integral role in this process [4]. Furthermore, proper imaging is vital to the accurate delineation of target volumes in radiotherapy (RT) planning, particularly when highly conformal RT techniques such as intensity modulated radiotherapy (IMRT) or volumetric arc therapy (VMAT) are utilized [9]. Initial reports have revealed that hybrid 18F-FDG PET/MRI offers higher sensitivity and specificity in the detection of HNC when compared to PET, CT and MRI used separately [10,11]. Moreover, PET/MRI has a higher correlation coefficient with pathological tumor size in comparison to contrast-enhanced CT (CECT), MR and PET/CT [10]. PET/MRI outperformed PET/CT by providing greater tumor conspicuity and higher sensitivity in determining the perineural spread in primary HNSCC. One study has demonstrated PET/MRI sensitivity to be 85% and specificity 92% in the detection of metastatic lymph nodes [3].

In HNSCC patient population, a group of younger, healthier individuals with limited or no tobacco exposure can be distinguished [12]. Prognosis in such cases is excellent as these patients are highly responsive to treatment [13]. Human papillomavirus (HPV)-related oropharyngeal cancers (OPC) are a frequent finding in this group of patients. Presence of HPV is an important prognostic factor, which is reflected in the 8th edition of the American Joint Committee on Cancer (AJCC) TNM (Tumor Nodes Metastases classification) staging system [13,14]. There is a limited number of studies on the relationship between PET imaging and HPV status in HNSCC [3,15–17]. Furthermore, very few studies concern the utility of PET/MRI in the characterization of HPV-related HNC [8,18]. According to our knowledge, there are no literature reports documenting the correlation between Epstein-Barr virus (EBV) status and PET/MRI features. Therefore, the aim of our study was to evaluate the correlation between PET/MR and CT parameters, biochemical parameters, Ki67 index, p16, HPV and EBV status as well as usefulness of PET/MRI in the preoperative staging of HNC patients.

2. Results

This section may be divided by subheadings. It should provide a concise and precise description of the experimental results, their interpretation as well as the experimental conclusions that can be drawn.

2.1. *Accuracy of T staging*

Agreement between T stages determined with CT, PET/MRI and histopathological (HP) examination, which is the clinical gold-standard technique used for cancer diagnosis, was evaluated. The T stage determined with CT was compatible with the HP stage in 56% of cases. T overstaging was observed in 11% of cases, downstaging in 33% of patients. PET/MRI results corresponded to HP staging in 67% of cases, were overstaged in 11%, downstaged in 22%.

2.2. Specificity, Sensitivity, Positive Predictive Value (PPV) and Negative Predictive Value (NPV) of Lymph Node Evaluation in CT and PET/MRI

The total number of detected lymph nodes in the HP examination of postoperative tissue material was 475, out of which 31 were metastatic. Twenty seven lymph nodes were described as malignant in CT scans and 24 in PET/MRI scans. Based on the CT and PET/MRI scans, lymph nodes of the neck were assigned into appropriate levels [19]. Results of the HP were referenced values. In regard to lymph node detection, PET/MRI sensitivity was 55%, specificity—98%, PPV—71%, NPV—97% and test reliability was 95%. Computed tomography sensitivity was 47%, specificity—97%, PPV—53%, NPV—96% and test reliability—94%.

2.3. Correlations between Clinical, Morphological and Metabolic Parameters

2.3.1. SUV Values in Relation to Tumor Geometrical Parameters, Biochemical Parameters and Ki67 Index

A high, statistically significant correlation between standardized uptake value (SUV)max and maximal tumor diameter determined with PET/MRI (r = 0.457, p = 0.036) (Figure 1) was revealed in comparison to the measurements obtained from CT images (r = 0.025, p = 0.913). On the other hand, poor and statistically insignificant correlations were observed between SUVmax values and tumor volume determined with PET/MRI (r = 0.309, p = 0.172), tumor volume determined with CT (r = 0.289, p = 0.203), Ki67 index (r = 0.04, p = 0.862), CRP concentration (r = 0.069, p = 0.764) and glucose levels (r = 0.308, p = 0.173).

A significant relationship was observed between SUVmean and CT tumor volume (r = 0.563, p = 0.007), PET/MRI tumor volume (r = 0.607, p = 0.003) and maximal tumor diameter determined with PET/MRI (r = 0.788, p = 0.00002) (Figure 1). Contrary to the aforementioned findings, correlations between SUVmean and maximal tumor diameter in CT (r = 0.165, p = 0.474), Ki67 index (r = 0.08, p = 0.728), CRP concentration (r = 0.138, p = 0.549) and glucose levels (r = 0.253, p = 0.268) were weak and insignificant.

2.3.2. Presence of p16, HPV and EBV in Relation to SUV Values, Tumor Geometrical Parameters

The average value of SUVmax in p16-positive patients was lower than in p16-negative patients. Despite substantial discrepancies in the obtained results, the difference between the p16-positive and the p16-negative groups was insignificant (p = 0.37). Maximal SUV was not significantly correlated with HPV and EBV status, and neither was maximal tumor diameter determined with CT or PET/MRI correlated with the presence of p16, HPV, EBV.

The average values of SUVmean in p16-, HPV- and EBV-positive patients were close to the values in p16-, HPV- and EBV-negative groups.

2.3.3. Number of Metastatic Lymph Nodes in Relation to SUV Values, Tumor Geometrical Parameters, Ki67 Index and Presence of p16, HPV, EBV

The correlation between CT-based tumor volume and the number of metastatic lymph nodes determined with CT was statistically significant (p = 0.006). The highest tumor volumes were found in the group of patients with 1 metastatic lymph node and the lowest in those without metastatic lymph nodes (p = 0.01). The number of metastatic lymph nodes determined with CT or PET/MRI and SUV values, PET/MRI-based tumor volume, maximal tumor diameter based on CT or PET/MR imaging, Ki67 index were insignificant.

No significant correlations were observed between the presence of p16 (p = 0.431, df = 2, Chi2 = 1.68), HPV (p = 0.623 df = 2, Chi2 = 0.946), EBV (p = 0.714 df = 2, Chi2 = 0.674) and the number of metastatic lymph nodes detected with CT, as well as between the positive status of p16 ($p = 0.24$ df = 2, Chi2 = 2.854), HPV ($p = 0.139$ df = 2, Chi2 = 3.94), EBV ($p = 0.414$ df = 2, Chi2 = 1.763) and the number of metastatic lymph nodes detected with PET/MRI.

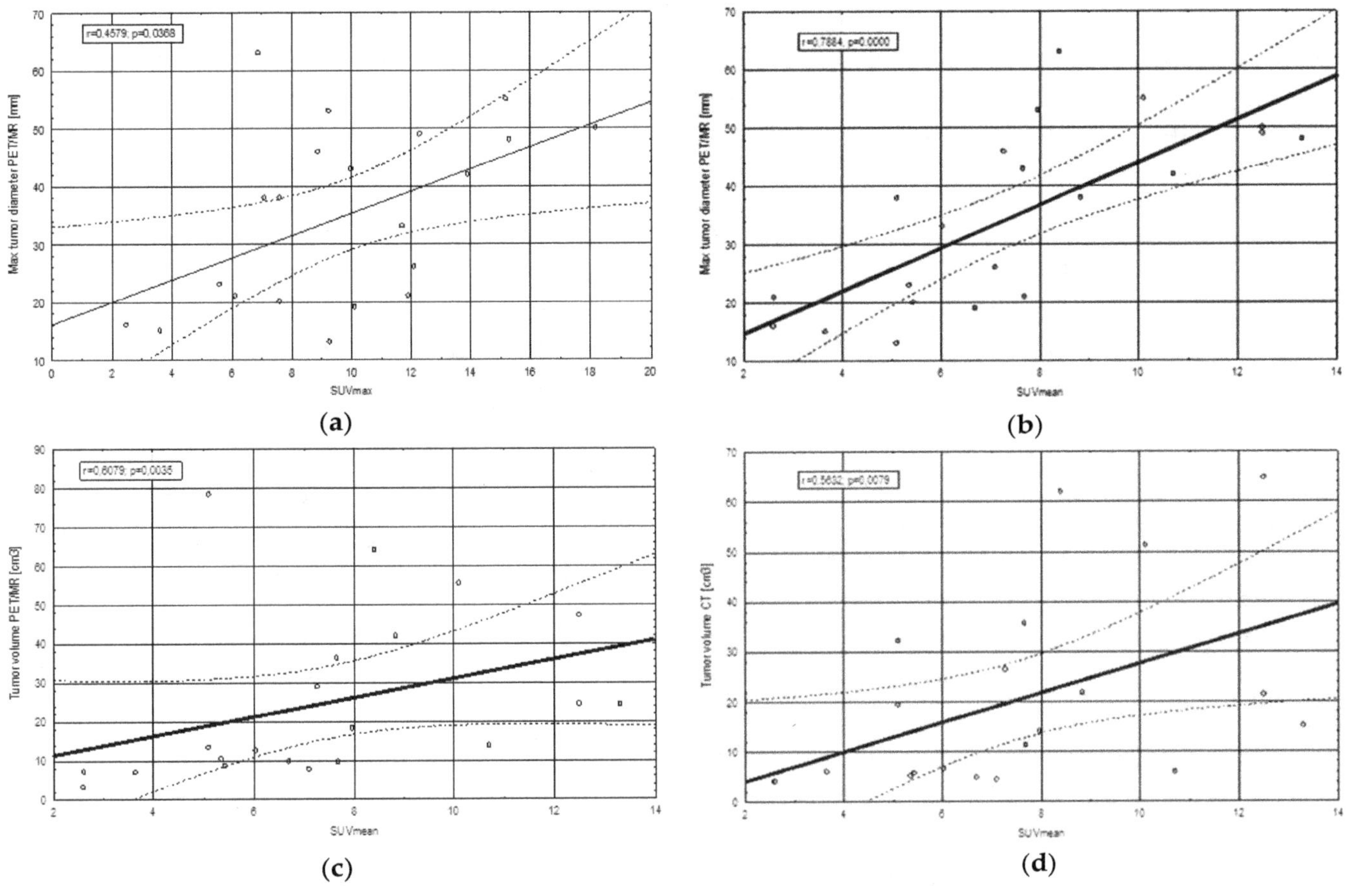

Figure 1. Statistically significant correlation between standardized uptake value (SUV) values and maximal tumor diameter (**a**,**b**) and tumor volume (**c**,**d**) obtained from positron emission tomography/magnetic resonance (PET/MR) or computed tomography (CT). Abbreviations: SUVmax—maximal standardized uptake value, SUVmean—mean standardized uptake value, r—correlation coefficient from Spearman's correlation test, *p*—statistical significance value.

3. Discussion

Hybrid PET/MRI imaging can play an important role in the initial staging of HNC patients. In our study, we compared the efficacy of PET/MRI with the routinely used CT scanning and HP examination, which is the clinical gold-standard technique used for cancer diagnosis, in primary tumor staging (T features) according to the AJCC TNM classification. Our results demonstrated that T staging based on PET/MRI images was compatible with HP outcomes in a higher number of patients (67%) in comparison with T staging based on CT images alone (56%). Similar results were obtained by other authors - T staging performed with PET/MRI was accurate in 75% of HNC cases compared to 59% with PET/CT and 50% with MRI alone [20]. Chan et al. demonstrated that greater accuracy in defining the extent of primary nasopharyngeal tumors was achieved with PET/MRI in comparison to PET/CT [21]. PET/MRI imaging offers more precision in depicting perineural infiltration, intracranial or inferior orbital fissure involvement. It should be mentioned that our study did not include nasopharyngeal cancer (NPC) patients. Other authors have demonstrated similar results: fused PET and MR imaging delivered more accurate T staging of HNC patients (74%) compared with PET/CT (63%) [22]. Tsujikawa et al. demonstrated that FDG PET/MRI with its greater soft tissue contrast, multiplanar image acquisition and functional imaging capability is useful in the evaluation of stages of oral cavity cancers and the assessment of oropharyngeal cancer patients based on the new AJCC TNM staging system [8].

Regional metastasis to the lymph nodes is one of the most important predictors of poor prognosis in HNC [23]. Based on the results of CT and PET/MRI scans, we calculated the sensitivity, specificity, PPV and NPV of both diagnostic tests. Positive predictive value expresses the probability that a positive diagnostic test result is reliable. Similarly, NPV determines the probability that a negative test result is reliable [24]. Our study revealed relatively low sensitivity of PET/MRI in metastatic lymph node detection. This could be associated with the fact that detecting small nodes with micrometastases remains a challenge for currently available diagnostic modalities, including PET/MRI [2]. Metastases can be present in unenlarged lymph nodes and not all enlarged nodes are malignant [25]. Another explanation for such results may be limited radiological expertise in interpreting PET/MRI images as this is a novel hybrid imaging technique. Our study has found that specificity, NPV and test reliability of PET/MR is marginally better than in CT results. On the other hand, PET/MR has 8% higher sensitivity and 18% higher PPV compared with CT. In a different study, the sensitivity, specificity and accuracy of PET/MRI-based evaluation of regional node status achieved a 99% rate each [21]. Based on lymph node levels, Schaarschmidt et al. demonstrated sensitivity, specificity, NPV and PPV of 81%, 99%, 98% and 89%, respectively, for PET/MRI [20]. On the other hand, Platzek et al. found that PET/MRI is capable of detecting 64% more metastatic lymph nodes, partly due to the fact that PET/MRI scans were performed following PET/CT scans without the additional FDG injection and the time interval between the FDG injection and PET/MR was longer, which contributed to an increase in FDG uptake by the lymph nodes [26]. Another study has highlighted a better diagnostic value of PET/MRI staging in primary tumors compared with cervical node classification in head and neck malignancies with 94% of primary tumors and 82% of regional nodes correctly classified in comparison to histopathology results [27].

Positron emission tomography with FDG as a radiotracer reflects the metabolic activity of tumor tissue which is expressed in SUV values [28]. Our study revealed a stronger correlation between SUVmean and tumor geometry, such as volume and maximal diameter, than between SUVmax and tumor geometry. PET complements anatomical imaging modalities, particularly in tumor volume determination. Therefore, our study demonstrated stronger correlations between SUV values and PET/MRI than between those values and CT [29]. Tumor volume and SUV values are considered prognostic factors—increased values of both are associated with a higher risk of death [30,31]. Biologically, larger tumors have higher metabolic activity and therefore, higher SUV values indicate a worse prognosis [32]. PET/MRI has an advantage over CT as it enables the measurements of tumor volume and SUV values to be obtained during one examination.

Poor and statistically insignificant correlations were found between SUVmax, SUVmean and KI67, CRP, glycemic parameters in our study. The authors of a meta-analysis concerning correlations between FDG uptake and Ki67 reported significant heterogeneity in HNC cases [33]. Furthermore, pretreatment SUVmax was significantly higher in patients with enhanced Ki67 expression in comparison to those with low Ki67 expression, but the study concerned diffuse large B-cell lymphoma [34]. Surov et al. reported that SUVmax was moderately correlated with Ki67 expression and therefore cannot be used as a surrogate marker for tumor proliferation [35]. A Chinese study on a group of lymphoma patients showed that post-treatment SUVmax values were significantly correlated with post-treatment CRP values [36]. By contrast, a previously mentioned study demonstrated that baseline SUVmax was weakly correlated with CRP ($r = 0.215$, $p = 0.011$) [34].

A recent meta-analysis investigating the effect of blood glucose levels on SUV values assessed with FDG-PET scans revealed positive correlations between glucose levels and SUVmax and SUVmean values in normal tissue such as brain, muscle, liver, but no significant correlations were found between blood glucose levels and SUVmax or SUVmean values in primary malignant tumors [37]. No evidence of a linear relationship between glycaemia and SUV has been reported by other authors [38].

However, it should be emphasized that high plasma glucose levels decrease FDG uptake, which might affect SUV values [39].

In the present study, differences between SUVmax or SUVmean and HPV or p16 presence were insignificant. Comparable results have been obtained in other studies, where no differences in SUVmax values between p16- and HPV-positive, and p16- and HPV-negative patients were reported [40–42]. By contrast, Schouten et al. demonstrated that SUVmax in HPV-positive tumors was significantly lower than in HPV-negative tumors [43]. This finding is in agreement with a study by Surov et al. which revealed that p16-negative tumors showed significantly higher SUVmax and SUVmean values in comparison to p16-positive carcinomas [44].

In our study, no correlation between SUV values and EBV infection status was observed. Literature data confirms our results [45,46].

Similarly, in the present study p16, HPV, EBV did not have a significant impact on the results of CT- or PET/MRI-determined tumor volume and maximal tumor diameter. However, according to the literature, in HNC patients, p16/HPV-positive tumors are usually smaller than p16/HPV-negative tumors [44,47]. Some studies have demonstrated that EBV status and primary tumor volume can be utilized in the prognostic stratification of NPC patients [48,49]. On the other hand, data confirming correlations between primary tumor volume and EBV-positivity is limited [50,51].

Maximal tumor diameter is an important primary tumor feature which is reflected in the TNM classification of HNC (e.g., T1 denotes a tumor size 2 cm or less in its largest dimension) [13]. There are a few studies demonstrating the prognostic value of maximal tumor diameter in OPC [52] and NPC [53], but there are no published papers concerning the influence of p16-, HPV- or EBV-positivity on maximal tumor diameter determined with CT or PET/MRI.

According to our knowledge, there are no literature reports examining the relationship between PET/MRI-based tumor volume and the number of metastatic lymph nodes in HNC patients. Our study did not find any correlations between tumor features obtained from PET/MRI scans and the number of metastatic lymph nodes. By contrast, correlations between tumor volume and the number of metastatic lymph nodes based on CT images were significant. The lowest tumor volumes determined with CT correlated with no metastases in the lymph nodes. This is normally the case in early stage HNC patients. We therefore expected to find significant correlations between the highest tumor volumes determined with CT and multiple metastatic lymph nodes. However, the highest CT-based tumor volumes were observed in patients with 1 metastatic lymph node. This can be explained by the highly inflammatory nature of HNSSC, particularly at advanced stages of the disease [54]. Large tumors investigated in the present study probably consisted not only of neoplastic tissue but also contained peritumoral inflammatory infiltrate. On the other hand, HNC has a high propensity to metastasize through the lymphatic pathway [55]. This could explain the occurrence of multiple metastases in the lymph nodes independently of tumor volumes presented in our study. Research concerning lung adenocarcinoma has demonstrated positive correlations between tumor size and the number of metastatic lymph nodes [56]. By contrast, Miller et al. reported that tumor volume in cervical cancer patients did not correlate with the presence of lymph node metastases [57].

In the present study, the correlation between the number of metastatic lymph nodes determined with PET/MRI and primary tumor SUV values was insignificant. Only few papers have explored this issue but the results obtained were contradictory. Some authors report that in lung cancer patients no statistically significant differences in SUVmax and SUVmean values between individuals with occult lymph nodes and those without have been found [58]. A different study has demonstrated that SUVmax and SUVmean are significantly associated with lymph node involvement in oesophageal cancer patients [59].

Correlations between the presence of HPV, p16 and EBV, and the number of metastatic lymph nodes determined with PET/MRI were insignificant in our study. Other authors have obtained similar results—HPV-positive patients were heterogenous in terms of nodal stages [60]. By contrast, in TROG 02.02 phase III trial, p16-positive patients were included in a more advanced nodal category in comparison with the p16-negative group [47]. The vast majority of NPC is linked to Epstein-Barr virus infection [61,62]. A lack of relationship between EBV status and the number of lymph nodes detected with PET/MRI is most probably associated with the inclusion of oropharyngeal and oral cavity cancer patients in our study.

Based on our results, further studies should include a larger number of HNC pts.

4. Materials and Methods

Thirty eight HNSCC patients underwent both CT and PET/MRI examinations. (Figure 2) Based on the CT and PET/MRI results, 21 patients underwent surgical treatment as first-line therapy and this group was subsequently included in the present study. The remaining patients received radiochemotherapy or palliative RT. Study inclusion criteria were as follows: age over 18 years old, informed consent for study participation, no unmanaged systemic diseases, no hypersensitivity or previous allergic reaction to intravenous iodine contrast or FDG, glucose blood level below 160mg/dL, no metal elements in the body (cardiac pacemakers, metal surgical stitches or clips, intrauterine contraceptive devices, metal shavings in the eyeball, cochlear implants, etc.). Clinical characteristics of the group are presented in Table 1. All pts had squamous cell carcinoma and in about 87% of cases histology grade score (G) was G2. The median age of study participants was 60 years (range of 36–74 years). Twelve of them were female, nine were male. Hypertension and diabetes were the most common comorbidities. In terms of laboratory parameters (Complete Blood Count, renal and liver function parameters, electrolyte blood concentration, thyroid hormones level), the group of patients was homogenous. Discrepancies were observed in C reactive protein (CRP) levels in the blood and its values ranged from 0.3 mg/mL to 120.5 mg/mL.

Prior to surgical treatment, contrast-enhanced (Ultravist 300, 1 mL/kg) CT was routinely performed in all study participants on the 64-detector row CT scanner (Aquilion CX, Canon Medical Systems Corporation, Otawara, Japan). Axial images were obtained with 3 mm slice thickness from the top of the cranium to manubrium sterni. The parameters included a 120 kV tube voltage, tube current 200 mA, 0.5 s rotation time, matrix size, 512×512 and a field of view of 250 mm. CT scans were interpreted by a radiologist experienced in the interpretation of head and neck region CT images.

All study participants also underwent PET/MRI scans on the 3 Tesla Siemens Biograph mMR scanner (Siemens Healthcare GmbH, Erlangen, Germany) after an average of 9 days (range 1 to 20 days) from the CT scans. The examination consisted of whole-body, low resolution MRI imaging, followed by a PET scan and a diagnostic MRI scan (T1- and T2-weighted sequences and contrast-enhanced sequences) of the head and neck region. MRI attenuation images were acquired using the Dixon approach with a coronal 2-point 3D T1-weighted volumetric interpolated breath hold examination (VIBE) (3.12 mm slice thickness, 20% interslice gap, integrated parallel acquisition technique factor 2, acquisition time 19s, 192×121 matrix, 500mm $\times$ 328 mm field of view (FOV), repetition time 3.6ms, echo time 1.23 and 2.46ms, scanning time 4 minutes 10 seconds). PET/MRI scans were obtained simultaneously with the patient remaining in the same position without specific head and neck immobilization (Orfit mask). All patients fasted for at least 6 hours prior to the test. Diagnostic scans were performed 1 hour after the intravenous administration of 18F-FDG (4 MBq/kg, range of 203–417 MBq 18F-FDG per patient). PET/MRI images were evaluated by both a radiologist and nuclear medicine specialist. Maximal and mean SUV of the primary volume were measured. Mean SUV was defined as the average SUV value in the voxel that showed $\geq$ 40% of SUVmax [63].

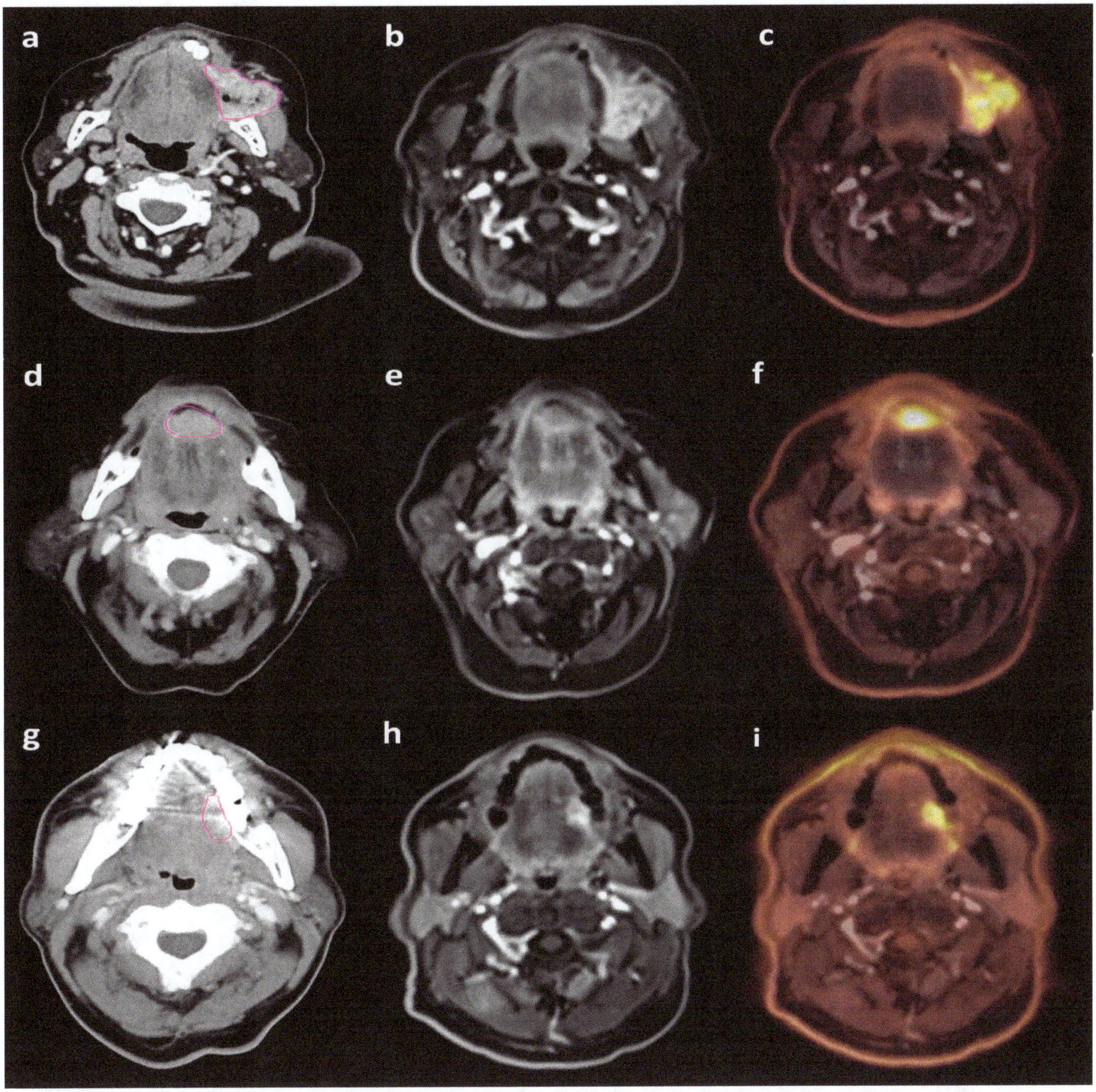

Figure 2. Contrast enhancement computed tomography (CT) (**a**,**d**,**g**), T1-weighted volumetric interpolated breath hold examination (VIBE) magnetic resonance (MR) (**b**,**e**,**h**) and positron emission tomography/MR (PET/MR) (**c**,**f**,**i**) imaging of head and neck cancer patients. (**a**,**b**,**c**)—patient with squamous cell carcinoma of the buccal mucosa in clinical stage T3N2b; (**d**,**e**,**f**)—patient with squamous cell carcinoma of the floor of the mouth in clinical stage T1N0; (**g**,**h**,**i**)—patient with squamous cell carcinoma of the oral tongue in clinical stage T2N0.

Table 1. Characterization of patient with head and neck squamous cell carcinoma (SSC) according to localization of the primary tumor, Ki67 expression, clinical stage (TNM classification, AJCC, ed. 8, 2017) based on postoperative histopathological (HP) examination, status of p16 protein, human papilloma virus (HPV) and Epstein-Barr virus (EBV) positivity, smoking status and biopsy performed before positron emission tomography/magnetic resonance (PET/MR) imaging.

No. of pts.	Localization of Primary Tumor	TNM Stage	Ki67 Index [%]	p16 Status	HPV Status	EBV Status	Smoking	Biopsy before PET/MR (days)
1	OT	T2 N1 M0	30	0	0	0	1	28
2	BM	T2 N1 M0	30	0	0	0	0	25
3	LG	T3 N2b M0	20	0	0	0	1	21
4	BoT	T2 N0 M0	20	0	0	0	1	20
5	BoT	T3 N2c M0	40	1	0	0	0	14
6	BoT	T2 N2c M0	30	0	0	0	1	18
7	OT	T1 N1 M0	50	1	1	1	0	14
8	FoM	T2 N2c M0	30	1	1	0	1	21
9	FoM	T1 N2b M0	20	0	0	0	0	18
10	OT	T2 N1 M0	40	1	1	0	0	16
11	MAR	T3 N0 M0	40	1	1	0	0	23
12	FoM	T3 N0 M0	20	0	0	0	1	20
13	FoM	T2 N2b M0	50	1	0	1	1	30
14	LG	T2 N0 M0	60	1	0	0	0	14
15	SSG	T3 N0 M0	30	0	0	0	0	15
16	OT	T1 N0 M0	30	0	0	0	0	15
17	OT	T3 N2b M0	30	0	0	0	1	21
18	FoM	T1 N0 M0	20	0	0	0	0	17
19	BM	T3 N2b M0	30	0	0	1	1	18
20	BoT	T1 N0 M0	20	0	0	0	0	28
21	FoM	T4a N2c M0	50	1	0	0	1	24

Abbreviations: OT—oral tongue, BM—buccal mucosa, LG—lower gingiva, BoT—base of tongue, FoM—floor of mouth, MAR—maxillary alveolar ridge, SSG—submandibular salivary gland, 0—absence of test feature, 1—presence of test feature.

Surgical treatment was performed an average of 19 days (range of 9 to 28 days) after the CT scans and an average of 13 days (range of 2 to 27 days) after the PET/MRI scans.

Tissue material obtained during surgery was subjected to routine histopathological examination (HP). Additionally, the HP protocol included the immunohistochemical evaluation of p16 protein expression as a surrogate marker for HPV infection, the latent membrane protein 1 (LMP1) expression as a surrogate marker for EVB as well as the detection of Ki67 protein indicating the proliferation rate of cancer cells. The immunohistochemical evaluation of p16 protein expression was conducted using a method described elsewhere [64,65]. Slides were considered positive for p16 protein if the specimen showed continuous staining of at least 50% of tumor cells. For the immunohistochemical detection (Dako, Poland) of EBV presence, antibodies against LMP1—monoclonal mouse anti-LMP protein (clone CS.1-4, Dako, Poland) were used. The expression of Ki67 protein was evaluated with an immunohistochemical method described in the literature [66]. Nuclear accumulation of Ki67 protein in neoplastic cells was assessed semiquantitatively and defined as a percentage of reaction-positive cells.

The presence of HPV genetic material was examined using the PCR method. A positive result (HPV presence in the analyzed material) was determined when at least one of the bands associated with a different HPV subtype was present on the strip along with the developing control line and the positive control. A negative result (no HPV presence) was determined when no bands associated with HPV were developed while the developing control line and the positive control band were both present.

Clinical and pathological stages of the disease were determined according to the 8th ed. of AJCC TNM classification [8]. Based on imaging tests, only round-shaped lymph nodes or nodes exceeding 10mm in the smallest transverse dimension with contrast enhancement on CT or MRI and/or increased 18F-FDG uptake in PET scans were taken into consideration. The results obtained from CECT, PET/MRI and HP were compared. HP results were referenced.

Agreement between CT- and PET/MRI-based T staging, sensitivity, specificity, PPV, NPV in metastatic lymph node detection were defined. Sensitivity was the proportion of patients with positive diagnostic test results (CT or PET/MRI scanning) who were correctly diagnosed in relation to referenced HP results. Specificity was the proportion of patients with negative imaging test results who were correctly diagnosed [67]. Positive predictive value is a proportion of true positive results among all positive findings (true positives and false positives). Similarly, negative predictive value is a proportion of true negative results among all negative results (true negatives and false negatives) [22].

Dependences between SUVmax and SUVmean values, the size and maximal diameter of the primary tumor, the number of metastatic lymph nodes detected with PET/MRI, HPV and EBV status, Ki67 index, glucose level and CRP concentration status were verified in the statistical analysis of the obtained results (Table 2). Considering the number of lymph nodes, study participants were divided into 3 groups: those without metastatic lymph nodes, those with 1 metastatic lymph node and those with 2 or more metastatic lymph nodes. The division was based on the 8th ed. of AJCC TNM classification of HNC, where N0 means no lymph node metastasis, N1–metastasis in single small lymph node and N2–among others, metastasis in multiple lymph nodes.

Table 2. Measurements of standardized uptake value (SUV) values, tumor geometrical parameters and number of metastatic lymph nodes obtained from positron emission tomography/magnetic resonance (PET/MR) and computed tomography (CT), as well as biochemical parameters in pts (patients) with head and neck squamous cell carcinoma.

No of pts	SUVmax [g/mL]	SUVmean [g/mL]	Maximal Tumor Diameter CT [mm]	Maximal Tumor Diameter PET/MR [mm]	Tumor Volume PET/MR [cm^3]	Tumor Volume CT [cm^3]	No of mts Lymph Nodes in CT	No of mts Lymph Nodes in PET/MR	CRP [mg/L]	Glucose [mg/dL]
1	11.7	6.03	34	33	12.63	6.65	0	1	1.9	92
2	11.9	7.68	15	21	9.62	11.24	2≤	0	0.5	110
3	9.25	7.96	45	53	18.23	13.97	2≤	2≤	3.1	99
4	12.1	7.09	27	26	7.76	4.35	0	1	9.1	139
5	15.2	10.1	50	55	55.48	51.26	2≤	2≤	1.1	88
6	9.26	5.09	28	13	13.38	19.51	2≤	2≤	0.9	99
7	10.1	6.7	24	19	9.76	4.78	0	1	0.4	93
8	7.08	5.1	51	38	78.35	32.12	2≤	2≤	1.1	117
9	15.3	13.3	10	48	24.27	15.06	0	2≤	4.2	122
10	5.59	5.35	25	23	10.31	5.09	0	1	1.2	104
11	7.59	8.84	35	38	41.97	21.82	2≤	2≤	44.4	91
12	10	7.65	41	43	36.2	35.65	0	0	0.9	83
13	3.62	3.64	18	15	6.91	6.07	2≤	2≤	0.7	92
14	13.9	10.7	18	42	13.79	5.89	2≤	1	3.6	118
15	12.3	12.5	39	49	47.08	64.8	1	0	0.3	93
16	6.11	2.61	25	21	7.16	4.08	0	0	16	85
17	8.9	7.26	0	46	28.85	26.4	2≤	2≤	120.5	98
18	7.59	5.43	19	20	8.71	5.66	0	0	17.4	122
19	18.2	12.5	39	50	24.37	21.34	2≤	2≤	2.1	104
20	2.5	2.6	20	16	3.28	4.12	0	0	0.6	87
21	6.9	8.41	60	63	64.14	62.03	1	0	5.1	101

Statistical analysis was performed using Microsoft Excel (version 2019, Microsoft Corporation, Washington, DC, USA) and Statistica 10 (Statsoft Inc., Tulsa, OK, USA). The level of statistical significance was established at $p < 0.05$. The Spearman's correlation test was used to analyze correlations between SUVmax/SUVmean values and maximal tumor diameter determined with CT or PET/MRI, CT or PET/MRI tumor volume, Ki67 index, CRP concentration, glucose level. The correlations between SUVmax, SUVmean, maximal tumor diameter determined with CT or PET/MRI and p16, HPV, EBV presence were analyzed using the t test. Correlation analysis between CT or PET/MRI tumor volume, Ki67 index, CRP concentration and p16, HPV, EBV status was performed with the Mann–Whitney U test. Correlations between the number of metastatic lymph nodes determined with CT or PET/MRI and features such as SUV values, maximal tumor diameter and tumor volume determined with CT or PET/MRI, KI67 index were established with the Kruskal–Wallis test. The Ch2 test was used to analyze the relationship between the number of metastatic lymph nodes determined with CT or PET/MRI and the positivity of p16, HPV and EBV.

5. Conclusions

Hybrid PET/MRI imaging is useful in the preoperative staging of HNC patients. Compared with CT scanning, the outcomes obtained using this imaging modality are more consistent with histopathology results, the gold-standard technique in cancer diagnosis, in regard to T staging. This novel imaging tool also offers higher specificity, sensitivity, PPV and NPV of lymph node evaluation in comparison with CT scanning. Statistically important correlations between SUVmax and maximal tumor diameter as well as between SUV mean and tumor volume and maximal tumor diameter evaluated with PET/MRI were revealed in the present study, which suggests that these parameters may be useful in clinical practice. The presence of p16, HPV, EBV did not correlate with SUV values, geometrical parameters of the tumor or the number of metastatic lymph nodes. Further studies on a larger group of patients are required.

Author Contributions: N.S.-K.—conceptualization, data curation, formal analysis, investigation, methodology, project administration, resources, visualization, writing-original draft, writing—review and editing, E.S.—conceptualization, data curation, funding acquisition, investigation, methodology, project administration, supervision, writing-original draft, writing—review and editing, D.D.-P.—investigation, methodology, K.B.N.—data curation, investigation, methodology, M.L.—formal analysis, investigation, methodology, J.R.—investigation, methodology, project administration, supervision, visualization. All authors have read and agreed to the published version of the manuscript.

Acknowledgments: The authors would like to express their thanks for fruitful help for Dorota Jurgilewicz, Malgorzata Mojsak, Piotr Szumowski, Marcin Hladunski, from Laboratory of Molecular Imaging, Medical University of Bialystok, Poland.

References

1. Burela, N.; Soni, T.; Patni, N.; Bhagat, J.; Kumar, T.; Natarajan, T. A quantitative comparison of gross tumor volumes delineated on [18F]-FDG-PET/CT scan and contrast-enhanced computed tomography scan in locally advanced head and neck carcinoma treated with intensity modulated radiotherapy. *Adv. Mod. Oncol. Res.* **2017**, *3*, 143–151. [CrossRef]
2. Kim, S.G.; Friedman, K.; Patel, S.; Hagiwara, M. Potential role of PET/MRI for imaging metastatic lymph nodes in head and neck cancer. *Am. J. Roentgenol.* **2016**, *207*, 248–256. [CrossRef] [PubMed]
3. Szyszko, T.A.; Cook, G.J.R. PET/CT and PET/MRI in head and neck malignancy. *Clin. Radiol.* **2018**, *73*, 60–69. [CrossRef] [PubMed]
4. Goel, R.; Moore, W.; Sumer, B.; Khan, S.; Sher, D.; Subramaniam, R.M. Clinical practice in PET/CT for the management of head and neck squamous cell cancer. *Am. J. Roentgenol.* **2017**, *209*, 289–303. [CrossRef]

5. Zheng, E.; Khariwala, S.S. Do All Patients with Head and Neck Cancer Require a Positron Emission Tomography Scan at Diagnosis? *Laryngoscope* **2018**. [CrossRef]
6. Leclerc, M.; Lartigau, E.; Lacornerie, T.; Daisne, J.F.; Kramar, A.; Grégoire, V. Primary tumor delineation based on 18FDG PET for locally advanced head and neck cancer treated by chemo-radiotherapy. *Radiother. Oncol.* **2015**, *116*, 87–93. [CrossRef]
7. Ligtenberg, H.; Jager, E.A.; Caldas-Magalhaes, J.; Schakel, T.; Pameijer, F.A.; Kasperts, N.; Philippens, M.E. Modality-specific target definition for laryngeal and hypopharyngeal cancer on FDG-PET, CT and MRI. *Radiother. Oncol.* **2017**, *123*, 63–70. [CrossRef]
8. Tsujikawa, T.; Narita, N.; Kanno, M.; Takabayashi, T.; Fujieda, S.; Okazawa, H. Role of PET/MRI in oral cavity and oropharyngeal cancers based on the 8th edition of the AJCC cancer staging system: A pictorial essay. *Ann. Nucl. Med.* **2018**, *32*, 239–249. [CrossRef]
9. Differding, S.; Hanin, F.X.; Grégoire, V. PET imaging biomarkers in head and neck cancer. *Eur. J. Nucl. Med. Mol. Imaging* **2015**, *42*, 613–622. [CrossRef]
10. Huang, S.H.; Chien, C.Y.; Lin, W.C.; Fang, F.M.; Wang, P.W.; Lui, C.C.; Chang, C.C. A comparative study of fused FDG PET/MRI, PET/CT, MRI, and CT imaging for assessing surrounding tissue invasion of advanced buccal squamous cell carcinoma. *Clin. Nucl. Med.* **2011**, *36*, 518–525. [CrossRef]
11. Loeffelbein, D.J.; Souvatzoglou, M.; Wankerl, V.; Dinges, J.; Ritschl, L.M.; Mücke, T.; Beer, A.J. Diagnostic value of retrospective PET-MRI fusion in head-and-neck cancer. *BMC Cancer* **2014**, *14*, 846. [CrossRef] [PubMed]
12. Mehanna, H.; Jones, T.M.; Gregoire, V.; Ang, K.K. Oropharyngeal carcinoma related to human papillomavirus. *BMJ Br. Med. J.* **2010**, 340. [CrossRef] [PubMed]
13. Lydiatt, W.M.; Patel, S.G.; O'Sullivan, B.; Brandwein, M.S.; Ridge, J.A.; Migliacci, J.C.; Shah, J.P. Head and neck cancers—Major changes in the American Joint Committee on cancer eighth edition cancer staging manual. *CA Cancer J. Clin.* **2017**, *67*, 122–137. [CrossRef] [PubMed]
14. O'Sullivan, B.; Huang, S.H.; Su, J.; Garden, A.S.; Sturgis, E.M.; Dahlstrom, K.; Adelstein, D. Development and validation of a staging system for HPV-related oropharyngeal cancer by the International Collaboration on Oropharyngeal cancer Network for Staging (ICON-S): A multicentre cohort study. *Lancet Oncol.* **2016**, *17*, 440–451. [CrossRef]
15. Tahari, A.K.; Alluri, K.; Quon, H.; Koch, W.; Wahl, R.L.; Subramaniam, R.M. FDG PET/CT imaging of Oropharyngeal SCC: Characteristics of HPV positive and negative tumors. *Clin. Nucl. Med.* **2014**, *39*, 225–231. [CrossRef]
16. Sharma, S.J.; Wittekindt, C.; Knuth, J.; Steiner, D.; Wuerdemann, N.; Laur, M.; Klussmann, J.P. Intraindividual homogeneity of 18F-FDG PET/CT parameters in HPV-positive OPSCC. *Oral Oncol.* **2017**, *73*, 166–171. [CrossRef]
17. Nesteruk, M.; Lang, S.; Veit-Haibach, P.; Studer, G.; Stieb, S.; Glatz, S.; Guckenberger, M. Tumor stage, tumor site and HPV dependent correlation of perfusion CT parameters and [18F]-FDG uptake in head and neck squamous cell carcinoma. *Radiother. Oncol.* **2015**, *117*, 125–131. [CrossRef]
18. Kim, Y.I.; Cheon, G.J.; Kang, S.Y.; Paeng, J.C.; Kang, K.W.; Lee, D.S.; Chung, J.K. Prognostic value of simultaneous 18 F-FDG PET/MRI using a combination of metabolo-volumetric parameters and apparent diffusion coefficient in treated head and neck cancer. *EJNMMI Res.* **2018**, *8*, 2. [CrossRef]
19. Grégoire, V.; Ang, K.; Budach, W.; Grau, C.; Hamoir, M.; Langendijk, J.A.; Lee, A.; Le, Q.T.; Maingon, P.; Nutting, C.; et al. Delineation of the neck node levels for head and neck tumors: A 2013 update. DAHANCA, EORTC, HKNPCSG, NCIC CTG, NCRI, RTOG, TROG consensus guidelines. *Radiother. Oncol.* **2014**, *110*, 172–181. [CrossRef]
20. Schaarschmidt, B.M.; Heusch, P.; Buchbender, C.; Ruhlmann, M.; Bergmann, C.; Ruhlmann, V.; Schlamann, M.; Antoch, G.; Forsting, M.; Wetter, A. Locoregional tumour evaluation of squamous cell carcinoma in the head and neck area: A comparison between MRI, PET/CT and integrated PET/MRI. *Eur. J. Nucl. Med. Mol. Imaging* **2016**, *43*, 92–102. [CrossRef]
21. Chan, S.C.; Yeh, C.H.; Yen, T.C.; Ng, S.H.; Chang, J.T.; Lin, C.Y.; Yen-Ming, T.; Fan, K.H.; Huang, B.S.; Hsu, C.L.; et al. Clinical utility of simultaneous whole-body 18 F-FDG PET/MRI as a single-step imaging modality in the staging of primary nasopharyngeal carcinoma. *Eur. J. Nucl. Med. Mol. Imaging* **2018**, *45*, 1297–1308. [CrossRef] [PubMed]

22. Sekine, T.; de Galiza Barbosa, F.; Kuhn, F.P.; Burger, I.A.; Stolzmann, P.; Huber, G.F.; Kollias, S.S.; von Schulthess, G.K.; Veit-Haibach, P.; Huellner, M.W. PET+ MR versus PET/CT in the initial staging of head and neck cancer, using a trimodality PET/CT+ MR system. *Clin. Imaging* **2017**, *42*, 232–239. [CrossRef] [PubMed]
23. De Bondt, R.B.; Nelemans, P.J.; Hofman, P.A.; Casselman, J.W.; Kremer, B.; van Engelshoven, J.M.; Beets-Tan, R.G. Detection of lymph node metastases in head and neck cancer: A meta-analysis comparing US, USgFNAC, CT and MR imaging. *Eur. J. Radiol.* **2007**, *64*, 266–272. [CrossRef] [PubMed]
24. Altman, D.G.; Bland, J.M. Statistics Notes: Diagnostic tests 2: Predictive values. *BMJ* **1994**, *309*, 102. [CrossRef]
25. Torabi, M.; Aquino, S.L.; Harisinghani, M.G. Current concepts in lymph node imaging. *J. Nucl. Med.* **2004**, *45*, 1509–1518.
26. Platzek, I.; Beuthien-Baumann, B.; Schneider, M.; Gudziol, V.; Langner, J.; Schramm, G.; Laniado, M.; Kotzerke, J.; van den Hoff, J. PET/MRI in head and neck cancer: Initial experience. *Eur. J. Nucl. Med. Mol. Imaging* **2013**, *40*, 6–11. [CrossRef]
27. Geraldine, B.E.; Pyatigorskaya, N.; De Laroche, R.; Herve, G.; Zaslavsky, C.; Bertaux, M.; Giron, A.; Soret, M.; Bertolus, C.; Sahli-Amor, M.; et al. Diagnostic performance of 18F-FDG PET/MR in head and neck malignancies. *J. Nucl. Med.* **2017**, *58*, 280.
28. Grégoire, V.; Thorwarth, D.; Lee, J. Molecular imaging-guided radiotherapy for the treatment of head-and-neck squamous cell carcinoma: Does it fulfill the promises? *Semin. Radiat. Oncol.* **2018**, *28*, 35–45. [CrossRef]
29. Samołyk-Kogaczewska, N.; Sierko, E.; Zuzda, K.; Gugnacki, P.; Szumowski, P.; Mojsak, M.; Burzyńska-Śliwowska, J.; Wojtukiewicz, M.Z.; Szczecina, K.; Jurgilewicz, D.H. PET/MRI-guided GTV delineation during radiotherapy planning in patients with squamous cell carcinoma of the tongue. *Strahlenther. Onkol.* **2019**, *195*, 780–791. [CrossRef]
30. Kocher, M.R.; Sharma, A.; Garrett-Mayer, E.; Ravenel, J.G. Pretreatment 18F-Fluorodeoxyglucose Positron Emission Tomography Standardized Uptake Values and Tumor Size in Medically Inoperable Nonsmall Cell Lung Cancer Is Prognostic of Overall 2-Year Survival after Stereotactic Body Radiation Therapy. *J. Comput. Assist. Tomo.* **2018**, *42*, 146–150. [CrossRef]
31. Rutkowski, T. The role of tumor volume in radiotherapy of patients with head and neck cancer. *Radiat. Oncol.* **2014**, *9*, 23. [CrossRef] [PubMed]
32. Paul, A.G.; Heilbrun, L.K.; Smith, D.W.; Miller, S.R. Association of 18F-FDG-PET SUV and Tumor Size in Cervical Cancer. *Int. J. Radiat. Oncol.* **2018**, *102*, e632. [CrossRef]
33. Deng, S.M.; Zhang, W.; Zhang, B.; Chen, Y.Y.; Li, J.H.; Wu, Y.W. Correlation between the uptake of 18F-fluorodeoxyglucose (18F-FDG) and the expression of proliferation-associated antigen Ki-67 in cancer patients: A meta-analysis. *PLoS ONE* **2015**, *10*. [CrossRef]
34. Huang, H.; Xiao, F.; Han, X.; Zhong, L.; Zhong, H.; Xu, L.; Zhu, J.; Ni, B.; Liu, J.; Fang, Y.; et al. Correlation of pretreatment 18F-FDG uptake with clinicopathological factors and prognosis in patients with newly diagnosed diffuse large B-cell lymphoma. *Nucl. Med. Commun.* **2016**, *37*, 689–698. [CrossRef] [PubMed]
35. Surov, A.; Meyer, H.J.; Wienke, A. Associations between PET parameters and expression of Ki-67 in breast cancer. *Transl. Oncol.* **2019**, *12*, 375–380. [CrossRef] [PubMed]
36. Ucar, E.; Yalcin, H.; Kavvasoglu, G.H.; Ilhan, G. Correlations between the maximum standard uptake value of positron emission tomography/computed tomography and laboratory parameters before and after treatment in patients with lymphoma. *Chin. Med. J.* **2018**, *131*, 1776–1779. [CrossRef]
37. Eskian, M.; Alavi, A.; Khorasanizadeh, M.; Viglianti, B.L.; Jacobsson, H. Effect of blood glucose level on standardized uptake value (SUV) in 18 F-FDG PET-scan: A systematic review and meta-analysis of 20, 807 individual SUV measurements. *Eur. J. Nucl. Med. Mol. Imaging* **2019**, *46*, 224–237. [CrossRef]
38. Higashi, T.; Saga, T.; Nakamoto, Y.; Ishimori, T.; Fujimoto, K.; Doi, R.; Imamura, M.; Konishi, J. Diagnosis of pancreatic cancer using fluorine-18 fluorodeoxyglucose positron emission tomography (fdg pet)—Usefulness and limitations in "clinical reality". *Ann. Nucl. Med.* **2003**, *17*, 261–279. [CrossRef]
39. Westerterp, M.; Sloof, G.W.; Hoekstra, O.S.; ten Kate, F.J.; Meijer, G.A.; Reitsma, J.B.; Boellaard, R.; van Lanschot, J.J.; Molthoff, C.F. 18 FDG uptake in oesophageal adenocarcinoma: Linking biology and outcome. *J. Cancer Res. Clin.* **2008**, *134*, 227–236.
40. Fleming, J.C.; Woo, J.; Moutasim, K.; Mellone, M.; Frampton, S.J.; Mead, A.; Woelk, C.H. HPV, tumour metabolism and novel target identification in head and neck squamous cell carcinoma. *Br. J. Cancer* **2019**, *120*, 356–367. [CrossRef]

41. Han, M.; Lee, S.J.; Lee, D.; Kim, S.Y.; Choi, J.W. Correlation of human papilloma virus status with quantitative perfusion/diffusion/metabolic imaging parameters in the oral cavity and oropharyngeal squamous cell carcinoma: Comparison of primary tumour sites and metastatic lymph nodes. *Clin. Radiol.* **2018**, *73*, 757.e21–757.e27. [CrossRef]
42. Noij, D.P.; Martens, R.M.; Zwezerijnen, B.; Koopman, T.; de Bree, R.; Hoekstra, O.S.; Castelijns, J.A. Diagnostic value of diffusion-weighted imaging and 18F-FDG-PET/CT for the detection of unknown primary head and neck cancer in patients presenting with cervical metastasis. *Eur. J. Radiol.* **2018**, *107*, 20–25. [CrossRef]
43. Schouten, C.S.; Hakim, S.; Boellaard, R.; Bloemena, E.; Doornaert, P.A.; Witte, B.I.; de Bree, R. Interaction of quantitative 18F-FDG-PET-CT imaging parameters and human papillomavirus status in oropharyngeal squamous cell carcinoma. *Head Neck* **2016**, *38*, 529–535. [CrossRef] [PubMed]
44. Surov, A.; Meyer, H.J.; Höhn, A.K.; Winter, K.; Sabri, O.; Purz, S. Associations between [18 F] FDG-PET and complex histopathological parameters including tumor cell count and expression of KI 67, EGFR, VEGF, HIF-1α, and p53 in head and neck squamous cell carcinoma. *Mol. Imaging Biol.* **2019**, *21*, 368–374. [CrossRef] [PubMed]
45. Ahmedova, A.; Ozkaya, K.; Tambas, M.; Gezer, U.; Ozgur, E.; Sahin, D.; Altun, M. Is there a correlation between serum Epstein-Barr virus DNA level and tumor metabolic activity, TNM staging and tumor load in nasopharyngeal cancer patients? *J. Clin. Oncol.* **2017**, *35*, e17543. [CrossRef]
46. Alessi, A.; Lorenzoni, A.; Cavallo, A.; Padovano, B.; Iacovelli, N.A.; Bossi, P.; Alfieri, S.; Serafini, G.; Colombo, C.B.; Cicchetti, A.; et al. Role of pretreatment 18F-FDG PET/CT parameters in predicting outcome of non-endemic EBV DNA-related nasopharyngeal cancer (NPC) patients treated with IMRT and chemotherapy. *La Radiologia Medica* **2019**, *124*, 414–421. [CrossRef] [PubMed]
47. Rischin, D.; Young, R.J.; Fisher, R.; Fox, S.B.; Le, Q.T.; Peters, L.J.; Solomon, B.; Choi, J.; O'Sullivan, B.; Kenny, L.M.; et al. Prognostic significance of p16INK4A and human papillomavirus in patients with oropharyngeal cancer treated on TROG 02.02 phase III trial. *J. Clin. Oncol.* **2010**, *28*, 4142–4148. [CrossRef] [PubMed]
48. Chen, Q.Y.; Guo, S.Y.; Tang, L.Q.; Lu, T.Y.; Chen, B.L.; Zhong, Q.Y.; Liu, L.T. Combination of tumor volume and Epstein-Barr virus DNA improved prognostic stratification of stage II nasopharyngeal carcinoma in the intensity modulated radiotherapy era: A large-scale cohort study. *Cancer Res. Treat.* **2018**, *50*, 861–871. [CrossRef]
49. Lu, L.; Li, J.; Zhao, C.; Xue, W.; Han, F.; Tao, T.; Lu, T. Prognostic efficacy of combining tumor volume with Epstein-Barr virus DNA in patients treated with intensity-modulated radiotherapy for nasopharyngeal carcinoma. *Oral. Oncol.* **2016**, *60*, 18–24. [CrossRef]
50. Peng, L.; Yang, Y.; Guo, R.; Mao, Y.P.; Xu, C.; Chen, Y.P.; Tang, L.L. Relationship between pretreatment concentration of plasma Epstein-Barr virus DNA and tumor burden in nasopharyngeal carcinoma: An updated interpretation. *Cancer Med.* **2018**, *7*, 5988–5998. [CrossRef]
51. Zhong, Q.; Xiao, Z.Y.; Wu, R.R. The correlation of EBV in plasma and primary tumor volume of NPC. *J. Gannan Med Univ.* **2010**, *4*, 5–11.
52. Gletsou, E.; Papadas, T.A.; Baliou, E.; Tsiambas, E.; Ragos, V.; Armata, I.E.; Fotiades, P.P. HPV infection in oropharyngeal squamous cell carcinomas: Correlation with tumor size. *J. BUON* **2018**, *23*, 433–438. [PubMed]
53. Liang, S.B.; Deng, Y.M.; Zhang, N.; Lu, R.L.; Zhao, H.; Chen, H.Y.; Chen, Y. Prognostic significance of maximum primary tumor diameter in nasopharyngeal carcinoma. *BMC Cancer* **2013**, *13*, 260. [CrossRef] [PubMed]
54. Kågedal, Å.; Rydberg Millrud, C.; Häyry, V.; Kumlien Georén, S.; Lidegran, M.; Munck-Wikland, E.; Cardell, L.O. Oropharyngeal squamous cell carcinoma induces an innate systemic inflammation, affected by the size of the tumour and the lymph node spread. *Clin. Otolaryngol.* **2018**, *43*, 1117–1121. [CrossRef] [PubMed]
55. De Bree, R.; Takes, R.P.; Castelijns, J.A.; Medina, J.E.; Stoeckli, S.J.; Mancuso, A.A.; Hunt, J.L.; Rodrigo, J.P.; Triantafyllou, A.; Teymoortash, A.; et al. Advances in diagnostic modalities to detect occult lymph node metastases in head and neck squamous cell carcinoma. *Head Neck* **2015**, *37*, 1829–1839. [CrossRef] [PubMed]
56. Chen, C.; Chen, Z.; Cao, H.; Yan, J.; Wang, Z.; Le, H.; Weng, J.; Zhang, Y. A retrospective clinicopathological study of lung adenocarcinoma: Total tumor size can predict subtypes and lymph node involvement. *Clin. Imaging* **2018**, *47*, 52–56. [CrossRef] [PubMed]

57. Miller, T.R.; Grigsby, P.W. Measurement of tumor volume by PET to evaluate prognosis in patients with advanced cervical cancer treated by radiation therapy. *Int. J. Radiat. Oncol.* **2002**, *53*, 353–359. [CrossRef]
58. Ouyang, M.L.; Xia, H.W.; Xu, M.M.; Lin, J.; Wang, L.L.; Zheng, X.W.; Tang, K. Prediction of occult lymph node metastasis using SUV, volumetric parameters and intratumoral heterogeneity of the primary tumor in T1-2N0M0 lung cancer patients staged by PET/CT. *Ann. Nucl. Med.* **2019**, *33*, 671–680. [CrossRef]
59. Kim, S.J.; Pak, K.; Chang, S. Determination of regional lymph node status using 18F-FDG PET/CT parameters in oesophageal cancer patients: Comparison of SUV, volumetric parameters and intratumoral heterogeneity. *Br. J. Radiol.* **2016**, *89*. [CrossRef]
60. Raman, A.; Sen, N.; Ritz, E.; Fidler, M.J.; Revenaugh, P.; Stenson, K.; Al-khudari, S. Heterogeneity in the clinical presentation, diagnosis, and treatment initiation of p16-positive oropharyngeal cancer. *Am. J. Otol.* **2019**, *40*, 626–630. [CrossRef]
61. Mirzamani, N.; Salehian, P.; Farhadi, M.; Amin Tehran, E. Detection of EBV and HPV in nasopharyngeal carcinoma by in situ hybridization. *Exp. Mol. Pathol.* **2007**, *81*, 231–234. [CrossRef] [PubMed]
62. Niedobitek, G. Epstein-Barr virus infection in the pathogenesis of nasopharyngeal carcinoma. *Mol. Pathol.* **2000**, *53*, 248–254. [CrossRef] [PubMed]
63. Higuchi, T.; Fujimoto, Y.; Ozawa, H.; Bun, A.; Fukui, R.; Miyagawa, Y.; Imamura, M.; Kitajima, K.; Yamakado, K.; Miyoshi, Y. Significance of Metabolic Tumor Volume at Baseline and Reduction of Mean Standardized Uptake Value in 18 F-FDG-PET/CT Imaging for Predicting Pathological Complete Response in Breast Cancers Treated with Preoperative Chemotherapy. *Ann. Surg. Oncol.* **2019**, *26*, 2175–2183. [CrossRef] [PubMed]
64. Śnietura, M.; Jaworska, M.; Pigłowski, W.; Goraj-Zając, A.; Woźniak, G.; Lange, D. High-risk HPV DNA status and p16 (INK4a) expression as prognostic markers in patients with squamous cell cancer of oral cavity and oropharynx. *Pol. J. Pathol.* **2010**, *61*, 133–139. [PubMed]
65. Begum, S.; Gillison, M.L.; Ansari-Lari, M.A.; Shah, K.; Westra, W.H. Detection of human papillomavirus in cervical lymph nodes: A highly effective strategy for localizing site of tumor origin. *Clin. Cancer Res.* **2003**, *9*, 6469–6475. [PubMed]
66. Guzińska-Ustymowicz, K.; Pryczynicz, A.; Kemona, A.; Czyżewska, J. Correlation between proliferation markers: PCNA, Ki-67, MCM-2 and antiapoptotic protein Bcl-2 in colorectal cancer. *Anticancer Res.* **2009**, *29*, 3049–3052.
67. Altman, D.G.; Bland, J.M. Diagnostic tests. 1: Sensitivity and specificity. *BMJ Br. Med. J.* **1994**, *308*, 1552. [CrossRef]

6

Ovarian Cancer Incidence Corrected for Oophorectomy

Lauren A. Baldwin [1,*], Quan Chen [2], Thomas C. Tucker [3], Connie G. White [4], Robert N. Ore [1] and Bin Huang [2]

1. The Division of Gynecologic Oncology, Department of Obstetrics and Gynecology, The University of Kentucky College of Medicine, 800 Rose Street, 330 Whitney-Hendrickson Building, Lexington, KY 40536, USA; robert.ore@uky.edu
2. Division of Cancer Biostatistics, College of Public Health & Biostatistics Shared Resource Facility, Markey Cancer Center, University of Kentucky, Lexington, KY 40506, USA; quan.chen@uky.edu (Q.C.); bhuang@kcr.uky.edu (B.H.)
3. Department of Epidemiology, College of Public Health & Kentucky Cancer Registry, Markey Cancer Center, University of Kentucky, Lexington, KY 40506, USA; tct@kcr.uky.edu
4. Kentucky Department for Public Health, Frankfort, KY 40601, USA; Connie.White@ky.gov

* Correspondence: labald1@uky.edu

Academic Editor: Tanya W. Moseley

Abstract: Current reported incidence rates for ovarian cancer may significantly underestimate the true rate because of the inclusion of women in the calculations who are not at risk for ovarian cancer due to prior benign salpingo-oophorectomy (SO). We have considered prior SO to more realistically estimate risk for ovarian cancer. Kentucky Health Claims Data, International Classification of Disease 9 (ICD-9) codes, Current Procedure Terminology (CPT) codes, and Kentucky Behavioral Risk Factor Surveillance System (BRFSS) Data were used to identify women who have undergone SO in Kentucky, and these women were removed from the at-risk pool in order to re-assess incidence rates to more accurately represent ovarian cancer risk. The protective effect of SO on the population was determined on an annual basis for ages 5–80+ using data from the years 2009–2013. The corrected age-adjusted rates of ovarian cancer that considered SO ranged from 33% to 67% higher than age-adjusted rates from the standard population. Correction of incidence rates for ovarian cancer by accounting for women with prior SO gives a better understanding of risk for this disease faced by women. The rates of ovarian cancer were substantially higher when SO was taken into consideration than estimates from the standard population.

Keywords: ovarian cancer; prevalence; incidence; oophorectomy; screening

1. Introduction

Cancer incidence rates are calculated by dividing new primary cancer cases of a disease by the population at risk in the same time period adjusted by the US standard population [1]. This assessment has great importance clinically, especially for gynecologic oncology with regard to training a sufficient number of physician specialists. Cancer incidence rates help physicians and researchers assess risk levels, which can be used for public health and individual patient education, to prioritize prevention and research efforts, and to guide assessment of the cost and efficacy of cancer screening. Thus, the accuracy of this risk assessment is very important.

There is an inherent problem in the incidence calculation for some malignancies due to the inclusion of patients in the denominator who are not at risk for the disease [2]. In gynecologic oncology, this has been most thoroughly evaluated in the case of endometrial cancer and hysterectomy. Many women will undergo hysterectomy in their lifetime for a variety of benign conditions [3,4]. These women are not at risk for developing endometrial cancer after uterine removal and should not be included in the population at risk for incidence rate calculation. There have been multiple publications that have evaluated methods of correcting risk calculations for endometrial cancer. In 2012, Siegel et al. reported on age-adjusted, hysterectomy-corrected uterine cancer rates stratified by race and geography and found that failure to adjust rates for hysterectomy leads to distortion of racial and geographic patterns and underestimates disease burden [5].

There is less guidance in the literature concerning the impact of oophorectomy rates on ovarian cancer incidence. Many women have salpingo-oophorectomy (SO) performed alone due to benign ovarian disease, or have SO performed at the time of hysterectomy for benign conditions. There has been new evidence linking the origin of serous ovarian cancer to the fimbriated end of the fallopian tube [6–17]. During adnexal surgeries, the tube is usually removed concurrently with the ovary. Whether the pathogenesis for the most common type of ovarian cancer truly arises from the distal tube or the ovary itself, those who have undergone SO should have drastically reduced risk of this type of malignancy. This reduction has been demonstrated in high risk women with Breast Cancer Susceptibility (*BRCA*) mutations who undergo risk-reducing salpingo-oophorectomy and have dramatically lower risk of ovarian malignancy [16–19].

The current reported incidence of ovarian cancer from 2005–2009 is 12.7 per 100,000 women [20]. Incidence rates are higher in whites and the average age at diagnosis is 63 [20]. Lifetime risk of developing ovarian cancer in the United States is 1.4% [20]. In 2016, 22,280 new cases were expected and 14,240 deaths anticipated from this disease [21]. Ovarian cancer is the 5th leading cause of death from malignancy in women in this country due to the fact that the majority of cases are diagnosed at an advanced stage. Research into prevention and screening for ovarian cancer is hampered by this low prevalence, which negatively affects accurately estimating the positive predictive value for these tests. We hypothesize that when incidence rates are corrected for prior SO, incidence of this disease will be higher than in commonly reported statistics which currently underestimate the risk of ovarian cancer for women whose ovaries and/or tubes remain intact.

2. Materials and Methods

2.1. Cancer Incidence Data

To calculate the cancer incidence rates, the most recent five-year ovary cancer cases diagnosed in years 2009–2013 from the Kentucky Cancer Registry (KCR) were extracted. Ovary cancer cases were defined as ICD-O-3 site codes C569 excluding ICD-O-3 histology codes 9050–9055, 9140, 9590–9992. Only invasive cancer cases were included for the analysis.

The KCR is a population-based registry, and has been awarded the highest level of certification by the North American Association of Central Cancer Registries for an objective evaluation of completeness, accuracy, and timeliness every year since 1997. The KCR is part of both the CDC National Program of Cancer Registries and the NCI Surveillance, Epidemiology, and End Results (SEER) program, which are considered among the most accurate and complete population-based cancer registries in the world. The KCR also links its database annually with the National Death Index (NDI) to capture the most accurate survival information. No new data was collected from subjects specifically for this study and no contact with any patients was required. All data was previously de-identified.

2.2. Kentucky Health Claims Data (KHCD)

In order to correctly calculate the age-adjusted rates for ovary cancer incidence, the underlying risk population needs to be modified to reflect the fact that women who had SO will have minimal risk of having ovarian cancer. To estimate the prevalence of women who had prior SO for years 2009–2013 in Kentucky, the Kentucky health claims data (KHCD) 2000–2014 data sets were acquired from the Office of Health Policy in the Kentucky Cabinet for Health and Family Services (KCHFS).

The KHCD data include hospital discharge reports from all Kentucky hospitals, Medicare provider-based entities and ambulatory facilities (http://lrc.ky.gov/KAR/900/007/030.htm). The data include in-patient and out-patient files containing de-identified individual records. Key elements, such as ICD-9 procedure codes, CPT codes, and demographics are included in the files. Age is presented in the format of age groups.

2.3. Kentucky Behavioral Risk Factor Surveillance System (BRFSS) Data

The Behavioral Risk Factor Surveillance System (BRFSS) data is the annual telephone survey that collects state data related to health risk behavior, chronic health conditions, and use of preventive services for all 50 states, the District of Columbia, and three territories in the U.S (https://www.cdc.gov/brfss/). For women aged 18 and older, responses to the question "Have you had a hysterectomy?" are included. The data related to this question was used to estimate the prevalence of prior hysterectomy by age group. Since the hysterectomy question was presented every other year, the Kentucky BRFSS data 2008–2012 was acquired from the KCHFS to match the ovary cancer incidence data 2009–2013.

2.4. Estimating Oophorectomy Prevalence

To estimate the prevalence of prior SO for Kentucky women in 2009–2013, two approaches were used. The first method estimated the full SO prevalence rates directly from the KHCD data and the second method estimated the SO prevalence rates based on both BRFSS data and KHCD data.

In the first method, SO cases were identified by ICD-9 procedure codes and CPT codes from the KHCD data for the years 2000–2014. Since the KHCD data in 2000–2003 did not include age or CPT codes and 2014 data were beyond the study period, only data for years 2004–2013 were used for the data analysis. The combined counts of SO cases by year and age group from both in-patient and out-patient files were considered as the total SO incidence. The age groups in KHCD data were categorized as 0, 1–5, 6–10, ... , 76–80, 81+ years. Statistical approaches to estimating prevalence from incidence data commonly involves mortality and survival data, and can be either parametric or non-parametric [22–25]. Counting Method, a non-parametric approach, was used to estimate prevalence of prior SO based on the SO incidence data from the KHCD [23]. This approach counts cases of 'still alive' individuals on the desired prevalence date while making adjustment based on the estimates of cases lost to follow-up. For example, the number of prevalence case in age i and calendar year j was estimated as

$$N_{ij} = \int_0^i I(t)S(t, i-t)dt$$

where $I(t)$ is the number of incidence in age t, and $S(t, i-t)$ is the survival probability from all causes from age t to $i-t$. Since the KHCD data do not include survival and mortality data, the US 2010 female life tables were used to estimate the survival probabilities from all causes in the specific years and age groups. Bridged life tables to match the age group defined in the KHCD were calculated from the complete US 2010 female life table [26]. Because no SO incidence data by age group were available prior to 2004, it was assumed that the incidence data prior to 2004 were same as in the average of 2004–2013. To understand the impact of the assumption, the same calculation was also done while assuming incidence data prior to 2004 was the same as in the year 2004 and the year 2012, as the highest count of prevalence was identified in year 2004 and the lowest in 2012. To reflect the fact that the US life expectancies have increased over time and that women with oophorectomy had lower life expectancies than the general population [27], the probability of survival estimates were lowered from values in the US life tables by 0.5% when calculating the complete prevalence rates for prior SO.

To validate the prevalence estimates from the first method, we also used the BRFSS data to estimate the prevalence rates. In previous published studies, prevalence rates of prior SO were estimated by multiplying the prevalence rates of hysterectomy from the BRFSS data by the proportion of hysterectomy incidences with bilateral oophorectomy [2]. Similarly, we calculated the ratio of SO vs.

hysterectomy by age group from the KHCD data for years 2004–2013 and the weighted prevalence rates of prior hysterectomy by age group for those aged 20+ from the BRFSS data for 2008, 2010 and 2012. The prior SO prevalence estimates by age groups were the product of the ratio of SO vs. hysterectomy and the prevalence of prior hysterectomy from the BFRSS data.

2.5. Age-Adjusted Incidence Rates for Ovary Cancer

All age-adjusted rates were calculated based on the standard 2000 US population. To examine how the different formats of age groups in the background population impact age-adjusted rates, the traditional age-adjusted rates based on the 19 age groups in the standard Kentucky population were calculated along with the traditional age-adjusted rates based on the 18 age groups defined in the KHCD data. To calculate the corrected age-adjusted rates for ovary cancer, the standard Kentucky population data were corrected by deducting the number of women with SO derived through the prevalence estimates from the two approaches previously discussed.

All analyses were done using SAS Statistical software version 9.4. SAS (SAS Institute, Cary, NC, USA) was also used to develop programs to calculate the complete prevalence rates from the KHCD data. Statistical tests were two sided with a p-value ≤ 0.05 used to identify statistical significance.

3. Results

There was a total of 81,359 SO cases identified from the KHDC data during 2004–2013 (Table 1). The highest frequencies were found in the age groups 41–45 and 46–50. Very few cases were found in women with ages younger than 20 or ages older than 80. The number of SO cases from the inpatient files had dropped steadily over the study period and the number of cases from the outpatient files had increased. The overall SO cases had consistently dropped since 2003 (Figure 1).

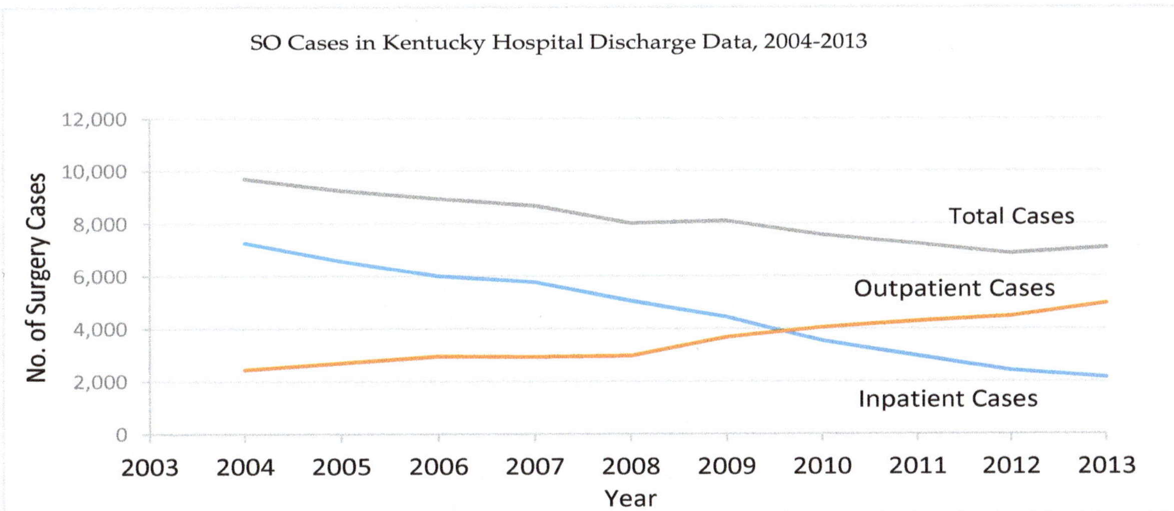

Figure 1. Trend of salpingo-oophorectomy (SO) cases from the Kentucky Hospital Discharge Data, 2004–2013.

Using the Counting Method, estimates of annual prevalence counts and rates by age group for the years 2009 to 2013 were calculated from the KHCD. Only results from the years 2009 and 2013 based on the assumption that SO incidences prior 2004 are same as the average in 2004–2013 are shown in Table 2. The results based on the assumptions that SO incidences prior 2004 are same as in 2004 or 2012 can be found in Tables S1 and S2. The prevalence rates increased by age and peaked at the oldest age groups of 76–80 and 81+. Because of the decreasing trend of SO cases, the prevalence rates had dropped from year 2009 to 2013. For example, the rates dropped from 27.4% to 24.4% in the age group 61–65 and from 42.1% to 38.1% in the age group 71–75 (Table 2).

Table 1. Salpingo-oophorectomy (SO) cases in Kentucky Hospital Discharge Data by age group, 2004–2013.

Year	Age Group																		
	0	1–5	6–10	11–15	16–20	21–25	26–30	31–35	36–40	41–45	46–50	51–55	56–60	61–65	66–70	71–75	76–80	81 and over	Total
2004	1	1	0	6	24	179	561	966	1482	2077	1919	987	445	356	265	202	142	79	9692
2005	0	1	1	7	24	191	542	887	1342	1999	1874	935	501	323	242	179	121	80	9249
2006	0	0	0	6	24	184	536	954	1308	1798	1662	894	500	365	277	201	142	87	8938
2007	1	0	1	5	31	193	500	833	1299	1669	1625	923	574	371	233	200	119	96	8673
2008	0	0	1	6	26	172	462	769	1119	1549	1512	832	486	382	306	179	124	86	8011
2009	1	2	0	8	38	147	500	771	1123	1530	1509	851	500	436	291	182	119	89	8097
2010	0	0	0	10	32	162	454	783	1075	1327	1373	828	479	384	265	198	112	75	7557
2011	2	1	2	12	40	155	411	764	1008	1241	1288	777	473	416	310	182	72	67	7221
2012	0	0	0	6	31	130	363	699	941	1185	1205	781	488	391	274	191	94	72	6851
2013	0	0	0	9	27	122	366	726	1031	1256	1188	748	518	425	307	186	103	63	7075
Total	5	5	5	75	297	1635	4695	8152	11,728	15,631	15,155	8556	4964	3849	2770	1900	1148	794	81,364

Table 2. Estimated SO Prevalence in Kentucky for year 2009 and 2013, by age groups *.

Age Group	Prob. of Survival	2009			2013		
		Population	Prevalence Count	Prevalence Rate	Population	Prevalence Count	Prevalence Rate
0	0.989	27,302	1.0	0.000	26,905	0.0	0.000
1–5	0.995	138,333	2.2	0.000	135,862	1.0	0.000
6–10	0.995	137,647	4.8	0.000	138,692	3.8	0.000
11–15	0.995	137,317	23.2	0.000	139,204	32.4	0.000
16–20	0.995	146,960	128.7	0.001	138,987	134.5	0.001
21–25	0.995	139,412	689.7	0.005	154,076	596.8	0.004
26–30	0.994	143,447	2624.1	0.018	137,250	2201.0	0.016
31–35	0.994	135,456	6206.3	0.046	142,561	5680.1	0.040
36–40	0.994	145,489	11,649.2	0.080	135,750	10,662.2	0.079
41–45	0.993	150,939	19,138.6	0.127	146,947	17,331.1	0.118
46–50	0.992	164,356	27,186.7	0.165	154,584	25,180.5	0.163
51–55	0.991	159,697	31,613.2	0.198	163,369	31,226.4	0.191
56–60	0.989	142,234	32,472.1	0.228	153,709	33,146.2	0.216
61–65	0.987	118,111	32,339.0	0.274	134,958	32,887.2	0.244
66–70	0.982	92,015	31,612.5	0.344	106,051	31,852.8	0.300
71–75	0.974	71,219	30,014.6	0.421	78,893	30,093.7	0.381
76–80	0.960	58,333	27,272.4	0.468	58,703	27,192.7	0.463
81+	0.911	84,869	39,805.1	0.469	87,494	39,812.0	0.455

* Assume SO incidence prior 2004 same as the average of incidence between years 2004–2013.

In Table 3, hysterectomy prevalence rates by age group were calculated from the BRFSS data for 2008, 2010, and 2012. The highest rates appeared in the age group 76–80. Ratios of SO vs. hysterectomy from the KHCD data varied from 65% to 103% by age group. The prior SO prevalence rates modified from the hysterectomy rates from the BRFSS data peaked in the age group 66–70 (50.7%) and were considerably smaller in the age group 81+ (42.5%) compared to the prevalence rates from the Counting Method.

Table 3. Estimated hysterectomy and oophorectomy prevalence based on the Kentucky BRFSS data and discharge data.

Age Group	Hysterectomy Prevalence Rate by BRFSS ^	Ratio of SO vs. Hysterectomy *	SO Prevalence Rate by BRFSS
21–25	0.000	0.902	0.000
26–30	0.024	0.723	0.018
31–35	0.076	0.665	0.051
36–40	0.120	0.649	0.078
41–45	0.196	0.719	0.141
46–50	0.256	0.879	0.225
51–55	0.379	1.010	0.383
56–60	0.415	1.033	0.429
61–65	0.461	1.021	0.471
66–70	0.513	0.988	0.507
71–75	0.517	0.963	0.498
76–80	0.532	0.900	0.479
81+	0.512	0.829	0.425

^ Estimated hysterectomy prevalence based on the KY BRFSS data, 2008–2012; * Ratio of SO vs. hysterectomy in Kentucky discharge data from year 2004 to 2013.

A total of 1403 invasive ovary cancer cases for years 2009–2013 were extracted from the KCR database. The age-adjusted rates from the standard Kentucky population show the rates 10.7 per 100,000 (95% Confidence Interval (CI) 10.2–11.3) for all ages (Table 4). To match the age groups defined in the KHCD data, the age adjusted rates based on the standard Kentucky population with modified age groups were also calculated. The corrected age-adjusted rates from adjusting the population under risk based on the prevalence estimates of prior SO from the KHCD data were 15.5 (95% CI 14.7–16.3) per 100,000 assuming SO incidences prior 2004 were the same as the average of the incidence in the years 2004–2013, 16.9 (95% CI 16.0–17.8) per 100,000 assuming the SO incidences prior to 2004 were the same as in 2004 (highest incidence), and 14.3 (95% CI 13.6–15.1) per 100,000 assuming the SO incidences prior to 2004 were the same as in 2012 (lowest incidence). The corrected age-adjusted rate from the BRFSS prevalence estimates of SO was 17.7 (95% CI 16.8–18.7), which is higher than the highest estimates from the KHCD data (16.9 per 100,000). Overall, risk population adjusted SO age-adjusted rates ranged from 33% to 65% higher than the rates from the standard population. We also included the age-specific rates for ovary cancer by various approaches in Table S3.

Table 4. Age adjusted rates for invasive ovary cancer in Kentucky, 2009–2013.

Type of Population Under Risk	All Ages				
	Population under Risk	*N*	Adj Rate	95% CI	
Standard Population ^	11,083,781	1403	10.73	10.16	11.32
Standard Population with Modified Age Group *	11,083,781	1403	10.73	10.17	11.32
Modified Population based on KCHD-Assumption 1 ~	9,630,865	1403	15.47	14.65	16.32
Modified Population based on KCHD-Assumption 2 ~	9,414,282	1403	16.88	15.98	17.82
Modified Population based on KCHD-Assumption 3 ~	9,847,449	1403	14.34	13.58	15.12
Modified Population based on BRFS †	9,009,436	1387	17.72	16.78	18.69

^ The standard 19 population age groups, 0, 1–4, 5–9, . . . , 80–84, 85+; * Use the 18 age groups in the hospital discharge data, 0, 1–5, 6–10, . . . , 76–80, 81+; ~Adjusted the standard population based on the prevalence rates from the Kentucky Health Claims Data; Assumption 1: Assume incidence prior to2004 same as the average in year 2004–2013; Assumption 2: Assume incidence prior to 2004 same as the average in year 2004; Assumption 3: Assume incidence prior to 2004 same as the average in year 2012; † Adjusted the standard population based on the prevalence rates from BRFSS data.

4. Discussion

In the efforts reported here, the rates of ovarian cancer were 33% to 65% higher when prior SO was taken into consideration than estimates from the standard population. Due to the limitation of data availability, the risk-population adjusted prior SO rates have rarely been calculated previously. In the current study, we used the KHCD data and the Counting Method, a modern statistical approach, to estimate the prior SO prevalence rates based on various assumptions and the risk-population adjusted SO rates. We also estimated the SO rates using estimated SO prevalence rates from the BRFSS data. The prevalence rates of prior SO from the Counting Method and the BRFSS data are different because of various assumptions and different data sources, hence leading to the variation of the risk-population adjusted SO rates. The results demonstrate the challenge to correctly estimate the rates because of the data limitations.

Compared to previous published studies with only one type of estimate [2], our study is able to provide a range of estimates that gives a more comprehensive view of the estimates. It is possible that the 0.5% survival deduction of probability of annul survival from the standard US life table was too harsh and caused the lower estimates of SO prevalence rates compared to the estimates from the BRFSS data. Using the ratio of SO vs. hysterectomy from the KHCD data to estimate SO prevalence rates from the BRFSS was likely biased as the ratio was based on incidence data, not prevalence data.

Ovarian cancer remains the deadliest gynecologic malignancy in the United States, being the 5th most common cause of cancer death in women. Over 14,000 deaths from ovarian cancer are expected for the US in 2016 [20]. Despite advances in operative care and chemotherapy, including the recent use of targeted agents for this disease, overall survival remains poor [20,28–30]. While ongoing research efforts continue to search for better treatments with which to combat this disease, another approach to improve survival is through screening and earlier detection of disease. The majority of ovarian cancer cases are diagnosed at advanced stage prior to the onset of symptoms. Pelvic exam has been shown to have limited value in detecting ovarian abnormalities, especially in postmenopausal and obese women [31]. Only 15% of cases are confined to the ovary at the time of diagnosis [32]. However, survival is much improved for women who are diagnosed at an early stage [26]. Therefore, efforts to increase the detection of early stage disease have a potential to greatly impact survival. Estimates that reveal the true risk of ovarian cancer will support efforts to screen for early stage disease.

Screening for malignancy has been highly effective for other common malignancies such as breast and cervix cancers [33,34]. Ovarian cancer meets criteria as a disease that could benefit from effective screening since it is the 5th leading cause of cancer mortality in women with proven improved survival when diagnosed at an earlier stage [20,26]. Screening has been studied in ovarian cancer, most commonly with serum Ca125 levels and transvaginal ultrasound (TVUS) or a combination of the two [35,36]. There have been four major trials that have evaluated ovarian cancer screening. The first of these is the prostate, lung, colorectal, and ovarian (PLCO) trial, which showed no benefit to screening [37]. There was a multicenter prospective randomized trial in Japan that compared screening with pelvic exam, serum Ca125, and ultrasound to routine care and saw an increase in the rate of optimal debulking in the screen detected cancers [38]. Optimal debulking has a known association with improved survival in ovarian cancer [39]. The University of Kentucky Ovarian Cancer Screening Trial (UKOCST) has been in progress since 1987 [40,41]. Over 45,000 women have been screened to date with TVUS. Detection of 47 ovarian cancers has been reported by the UKOCST and these women have improved five-year survival and are more likely to be early stage than women with clinically detected cancers [29,34,42]. Most recently, the results of the UKCTOCS randomized trial were published in the Lancet and have shown a survival benefit for screening [30].

Taken together, the available data from these four trials suggests screening works to detect disease at an earlier stage, which leads to improved survival. However, one of the most common criticisms of screening and the studies that have evaluated it is the lower positive predictive values, which are likely driven by the lower prevalence of this disease. Statistical calculations for predictive values vary greatly depending on the prevalence of the disease being studied, unlike sensitivity and specificity of a test, which remain constant. Thus, a test with inherently good sensitivity and specificity can be brought to improved predictive ability by narrowing the screening population to a high-risk group for which the prevalence is high.

One way to narrow threat risk population for ovarian cancer is by focusing on ages at which incidence is high. This has been commonly applied in previous screening trials and the results of the work reported here confirm the importance of age. In the present study, ovarian cancer incidence is highest for women over age 75, while the rate of hysterectomy peaks at age 65. Age continues to be one of the most important risk factors for ovarian cancer.

Given the importance of correct incidence to predictive calculations for screening programs and epidemiologic risk assessment, an accurate calculation of incidence is critical. An accurate assessment of risk is more easily determined in some diseases than others. If all subjects are at risk, then the calculation is a straight forward division of those diagnosed with disease by those at risk. This is not so clear in all diseases, however. For example, surgical interventions for unrelated problems can reduce the at-risk pool for certain disease sites. This has been demonstrated in the literature regarding endometrial cancer [5,43]. Correcting risk rates for endometrial cancer involves reducing threat risk pool (or denominator of the calculation) by removing those women who have undergone prior hysterectomy for a benign condition. Ignoring hysterectomy underestimates the risk for women who have not undergone that procedure and has also been shown to distort data regarding the distribution of disease [44]. Hysterectomy has recently been declining in nationwide statistics for the US, but remains one of the most common procedures performed in this country today, which alters the epidemiology significantly for uterine derived cancer risk [38]. Approximately 600,000 hysterectomies are performed each year in the United States, and around a third of all women have had the procedure by the time they turn 60 [45–47].

Salpingo-oophorectomy (SO) is even more difficult to quantify than hysterectomy. Many women elect to have their ovaries and tubes removed at the time of a hysterectomy that is performed for a variety of reasons related to primary uterine pathologies. Additionally, many women undergo bilateral SO either separate from a hysterectomy or at some time after a hysterectomy has been performed for a wide variety of primary ovarian or other conditions, many of which are benign. These include endometriosis, non-cancerous ovarian cysts or masses, risk reduction for genetic conditions, and for hormone reduction in breast cancer patients. The overall trend for SO in the US has been on the decline [48]. This decline coincides with the similar decline in hysterectomy rate. This decline may also be a result of data showing that surgical menopause prior to age 50 in women who never used estrogen is associated with increased all causes mortality [49]. Despite this, the rates of SO remain significant [42].

Given the robust number of women who have undergone SO, risk of ovarian cancer is greatly reduced for these women and importantly alters the epidemiology of risk for malignancy at this site on a population level. There are some important caveats to this reduction. Serous peritoneal cancers behave nearly identically to ovarian cancer and the risk for these cancers is unlikely to be altered by SO [50]. It should be noted that peritoneal cancer is quite rare. The protective effect of SO is illustrated in high risk women who have undergone prophylactic SO for BRCA mutation, and have achieved a drastically reduced risk of serous malignancy [16–19]. In one study, the relative risk of ovarian, fallopian tube or peritoneal carcinoma in women with known BRCA mutations after risk reducing bilateral SO was 0.04 (95% CI 0.01–0.16) [18]. Recent literature supports two separate types of ovarian malignancy, with separate pathogenesis [6–17]. Type 1 tumors are generally considered low grade malignancies that arise from the epithelium of the ovaries. Type 2 cancers generally include high grade serous malignancies that are felt to arise from the distal, fimbriated end of the fallopian tube. The fallopian tube is generally removed with the ipsilateral ovary in most procedures that are performed—few indications, if any, would preserve the tube if the ovary is being removed. Thus, protection from Type 2 ovarian malignancy is gained from ovarian removal in most cases since the tube is removed concomitantly (i.e., a salpingo-oophorectomy is typically performed rather than an oophorectomy alone).

An additional consideration is that there is a rising trend in bilateral salpingectomy rather than bilateral salpingo-oophorectomy, which allows ovarian preservation while still potentially reducing cancer risks [42]. The degree to which this procedure is as protective as SO has yet to be determined. The current study takes into account women having SO but not salpingectomy alone. An argument can be made to include these patients for future studies, which has the potential to further correct the underestimation of the prevalence of ovarian cancer for women who retain all portions of their adnexa.

Overall, the SO rate nationally has been reported to be declining. However, it is still common for women to undergo this procedure and greater than 40% of women still undergo bilateral SO at the time of hysterectomy [42,51]. This significant rate needs to be taken into account for estimating accurate ovarian cancer incidence. Failing to recognize and account for the population of women no longer at risk underestimates the incidence for the rest of the population. This was the driving motivation for the current study and the results confirm that incidence rates need to take surgical procedures into account. Incidence is certainly higher by all methods used for calculation in this study once SO was taken into account. This was true both with overall incidence across ages, as well as age-adjusted groups.

There is inherent difficulty in establishing the overall risk associated with SO. Prior studies have shown an overall mortality disadvantage for women who undergo premenopausal oophorectomy—prior to age 50—and never used estrogen therapy [43]. This decrease in lifespan may be attributed to changes in cardiovascular health and other important roles provided through the hormonal functions of the ovary. How this risk quantitatively translates to changes in expected lifespan on an annual statistical level is unclear. This study estimated decreased survival of 0.5% annually for women who had undergone premenopausal SO. However, these are estimates and the true annual change in expected survival is unknown. Even taking this into account though, all calculations still show that incidence is underestimated if SO is not taken into account when evaluating ovarian cancer.

The strengths of this study include the use of population level data and novel statistical evaluation to correct risk assessments in an important way for women with regard to ovarian cancer. A couple of limitations are worth noting. Most notably, this study is limited by the dependence on CPT and ICD codes for diagnosis. Actual operative reports or pathology reports were not available for confirmation of procedure performed. This introduces the possibility of inappropriate coding leading to incorrect inclusion (or exclusion) of patients in the analysis. In addition, newer ICD codes are more specific in that bilateral procedures are noted and were isolated for inclusion. This is important as unilateral procedures would not be expected to confer the same protection against ovarian cancer as the remaining ovary and/or tube could lead to a malignancy. Not all CPT codes separate unilateral from bilateral procedures and thus there is some uncertainty on the extent of adnexal removal with patients coded this way. Also, some hysterectomy codes are nonspecific as to inclusion of adnexal removal or not. Most notably, abdominal hysterectomy CPT codes can include patient "with or without" adnexal removal. Thus, using these codes can contribute uncertainty to the study as the true proportion of patient with adnexal removal with hysterectomy is not indicated by the code. About 30% of the procedures included in this study came from these questionable codes and the estimates for SO prevalence are likely over estimated because of their inclusion. Future studies can address these uncertainties by verifying procedures performed by complete chart review. This technique is time consuming and would limit the number of patients able to be studied, but is important for refining the exact risk estimates. The advancement of electronic medical records and more specific ICD coding will make this kind of confirmation more feasible in the future.

Additionally, because the KHCD data prior to 2004 are not available, the SO rates prior to 2004 were based on assumptions. This will certainly generate biases for the estimates. Although this study requires a range of assumptions, it is reasonable to assume the true estimate is captured within the variation of the estimates. There are no survival data available in the KHCD data, hence the 2010 US life table estimates with a 0.5% deduction were used to estimate the alive SO cases for specific prevalence date and age groups. How much bias is introduced and in which direction this bias goes is unknown. With increasing availability and reliability of health claims data, this approach will likely provide more accurate estimates in the future. The BRFSS data are limited by sampling biases, recall biases, and missing data. Overall, although we cannot provide specific rates for the SO estimates, we can conclude that the corrected rates of ovarian cancer were substantially higher when SO was taken into consideration than estimates from the standard population.

Finally, this study should be expanded to a broader national population as there may be important differences between the population in Kentucky versus other parts of the nation.

In conclusion, this study presents an important concept for correcting the underestimation of ovarian cancer risk for women who retain their ovaries and tubes. This correction has critical implications for the calculation of screening program performance in terms of predictive value. It is also critically important to refine the epidemiological assessment of the distribution of this disease and the populations at risk so that the highest risk groups can be identified, which will improve screening programs ability to reduce mortality from ovarian cancer while reducing harm from unnecessary interventions.

Acknowledgments: The University of Kentucky Biostatistics and Bioinformatics Shared Resource Facility was utilized for this project which are supported by the Markey Cancer Center (P30CA177558).

Author Contributions: Lauren Baldwin contributed to data summary review, abstract composition and manuscript construction; Lauren Baldwin, Bin Huang, Tom C. Tucker and Robert N. Ore contributed to concept development and manuscript organization; Tom C. Tucker and Connie White contributed to data access and collection; Bin Huang and Quan Chen contributed to statistical programming and performed statistical analysis; All authors contributed to manuscript preparation. The authors are solely responsible for subject development, data collection & analysis, and composition.

References

1. Ries, L.A.G.; Kosary, C.L.; Hankey, B.F.; Miller, B.A.; Edwards, B.K. (Eds.) SEER Cancer Statistics Review 1973–1996. National Cancer Institute, 1999. Available online: https://seer.cancer.gov/archive/csr/1973_1996/overview.pdf (accessed on 21 March 2017).
2. Merrill, R.M.; Feuer, E.J. Risk-adjusted cancer incidence rates (United States). *Cancer Causes Control* **1996**, *7*, 544–552. [CrossRef] [PubMed]
3. Wilcox, L.S.; Koonin, L.M.; Pokras, R.; Strauss, L.T.; Xia, Z. Hysterectomy in the United States, 1988–1990. *Obstet. Gynecol.* **1994**, *83*, 549–555. [CrossRef] [PubMed]
4. Lepine, L.A.; Hillis, S.D.; Marchbanks, P.A.; Koonin, L.M.; Morrow, B.; Kieke, B.A.; Wilcox, L.S. Hysterectomy Surveillance—United States, 1980–1993. *MMWR CDC Surveill. Summ.* **1997**, *46*, 1–15. [PubMed]

5. Siegel, R.L.; Devesa, S.S.; Cokkinides, V.; Ma, J.; Jemal, A. State-level Uterine Corpus Cancer Incidence Rates Corrected for Hysterectomy Prevalence, 2004 to 2008. *Cancer Epidemiol. Biomarkers Prev.* **2013**, *22*, 25–31. [CrossRef] [PubMed]
6. Alvarado-Cabrero, I.; Navani, S.S.; Young, R.H.; Scully, R.E. Tumors of the fimbriated end of the fallopian tube: A clinicopathologic analysis of 20 cases, including nine carcinomas. *Int. J. Gynecol. Pathol.* **1997**, *16*, 189–196. [CrossRef] [PubMed]
7. Colgan, T.J.; Murphy, J.; Cole, D.E.; Narod, S.; Rosen, B. Occult carcinoma in prophylactic oophorectomy specimens: Prevalence and association with BRCA germline mutation status. *Am. J. Surg. Pathol.* **2001**, *25*, 1283–1289. [CrossRef] [PubMed]
8. Cass, I.; Holschneider, C.; Datta, N.; Barbuto, D.; Walts, A.E.; Karlan, B.Y. BRCA-mutation-associated fallopian tube carcinoma: A distinct clinical phenotype? *Obstet. Gynecol.* **2005**, *106*, 1327–1334. [CrossRef] [PubMed]
9. Medeiros, F.; Muto, M.G.; Lee, Y.; Elvin, J.A.; Callahan, M.J.; Feltmate, C.; Garber, J.E.; Cramer, D.W.; Crum, C.P. The tubal fimbria is a preferred site for early adenocarcinoma in women with familial ovarian cancer syndrome. *Am. J. Surg. Pathol.* **2006**, *30*, 230–236. [CrossRef] [PubMed]
10. Kindelberger, D.W.; Lee, Y.; Miron, A.; Hirsch, M.S.; Feltmate, C.; Medeiros, F.; Callahan, M.J.; Garner, E.O.; Gordon, R.W.; Birch, C.; et al. Intraepithelial carcinoma of the fimbria and pelvic serous carcinoma: Evidence for a causal relationship. *Am. J. Surg. Pathol.* **2007**, *31*, 161–169. [CrossRef] [PubMed]
11. Crum, C.R.; Drapkin, R.; Miron, A.; Ince, T.A.; Muto, M.; Kindelberger, D.W.; Lee, Y. The distal fallopian tube: A new model for pelvic serous carcinogenesis. *Curr. Opin. Obstet. Gynecol.* **2007**, *19*, 3–9. [CrossRef] [PubMed]
12. Landen, C.N.; Birrer, M.J.; Sood, A.K. Early events in the pathogenesis of epithelial ovarian cancer. *J. Clin. Oncol.* **2008**, *26*, 995–1005. [CrossRef] [PubMed]
13. Lengyel, E. Ovarian cancer development and metastasis. *Am. J. Pathol.* **2010**, *177*, 1053–1064. [CrossRef] [PubMed]
14. Kurman, R.J.; Shih, L.-M. The origin and pathogenesis of epithelial ovarian cancer: A proposed unifying theory. *Am. J. Surg. Pathol.* **2010**, *34*, 433–443. [CrossRef] [PubMed]
15. Crum, C.P.; Mckeon, F.D.; Xian, X. The oviduct and ovarian cancer: Causality, clinical implications, and "targeted prevention". *Clin. Obstet. Gynecol.* **2012**, *55*, 24–35. [CrossRef] [PubMed]
16. Domchek, S.M.; Friebel, T.M.; Garber, J.E.; Isaacs, C.; Matloff, E.; Eeles, R.; Evans, D.G.; Rubinstein, W.; Singer, C.F.; Rubin, S.; et al. Occult ovarian cancers identified at risk-reducing salpingo-oophorectomy in a prospective cohort of BRCA1/2 mutation carriers. *Breast Cancer Res. Treat.* **2010**, *124*, 195–203. [CrossRef] [PubMed]
17. Sherman, M.E.; Piedmonte, M.; Mai, P.L.; Ioffe, O.B.; Ronnett, B.M.; van Le, L.; Ivanov, I.; Bell, M.C.; Blank, S.V.; DiSilvestro, P.; et al. Pathologic findings at risk-reducing salpingo-oophorectomy: Primary results from Gynecologic Oncology Group Trial GOG-0199. *J. Clin. Oncol.* **2014**, *32*, 3275–3283. [CrossRef] [PubMed]
18. Rebbeck, T.R.; Lynch, H.T.; Neuhausen, S.L.; Narod, S.A.; Van't Veer, L.; Garber, J.E.; Evans, G.; Isaacs, C.; Daly, M.B.; Matloff, E.; et al. Prevention and Observation of Surgical End Points Study Group. *N. Engl. J. Med.* **2002**, *346*, 1616. [CrossRef] [PubMed]
19. Kauff, N.D.; Satagopan, J.M.; Robson, M.E.; Scheuer, L.; Hensley, M.; Hudis, C.A.; Ellis, N.A.; Boyd, J.; Borgen, P.I.; Barakat, R.R.; et al. Risk-reducing salpingo-oophorectomy in women with a *BRCA1* or *BRCA2* mutation. *N. Engl. J. Med.* **2002**, *346*, 1609. [CrossRef] [PubMed]
20. Cancer of the Ovary: SEER Stat Fact Sheets. Available online: http://seer.cancer.gov/statfacts/html/ovary.html (accessed on 27 December 2016).
21. Siegel, R.L.; Miller, K.D.; Jemal, A. Cancer statistics, 2016. *CA Cancer J. Clin.* **2016**, *66*, 7–30. [CrossRef] [PubMed]
22. Capocaccia, R.; de Angelis, R. Estimating the completeness of prevalence based on cancer registry data. *Stat. Med.* **1997**, *16*, 425–440. [CrossRef]
23. Gail, M.H.; Kessler, L.; Midthune, D.; Scoppa, S. Two approaches for estimating disease prevalence from population-based registries of incidence and total mortality. *Biometrics* **1999**, *55*, 1137–1144. [CrossRef] [PubMed]

24. Marriotto, A.; Gigli, A.; Capocaccia, R.; Tavilla, A.; Clegg, L.X.; Depry, M.; Scoppa, S.; Ries, L.A.; Rowland, J.H.; Tesauro, G.; et al. Complete and Limited Duration Cancer Prevalence Estimates. SEER Cancer Statistics Review, 1973–1999, 2002. Available online: https://seer.cancer.gov/archive/csr/1973_1999/prevalence.pdf (accessed on 31 December 2016).
25. Verdecchia, A.; de Angelis, G.; Capocaccia, R. Estimation and projections of cancer prevalence from cancer registry data. *Stat. Med.* **2002**, *21*, 3511–3526. [CrossRef] [PubMed]
26. Arias, E. United States Life Tables, 2010. National Vital Statistics Reports, 2014; Volume 63. Available online: https://www.cdc.gov/nchs/data/nvsr/nvsr64/nvsr64_11.pdf (accessed on 31 December 2016).
27. Contemporary OB/GYN: Bilateral Oophorectomy: Solving the Risk/Benefit Equation—Choosing candidates, Monitoring Outcomes. Available online: http://contemporaryobgyn.modernmedicine.com/contemporary-obgyn/news/modernmedicine/modern-medicine-now/bilateral-oophorectomy-solving-riskbenefi?page=full (accessed on 31 December 2016).
28. Oza, A.M.; Cook, A.D.; Pfisterer, J.; Embleton, A.; Ledermann, J.A.; Pujade-Lauraine, E.; Kristensen, G.; Carey, M.S.; Beale, P.; Cervantes, A.; et al. Standard chemotherapy with or without bevacizumab for women with newly diagnosed ovarian cancer (ICON7): Overall survival results of a phase 3 randomised trial. *Lancet Oncol.* **2015**, *16*, 928–936. [CrossRef]
29. Burger, R.A.; Brady, M.F.; Bookman, M.A.; Fleming, G.F.; Monk, B.J.; Huang, H.; Mannel, R.S.; Homesley, H.D.; Fowler, J.; Greer, B.E.; et al. Incorporation of bevacizumab in the primary treatment of ovarian cancer. *N. Engl. J. Med.* **2011**, *365*, 2473–2483. [CrossRef] [PubMed]
30. Ledermann, J.; Harter, P.; Gourley, C.; Friedlander, M.; Vergote, I.; Rustin, G.; Scott, C.; Meier, W.; Shapira-Frommer, R.; Safra, T.; et al. Olaparib maintenance therapy in platinum-sensitive relapsed ovarian cancer. *N. Engl. J. Med.* **2012**, *366*, 1382–1392. [CrossRef] [PubMed]
31. Ueland, F.R.; Depriest, P.D.; Desimone, C.P.; Pavlik, E.J.; Lele, S.M.; Kryscio, R.J.; van Nagell, J.R., Jr. The accuracy of examination under anesthesia and transvaginal sonography in evaluating ovarian size. *Gynecol. Oncol.* **2005**, *99*, 400–403. [CrossRef] [PubMed]
32. Jelovac, D.; Armstrong, D.K. Recent progress in the diagnosis and treatment of ovarian cancer. *CA Cancer J. Clin.* **2011**, *61*, 183–202. [CrossRef] [PubMed]
33. Whitlock, E.P.; Vesco, K.K.; Eder, M.; Lin, J.S.; Senger, C.A.; Burda, B.U. Liquid-based cytology and human papillomavirus testing to screen for cervical cancer: A systematic review for the US Preventive Services Task Force. *Ann. Intern. Med.* **2011**, *155*. [CrossRef] [PubMed]
34. Myers, E.R.; Moorman, P.; Gierisch, J.M.; Havrilesky, L.J.; Grimm, L.J.; Ghate, S.; Davidson, B.; Mongtomery, R.C.; Crowley, M.J.; McCrory, D.C.; et al. Benefits and Harms of Breast Cancer Screening: A Systematic Review. *J. Am. Med. Assoc.* **2015**, *314*, 1615–1634. [CrossRef] [PubMed]
35. Nagell, J.R., Jr.; Miller, R.W.; DeSimone, C.P.; Ueland, F.R.; Podzielinski, I.; Goodrich, S.T.; Elder, J.W.; Huang, B.; Kryscio, R.J.; Pavlik, E.J. Long-term survival of women with epithelial ovarian cancer detected by ultrasonographic screening. *Obstet. Gynecol.* **2011**, *118*, 1212–1221. [CrossRef] [PubMed]
36. Jacobs, I.J.; Menon, U.; Ryan, A.; Gentry-Maharaj, A.; Burnell, M.; Kalsi, J.K.; Amso, N.N.; Apostolidou, S.; Benjamin, E.; Cruickshank, D.; et al. Ovarian cancer screening and mortality in the UK Collaborative Trial of Ovarian Cancer Screening (UKCTOCS): A randomised controlled trial. *Lancet* **2016**, *387*, 945–956. [CrossRef]
37. Buys, S.S.; Partridge, E.; Black, A.; Johnson, C.C.; Lamerato, L.; Isaacs, C.; Reding, D.J.; Greenlee, R.T.; Yokochi, L.A.; Kessel, B. Effect of screening on ovarian cancer mortality—The Prostate, Lung, Colorectal and Ovarian (PLCO) Cancer Screening Randomized Controlled Trial. *J. Am. Med. Assoc.* **2011**, *305*, 2295–2303. [CrossRef] [PubMed]
38. Kobayashi, H.; Yamada, Y.; Sado, T.; Sakata, M.; Yoshida, S.; Kawaguchi, R.; Kanayama, S.; Shigetomi, H.; Haruta, S.; Tsuji, Y.; et al. A randomized study of screening for ovarian cancer: A multicenter study in Japan. *Int. J. Gynecol. Cancer* **2008**, *18*, 414–420. [CrossRef] [PubMed]
39. Bristow, R.E.; Tomacruz, R.S.; Armstrong, D.K.; Trimble, E.L.; Montz, F.J. Survival effect of maximal cytoreductive surgery for advanced ovarian carcinoma during the platinum era: A meta-analysis. *J. Clin. Oncol.* **2002**, *20*, 1248–1259. [CrossRef] [PubMed]
40. Nagell, J.R., Jr.; Miller, R.W. Evaluation and Management of Ultrasonographically Detected Ovarian Tumors in Asymptomatic Women. *Obstet. Gynecol.* **2016**, *127*, 848–858. [CrossRef] [PubMed]

41. Ueland, F.R.; DePriest, P.D.; Pavlik, E.J.; Kryscio, R.J.; van Nagell, J.R., Jr. Preoperative differentiation of malignant from benign ovarian tumors: The efficacy of morphology indexing and Doppler flow sonography. *Gynecol. Oncol.* **2003**, *91*, 46–50. [CrossRef]
42. Pavlik, E.J.; Ueland, F.R.; Miller, R.W.; Ubellacker, J.M.; Desimone, C.P.; Elder, J.; Hoff, J.; Baldwin, L.; Kryscio, R.J.; Nagell, J.R., Jr. Frequency and disposition of ovarian abnormalities followed with serial transvaginal ultrasonography. *Obstet. Gynecol.* **2013**, *122*, 210–217. [CrossRef] [PubMed]
43. Sherman, M.E.; Carreon, J.D.; Lacey, J.V., Jr.; Devesa, S.S. Impact of hysterectomy on endometrial carcinoma rates in the United States. *J. Natl. Cancer Inst.* **2005**, *97*, 1700–1702. [CrossRef] [PubMed]
44. Temkin, S.M.; Minasian, L.; Noone, A.M. The End of the Hysterectomy Epidemic and Endometrial Cancer Incidence: What Are the Unintended Consequences of Declining Hysterectomy Rates? *Front. Oncol.* **2016**, *6*, 89. [CrossRef] [PubMed]
45. ACOG. ACOG Committee Opinion No. 444: Choosing the route of hysterectomy for benign disease. *Obstet. Gynecol.* **2009**. [CrossRef]
46. Whiteman, M.K.; Hillis, S.D.; Jamieson, D.J.; Morrow, B.; Podgornik, M.N.; Brett, K.M.; Marchbanks, P.A. Inpatient hysterectomy surveillance in the United States, 2000–2004. *Am. J. Obstet. Gynecol.* **2008**. [CrossRef] [PubMed]
47. Wright, J.D.; Herzog, T.J.; Tsui, J.; Ananth, C.V.; Lewin, S.N.; Lu, Y.-S.; Neugut, A.I.; Hershman, D.L. Nationwide trends in the performance of inpatient hysterectomy in the United States. *Obstet. Gynecol.* **2013**, *122*, 233–241. [CrossRef] [PubMed]
48. Mikhail, E.; Salemi, J.L.; Mogos, M.F.; Hart, S.; Salihu, H.M.; Imudia, A.N. National trends of adnexal surgeries at the time of hysterectomy for benign indication, United States, 1998–2011. *Am. J. Obstet. Gynecol.* **2015**. [CrossRef] [PubMed]
49. Parker, W.H.; Feskanich, D.; Broder, M.S.; Chang, E.; Shoupe, D.; Farquhar, C.M. Long-term mortality associated with oophorectomy versus ovarian conservation in the nurses' health study. *Obstet. Gynecol.* **2013**, *121*, 709–716. [CrossRef] [PubMed]
50. Bandera, C.A.; Muto, M.G.; Schorge, J.O.; Berkowitz, R.S.; Rubin, S.C.; Mok, S.C. BRCA1 gene mutations in women with papillary serous carcinoma of the peritoneum. *Obstet. Gynecol.* **1998**, *92*, 596–600. [CrossRef] [PubMed]
51. Howard, B.V.; Kuller, L.; Langer, R.; Manson, J.E.; Allen, C.; Assaf, A.; Cochrane, B.B.; Larson, J.C.; Lasser, N.; Rainford, M.; et al. Risk of cardiovascular disease by hysterectomy status, with and without oophorectomy: The Women's Health Initiative Observational Study. *Circulation* **2005**, *111*, 1462–1470. [CrossRef] [PubMed]

7

Psychological and Behavioral Impact of Participation in Ovarian Cancer Screening

Michael A. Andrykowski

Department of Behavioral Science, University of Kentucky College of Medicine, Lexington, KY 40536-0086, USA; mandry@uky.edu

Academic Editor: Andreas Kjaer

Abstract: Evaluation of costs and benefits associated with cancer screening should include consideration of any psychological and behavioral impact associated with screening participation. Research examining the psychological and behavioral impact of screening asymptomatic women for ovarian cancer (OC) was considered. Research has focused upon potential negative psychological (e.g., distress) and behavioral (e.g., reduced future screening participation) impact of false positive (FP) OC test results. Results suggest FP OC screening results are associated with greater short-term OC-specific distress. While distress dissipates over time it may remain elevated relative to pre-screening levels for several weeks or months even after clinical follow-up has ruled out malignancy. The likelihood of participation in future OC screening may also be reduced. Research focused upon identification of any beneficial impact of participation in OC screening associated with receipt of "normal" results was also considered. This research suggests that a "normal" screening test result can have psychological benefits, including increased positive affect and beliefs in the efficacy of screening. It is concluded that any psychological or behavioral harms attributable to OC screening are generally very modest in severity and duration and might be counterbalanced by psychological benefits accruing to women who participate in routine OC screening and receive normal test results.

Keywords: ovarian cancer; psychological; psychosocial; behavioral; screening; false positive test result

---

1. Introduction

For some cancers, participation in cancer screening can lead to early diagnosis and an associated improvement in five-year survival. Consequently, great effort has been expended to develop cost-effective screening tests and protocols for cancers of the breast, colon, rectum, cervix, prostate, lung, and ovary—cancers with a high likelihood of treatment success when diagnosed and treated at an early stage of disease. Furthermore, for those screening tests for which the evidence suggests cost-effectiveness, great effort has been expended to ensure widespread uptake and appropriate repeat screening by screening-eligible individuals.

While participation in cancer screening can improve prognosis for some cancers, cancer screening is not without its drawbacks. All cancer screening approaches yield some proportion of inconclusive or abnormal results. These results typically require additional clinical follow-up to determine if a malignancy is present. Clinical follow-up might include surgery or biopsy, performance of a second-line screening test, or perhaps simply a repeat of the original screening test. In most instances, follow-up indicates the original abnormal or inconclusive screening test result is benign—no malignancy is present. Such false positive (FP) results may not be psychologically or behaviorally benign, however. A survey of recipients of FP test results in the context of breast, prostate, cervical or colorectal cancer screening found 40% described the experience as "very scary" or "the scariest time of my life" [1]. In general, research has shown a FP cancer screening test result can negatively impact both psychological (e.g., distress) and behavioral (e.g., participation in future cancer screening) outcomes [2–6], although research suggesting no impact is also available (e.g., [7]).

Recommendation of any cancer screening test for routine use in asymptomatic, average-risk women is based on the relative balance of the benefits and costs associated with that screening test. Identification of the benefits of any cancer screening test is relatively straightforward. Whether a cancer screening test results in a significant reduction in the number of deaths due to that specific cancer (i.e., cancer-specific mortality) is the primary determinant of the benefits of a particular screening test. A broader view of the benefits of a screening test could include consideration of any psychological or behavioral benefits associated with a screening test. Though rarely considered, participation in cancer screening may yield positive outcomes including reductions in cancer worry or increases in feelings of reassurance and well-being [8,9].

As one might expect, calculation of the costs of a screening test include consideration of the monetary costs associated with testing. In addition, calculation of the costs of a screening test should also include the "costs" associated with FP screening test results. These costs include the monetary as well as physical morbidity costs associated with performance of additional follow-up procedures or unnecessary surgeries. In addition, a FP screening test result might also exact certain psychological or behavioral costs. Psychological costs include fear or anxiety, a heightened sense of personal risk for cancer, or reduced confidence in the efficacy of the screening test, all of which might result in a significant behavioral cost—a lessened likelihood of returning for repeat screening in the future. If the collective costs associated with a screening test exceed the collective benefits of screening, one might well conclude that a particular screening test does more harm than good.

The purpose of this paper is to consider the literature regarding the psychological and behavioral impact of participation in routine screening for ovarian cancer (OC). Evidence regarding the potential for OC screening to yield both positive and negative psychological and behavioral outcomes will be considered.

2. Screening for Ovarian Cancer

When diagnosed and treated at a localized stage, OC is associated with a good prognosis. The five-year relative survival rate is 92% [10]. Unfortunately, the majority of cases of OC (61%) are diagnosed with late stage disease where existing treatment approaches are less likely to be successful and five-year relative survival rates are correspondingly only 27% [10]. Given this state of affairs, considerable effort has been expended to develop cost-effective approaches to screening for OC [11–16]. For the most part, these approaches include transvaginal ultrasonography (TVS) and serum tests for cancer antigen 125 (CA125), alone or in combination. While demonstrating some value in promoting early detection of OC in average-risk, asymptomatic women, no approach to OC screening has been shown to significantly reduce OC-specific mortality in asymptomatic, average-risk women in a prospective, randomized trial. As a result, implementation of routine screening for OC in asymptomatic, average-risk women has been controversial. Currently, the US Preventive Services Task Force recommends against routine screening for OC in asymptomatic, average-risk women (D recommendation) [17]. However, despite this recommendation, screening for OC is widely available and utilized for asymptomatic women at either average or elevated risk for OC. A recent survey of primary care physicians and obstetrician-gynecologists in the USA found many (33%) believed TVS and CA125 were effective screening tests for OC and many would offer OC screening tests to low (28%) and medium risk (65%) women [18].

3. Impact of False Positive OC Screening Test Results

Similar to screening tests for other cancers, screening for OC yields a certain proportion of inconclusive or abnormal test results [19]. For asymptomatic women at average risk for OC, approximately 5%–10% of OC screening tests yield an inconclusive or abnormal result, necessitating clinical follow-up. Fortunately, the vast majority of inconclusive or abnormal OC screening test results are ultimately deemed benign. While clinically benign, however, a FP OC screening test result may not be psychologically or behaviorally benign. An inconclusive or abnormal OC test result requiring additional clinical follow-up could understandably cause a woman to consider the possibility of a diagnosis of OC, resulting in a heightened sense of personal vulnerability. This in turn could result in the experience of fear, anxiety, and/or distress as well as a reduced likelihood of returning for future OC screening.

What is the evidence for such reactions? To answer this question a group of 10 studies are considered [20–29]. While an attempt was made to use PubMed to identify all relevant studies, a systematic review of the literature was not conducted and consequently no guarantee is made regarding the completeness of the studies considered here. Each of the 10 studies considered involves comparison of two groups of women participating in OC screening: women receiving a "normal" screening test result (i.e., Normal group) and women receiving an abnormal test result with clinical follow-up revealing no malignancy present (i.e., FP group). Comparison of these two groups of women has the potential to shed light on the impact of a FP OC screening test result. The specific OC screening test(s) employed varies across these studies but each employed CA125 testing or ultrasonography, typically transvaginal sonography (TVS), either alone or in combination. The psychological and behavioral outcomes the Normal and FP groups are compared upon vary widely across studies. The most common outcomes being generic mental health outcomes (e.g., state anxiety, depression, distress), OC-specific measures of distress and worry, OC risk perception, and participation in future cancer screening, either actual or stated intention to participate. These studies also vary widely with regard to study design (e.g., cross sectional vs. longitudinal), sample size in both the Normal and FP groups, and the timing of the assessment of outcomes (e.g., short-term vs long-term). Finally, some of these studies focused upon OC screening for women at intermediate or high risk for OC, typically due to a strong family history of OC [23,25–28]. The remaining studies focused upon OC screening among asymptomatic women generally at average risk for OC [20–22,24,29].

3.1. Impact of FP Results on Women at Intermediate or High Risk for OC

In an early study, 266 women at risk for familial OC underwent either transabdominal or transvaginal ultrasonagraphy with color Doppler imaging [27]. Women with abnormal results on initial scan returned in six weeks for a repeat scan. Women with repeat abnormal results at the repeat scan were referred for surgery. All women completed a questionnaire 6–15 weeks before the initial scan and again after their initial scan. Women also completed the same questionnaire after a repeat scan. Psychological outcomes assessed included OC risk perception, cancer worry, coping style, depression and anxiety symptoms, and general distress. Results indicated that following an initial scan, before a repeat scan ruled out the presence of malignancy, women receiving an abnormal result ($n = 51$) reported greater cancer worry, general distress, and anxiety than women receiving a normal scan result (i.e., Normal group; $n = 189$). Of women receiving an abnormal result at the initial scan, 32 received a normal result at the repeat scan and thus constituted a FP group. In the FP group, distress returned to baseline levels but remained elevated relative to the Normal group. Overall, it was concluded FP results are associated with increased distress in the short-term but this adverse impact is neither severe nor persistent.

Participants in this initial study completed the same study questionnaire as in the initial study one year after their initial scan [28]. In general, one year after their initial scan, women in the FP group did not differ from women in the Normal group with regard to distress and anxiety. However, more women in the FP group described themselves as "more worried" about cancer than women in the Normal group. It was concluded while FP results may be associated with some increased worry about cancer in the longer term, there is little evidence to suggest severe and persistent adverse psychological effects.

Kauff et al. examined women at intermediate risk for OC due to a personal or family history of breast and/or ovarian cancer but no documented BRCA1/2 mutation [25]. Women were offered semi-annual OC screening using TVS, CA125 testing, and pelvic examination. Women completed a baseline assessment at enrollment in the screening program and follow-up assessments every six months thereafter in conjunction with OC screening. Impact on mental quality of life (QOL) was indexed by the Mental Component Score of the Medical Outcome Study Short Form-36. At least one follow-up assessment was completed by 135 women. During a mean of 19.8 months of follow-up, 52 women experienced ≥1 abnormal OC screening test result. None of these women were ultimately deemed to have OC and constituted the FP group. Women in the FP group evidenced a clinically and statistically significant mean 6.4 point decrease in their Mental Component Score between baseline and their most recent follow-up assessment. (Lower scores represent poorer mental QOL). Women with no abnormal OC screening test result constituted the Normal group (n = 83) and evidenced a statistically and clinically insignificant mean 0.67 point drop in their Mental Component Score. It was concluded for women at intermediate risk for OC, FP screening results are associated with a significant decline in mental QOL.

As part of the United Kingdom Familial Ovarian Cancer Screening Study (OKFOCSS), women at increased genetic risk for OC (estimated lifetime risk >10%) participated in an OC screening program involving thrice yearly CA125 testing coupled with annual TVS [23]. If an abnormal test result occurred for either type of testing, women were recalled for retesting within two months. Women (n = 1999) completed a baseline assessment (T1) one month prior to an initial CA125 test and a follow-up assessment one week after receiving the result of this initial test (T2). Women receiving an abnormal test result at any time completed an additional follow-up one week after repeat of the screening test ruled out malignancy and they were returned to routine screening (T3). These women constituted the FP group (n = 167). The remaining women who received only normal test results during participation in the screening program constituted the Normal group. Finally, all women completed a final follow-up assessment nine months after receiving a normal test result (n = 825) or nine months after return to routine screening after receiving a FP result (n = 87) (T4). Specific outcomes assessed at each assessment included OC-specific distress, anxiety and depression symptoms, and reassurance. Compared to the Normal group the FP group reported moderately elevated OC-specific distress one week after being notified of their abnormal result. No difference in OC-specific distress was evident at T3 or T4, after women with FP results returned to routine screening. No differences with regard to anxiety, depression, or reassurance were noted between the Normal screening and FP groups at any assessment point. Finally, women in the FP group were significantly more likely to withdraw from the screening program (primarily for risk-reducing salpingo oophorectomy) (OR = 4.38). It was concluded FP screening results are associated with transient OC-specific distress but are not associated with sustained psychological harm.

Finally, 111 female BRCA1/2 mutation carriers who had not undergone risk-reducing surgery (i.e., salpingo oophorectomy) participated in a screening program involving both annual breast cancer screening and OC screening involving both CA125 testing and TVS [26]. All abnormal screening test results were followed by additional imaging and biopsy when appropriate. All participants completed a questionnaire prior to a baseline screening visit, as well as 3 and 12 months post-baseline. Psychological outcomes assessed included general anxiety, perceived absolute and comparative risk for OC, and OC worry. Women receiving normal OC screening test results following baseline screening constituted the Normal group and those receiving abnormal results with no cancer subsequently detected constituted a FP group. No significant differences were found between the Normal and FP groups for any of the OC risk or worry outcomes at either the 3 or 12 month follow-ups. Furthermore, there were no differences between the two groups in the likelihood of undergoing risk-reducing surgery. It was concluded FP test results were not associated with large increases in risk perception, cancer worry, or uptake of risk-reducing surgery. Unfortunately, only two women received abnormal CA125 test results (<2% of the sample) while the number of women receiving FP TVS test results was not reported. As a result, it is unclear whether the lack of significant findings might be due to a true absence of effect or simply due to inadequate statistical power.

3.2. Summary: Impact of FP Results on Women at Intermediate or High Risk for OC

Each of the studies considered in this group examined the impact of a FP screening test result on one or more psychological outcomes. Overall, the evidence suggests that a FP result in screening programs targeted at women at intermediate or high risk for OC is associated with significantly poorer psychological status in the immediate aftermath of an abnormal OC screening test result. This appears particularly true with regard to cancer-specific worry and distress [23,25,27]. Little evidence suggests much impact on more general indices of depression, anxiety or mental health or on perceptions of OC risk. Any impact on psychological status appears to be short-lived, however, as differences between FP and Normal groups generally decline over time following determination no malignancy is present [23,28]. The study by Kauff et al. [25] appears to be an exception to this general conclusion, however, as they found FP results were associated with significant and long-term declines in a generic measure of mental health. However, their data analytic strategy did not account for when a FP result was experienced in the course of the mean nearly 20 months of observation. This makes it difficult to attribute any observed declines in mental health status to the experience of a FP screening test result. Finally, Brain et al. found women receiving FP results were over four times more likely to withdraw from their OC screening program [23]. Withdrawal was typically followed by risk-reducing surgery, however, eliminating the need for further OC screening. It was unclear, however, whether women in the FP group were more likely than women in the Normal group to discontinue participation in OC screening in the absence of risk-reducing surgery. This is a critical missing piece of information given any risk-reducing impact of a screening program is predicated upon continued, appropriate participation with the program [30].

3.3. Impact of FP Results on Women at Average Risk for OC

The studies considered here examined the psychological and behavioral impact of a FP OC screening test result on asymptomatic women generally at average risk for OC [20–22,24,29]. Andersen et al. examined women (n = 592) at "conventional" risk for OC (i.e., $\leq$1 first degree relative with OC) undergoing alternating CA125 and TVS testing every six months for 18 months [20]. Abnormal CA125 results were followed by TVS screening while abnormal TVS results required repeat TVS screening in six to eight weeks. Measures of QOL, worry about OC risk, and OC-specific distress were completed at a baseline assessment prior to the initial OC screening test and a follow-up two years post-baseline, after the screening program was concluded. At follow-up, women receiving a FP OC screening test result at some point during the two-year screening period (n = 32) were compared to similar women who received normal screening test results (i.e., Normal group). The FP group reported significantly greater worry about OC risk. Cancer-specific distress and quality of life did not differ between the FP and Normal screening groups. It was concluded FP screening test results may have long-term effects and increase worry about cancer risk.

Barrett et al. examined the psychological impact of a FP screening test in women participating in the United Kingdom Collaborative Trial of Ovarian Cancer Screening (UKCTOCS), a randomized trial of annual multimodal OC screening [21]. Women (n = 202,638) were randomized to one of three arms: (1) OC screening with CA125 testing followed, if necessary, by TVS (CA125+TVS) as a second line test; (2) OC screening with TVS; or (3) no OC screening. Following receipt of an abnormal screening test result women in the CA125+TVS arm underwent a repeat CA125 test with (Level 2) or without (Level 1) TVS testing. Women in the TVS group underwent a repeat TVS test by a senior ultrasonographer within three months (Level 1) or a repeat TVS test or biopsy within six weeks (Level 2). All women completed a baseline questionnaire prior to randomization. Women in the two screening groups who received an abnormal screening test result (n = 22,035) completed a questionnaire following each abnormal screen and annually thereafter. The questionnaire included measures of state anxiety as well as general psychological morbidity as assessed by the General Health Questionnaire (GHQ-12). Results indicated greater psychological morbidity in women after receipt of a FP test result but only for women receiving more intensive repeat screening (i.e., Level 2 repeat screening). In other words, women in the CA125+TVS screening group exhibited greater psychological morbidity only if repeat screening involved repeat of both the CA125 and TVS tests while women in the TVS screening group exhibited greater psychological morbidity only if repeat screening involved a TVS scan or biopsy (i.e., Level 2 repeat screening). No differences between the FP and Normal groups were found for state anxiety. It was concluded a FP test results in slightly increased psychological morbidity when an abnormal screening test result is followed by more intensive forms of repeat screening.

The remaining studies in this group examined asymptomatic, average-risk women participating in an ongoing trial of OC screening using annual TVS at the University of Kentucky [22,24,29]. In this trial, an abnormal TVS test result requires repeat of the TVS screening test in 2–16 weeks. In an initial study [22], women (n = 540) completed a baseline assessment immediately before undergoing a routine annual TVS screening test and follow-up assessments two weeks and four months post-baseline. A single-item measure of OC risk perception (i.e., perceived lifetime personal risk) as well as measures of general and OC-specific distress were completed at all assessments. Women receiving a FP screening test result (n = 33) at baseline were compared to women receiving a normal screening test result (i.e., Normal group; n = 507). Compared to women receiving a "normal" TVS test result, women receiving a FP result reported significantly elevated OC-specific distress at the two-week follow-up, before a repeat TVS test had clarified whether a malignancy was present. Distress returned to baseline levels at four-month follow-up, after repeat of the TVS test indicated no malignancy was present. No differences between the FP and Normal groups on mood disturbance, depression, or OC risk perception were found. It was concluded a FP test result is associated with a significant, but transient, increase in OC-specific distress.

As a follow-up to this initial study, a larger longitudinal study examining psychological and behavioral responses to receipt of a FP OC screening test result was implemented [29]. Women receiving a FP TVS test result (n = 375) in the course of routine, annual TVS screening were compared to women (n = 375) receiving a normal test result (i.e., Normal group). Women in the FP group were matched with women in the Normal group with regard to age, family history of OC, and OC screening history (prior FP result, number of prior TVS tests). Women in the FP group completed a baseline assessment immediately prior to undergoing a repeat TVS test, required to clarify the nature of a recent abnormal TVS test 2 to 16 weeks earlier. Women in the Normal group completed a baseline assessment immediately prior to a routine, annual TVS screening test. Both groups completed follow-up assessments one and four months after baseline. Results indicated FP test results were associated with clinically significant increases in OC-specific distress with distress remaining elevated through the four month follow-up. Women receiving a FP result also reported significantly higher perceptions of OC risk on two different, two-item composite measures of risk (Personal OC Risk and Comparative OC Risk) and fewer perceived positive consequences of screening participation. A FP test result also impacted screening intentions as the FP group reported at one month follow-up significantly weaker intentions to return for future OC screening. No differences between the FP and Normal groups were found with regard to depressive symptoms, benefit finding, or beliefs in the effectiveness of OC screening at any of the study assessments. It was concluded FP results negatively impact both affective (OC-specific distress) and cognitive (risk perception) outcomes in both the short and intermediate term. The negative psychological impact of a FP test is still evident for several months after repeat testing has ruled out malignancy and may serve to reduce motivation to participate in future routine OC screening.

Finally, Floyd et al. examined the impact of a FP test result on women's interest in receiving health-related information [24]. Based on the possibility a FP screening test result could be experienced as a very scary and threatening event [1], it was hypothesized a FP result may serve as a "teachable moment" [31] and enhance interest in obtaining additional information about OC as well as other health-related topics. A Normal screening group (n = 124) consisted of women undergoing a routine, annual TVS test with receipt of normal results. This group completed a baseline assessment prior to undergoing routine TVS screening. A FP screening group (n = 279) consisted of women who had received an abnormal TVS test result 2–16 weeks earlier and were returning for a repeat TVS test to clarify whether a malignancy was present. These women completed a baseline assessment prior to undergoing this repeat TVS screening test. All women completed a follow-up assessment one month post-baseline where interest in receiving information about 10 different health- and cancer-related topics was assessed. Contrary to hypothesis, results indicated women receiving FP screening test results were significantly less interested in receiving health- and cancer-related information than women receiving normal screening results. It was concluded receipt of a FP result does not represent a teachable moment when women may be more receptive to health information and health behavior change. Rather receipt of a FP screening test result appears to make women less interested in health-related information, including information regarding OC.

3.4. Summary: Impact of FP Results on Women at Average Risk for OC

Most studies in this group examined the impact of a FP screening test result on one or more psychological outcomes [20–22,29]. In each of these studies, a negative impact on psychological outcomes was observed. Receipt of a FP result was associated with poorer psychological status, particularly OC-specific worry [20] and OC-specific distress [22,29]. Little evidence suggests FP results exert a significant impact on more general measures of psychological morbidity or distress, although one study did find elevated psychological morbidity in women receiving a FP result requiring more intense, invasive repeat testing after an abnormal result [21]. While it is clear FP results impact OC-specific distress, the duration of this impact is not completely clear. It is quite apparent receipt of an abnormal screening test result is associated with an immediate and pronounced spike in OC-specific distress [22,29] which remains elevated for at least several weeks or months even after repeat OC screening rules out malignancy [29]. Overall, the evidence suggests that receipt of a FP screening test result increases OC-specific distress and worry in the short term and quite possibly in the intermediate term. As for other outcomes, the data are sparse or mixed. The two studies that examined the impact of a FP test result on perceptions of OC risk yielded mixed results [22,29]. While one study found no impact upon OC risk perception [22], a larger and better designed study found a FP result resulted in higher perceptions of OC risk up to four months after repeat TVS testing ruled out malignancy [29]. The failure to find a significant impact on OC risk perception in the earlier study [22] could be due to a lack of statistical power as well as use of a relatively crude measure of OC risk perception. The earlier study [22] included only 33 women in the FP result group compared to 375 women in the later study [29], making it less likely a "true" impact on OC risk perception could be detected in the earlier study. Additionally, the earlier study indexed OC risk perception using only a single, single-item measure of risk perception. In contrast, the later study [29] found significant effects on two separate, two-item composite measures of OC risk perception. Finally, a FP result may impact the likelihood of participation in future screening as receipt of a FP result was associated with significantly weaker intentions to return for future OC screening [29].

4. Impact of Normal OC Screening Test Results

As might be expected, an abnormal or FP test result appears to have at least some negative impact on psychological and behavioral outcomes. Might the opposite be true? Does receipt of a "normal" OC screening test result yield a positive impact on psychological or behavioral outcomes? In contrast to the attention focused upon the impact of abnormal or FP results, it appears the impact of a "normal" test result on psychological and behavioral outcomes has received less attention. In an initial study, high-risk women (n = 275) underwent ultrasound screening for OC [32]. Nearly $\frac{3}{4}$ reported feeling reassured after screening. In a more recent and comprehensive study, asymptomatic, average-risk women (n = 560) completed a baseline assessment immediately prior to undergoing routine, annual TVS screening for OC as well as follow-up assessment two weeks and four months post-baseline [33]. All women received a "normal" screening test result. Growth curve modeling revealed receipt of a "normal" test result was associated with a significant decrease in OC-specific distress and significant increases in positive affect, belief in the efficacy of OC screening, and knowledge of OC risk factors between the baseline and four-month follow-up assessment. No effect was observed on OC risk perceptions, negative affect, or more generic measures of distress (i.e., depression, mood disturbance). It was concluded participation in routine OC screening with receipt of a normal result can positively impact affective and cognitive psychological outcomes that can serve to promote continued participation in OC screening.

5. Summary and Recommendations

Determination of the value of any cancer screening test requires careful consideration of the costs and benefits associated with that screening test. Obviously, certain types of costs and benefits are weighed more heavily than others. The paramount benefit of a screening test is the extent to which it reduces cancer-related mortality. On the cost side of the ledger, the economic and physical morbidity costs (e.g., surgeries) associated with a screening test are weighed most heavily. Less frequently considered are any psychological and behavioral costs and benefits associated with a cancer screening test.

The purpose of this paper was to consider the psychological and behavioral impact, both costs and benefits, associated with participation in OC screening. The studies we considered are diverse in methodology and design. Most of these studies focused upon documenting the psychological "costs" associated with abnormal, ultimately FP, OC screening test results. In general, these studies clearly suggest that women who experience a FP OC screening test result report more OC-specific worry and distress in the short-term [22,23,27,29]. This is unsurprising, of course, given receipt of an abnormal result raises at least the possibility of a subsequent diagnosis of OC. This distress appears to dissipate over time, but may still be present to a degree four months to a year or more after receipt of an abnormal result and after clinical follow-up has ruled out a malignancy [20,28,29]. This general conclusion appears to be true regardless of the OC risk status of the asymptomatic women being screened.

In contrast to the findings for OC-specific distress and worry, the impact of a FP screening test result on other psychological outcomes is less clear. The impact on generic measures of mental health, depression and anxiety is mixed with some research showing a negative impact [21,25,27] and other research showing no impact [20,22,23,29]. Similarly, the impact of a FP result on perceptions of OC risk is also mixed with some studies finding no impact [22,27] but another, larger, better-designed study finding increased perceptions of OC risk in women experiencing a FP result [29].

With regard to behavioral costs associated with a FP OC screening test result, FP test results may be associated with reduced future participation in OC screening [23] or reduced intentions to return for routine screening in the future [29]. Given the effectiveness of any cancer screening modality is predicated upon continued screening uptake at appropriate intervals, this is a significant potential cost associated with FP results in the OC screening setting.

In contrast to the negative impact of a FF OC screening test result, it appears woman may benefit from participation in routine OC screening when a "normal" screening test result is received. For asymptomatic, average-risk women, participation in OC screening with receipt of a "normal" test result was associated with a significant decrease in OC-specific distress and significant increases in positive affect, belief in the efficacy of OC screening, and knowledge of OC risk factors over a four month period following screening [33]. Additionally, comparison of women receiving FP and normal results found women receiving normal screening test results attributed more positive consequences to their screening experience such as greater feelings of well-being and reassurance [29]. This data is provocative in its suggestion that participation in screening may not be a completely benign experience from a psychological and behavioral standpoint. Rather, participation in screening may create affective and cognitive conditions that may not only be inherently positive and reinforcing, but may also serve to further promote continued participation in OC screening.

While showing some ability to detect OC at an earlier stage, randomized trials have failed to show a reduction in cancer-specific mortality in asymptomatic, average-risk women participating in OC screening programs. Coupled with consideration of the monetary costs of OC screening and the potential physical morbidity costs (e.g., surgery) associated with FP test results, the US Preventive Services Task Force recommends against routine screening for OC in asymptomatic, average-risk women (D recommendation) [17]. Despite this negative recommendation, routine screening of asymptomatic women at average risk for OC is unlikely to go away. OC screening is well accepted by many physicians [18] as well as by the public. An overwhelming majority of women participating in the University of Kentucky OC screening program indicated they agreed or strongly agreed that TVS screening is effective in the early diagnosis of OC [29]. As a result, further research on the psychological and behavioral impact of participation in OC screening is warranted. While more research is needed, what is particularly needed is better research. Future research examining the impact of FP screening test results should be characterized by (1) sufficient numbers of women receiving abnormal or FP results to ensure adequate statistical power and the ability to interpret null findings; (2) longitudinal assessment to enable identification of the duration of impact of a specific abnormal or FP test result on key psychological and behavioral outcomes; and (3) removal of women who undergo risk-reducing oophorectomy from analyses focused upon understanding the impact of FP results on future screening participation.

In addition, there is likely benefit from expanding the focus of research regarding the psychological and behavioral impact of participation in OC screening. In particular, more research is needed regarding the potential impact of participation in routine OC screening with receipt of a "normal" test result. While research has examined the potential positive impact of a normal test result [33] the potential negative impact of a normal test result has received scant, if any, attention. Potential negative impact might involve delay in help-seeking following any subsequent onset of symptoms related to OC or a general complacency about health. Two other areas are also largely unexamined: the psychological and behavioral impact of false negative OC screening test results—receipt of a normal screening test result when OC is present—and the impact of true positive OC screening test results. In the latter case, the psychological and behavioral impact of a diagnosis of OC may differ depending on whether OC was screening- or symptomatically-detected.

In conclusion, the research considered here does not suggest that FP test results in the course of screening asymptomatic women for OC result in significant, durable psychological harm. In addition, there is some suggestion that participation in routine screening for OC may confer psychological benefits. Some have contended OC screening "does more harm than good" [34]. If true, this contention is true based largely on consideration of the physical harms associated with surgeries performed for diagnostic or preventive purposes following abnormal OC screening results. Any psychological or behavioral harms attributable to OC screening appear to be, at worst, rather modest in severity and duration and might well be counterbalanced by psychological benefits accruing to women who participate in routine OC screening and who receive normal test results.

References

1. Schwartz, L.M.; Woloshin, S.; Fowler, F.J., Jr.; Welch, H.G. Enthusiasm for cancer screening in the United States. *J. Am. Med. Assoc.* **2004**, *291*, 71–78. [CrossRef] [PubMed]
2. Brewer, N.T.; Salz, T.; Lillie, S.E. Systematic review: The long-term effects of false-positive mammograms. *Ann. Intern. Med.* **2007**, *146*, 502–510. [CrossRef] [PubMed]
3. Lin, K.; Lipsitz, R.; Miller, T.; Janakiraman, S. Benefits and harms of prostate-specific antigen screening for prostate cancer: An evidence update for the U.S. Preventive services task force. *Ann. Intern. Med.* **2008**, *149*, 192–199. [CrossRef] [PubMed]
4. Slatore, C.G.; Sullivan, D.R.; Pappas, M.; Humphrey, L.L. Patient-centered outcomes among lung cancer screening recipients with computed tomography: A systematic review. *J. Thorac. Oncol.* **2014**, *9*, 927–934. [CrossRef] [PubMed]

5. Taylor, K.L.; Shleby, R.; Gelmann, E.; McGuire, C. Quality of life and trial adherence among participants in the prostate, lung, colorectal, and ovarian cancer screening trial. *J. Natl. Cancer Inst.* **2004**, *96*, 1083–1094. [CrossRef] [PubMed]
6. Wardle, J.; Pope, R. The psychological costs of screening for cancer. *J. Psychosom. Res.* **1992**, *36*, 609–624. [CrossRef]
7. O'Sullivan, I.; Sutton, S.; Dixon, S.; Perry, N. False positive results do not have a negative effect on reattendance for subsequent breast screening. *J. Med. Screen* **2001**, *8*, 145–148. [CrossRef] [PubMed]
8. Cockburn, J.; de Luise, T.; Hurley, S.; Clover, K. Development and validation of the PCQ: A questionnaire to measure the psychological consequences of screening mammography. *Soc. Sci. Med.* **1992**, *34*, 1129–1134. [CrossRef]
9. Tyndel, S.; Austoker, J.; Henderson, B.J.; Brain, K.; Bankhead, C.; Clements, A.; Watson, E.K. What is the psychological impact of mammographic screening on younger women with a family history of breast cancer? Findings from a prospective cohort study by the PIMMS Management Group. *J. Clin. Oncol.* **2007**, *25*, 3823–3830. [CrossRef] [PubMed]
10. *Cancer Facts and Figures*; American Cancer Society: Atlanta, GA, USA, 2015.
11. Buys, S.S.; Partridge, E.; Black, A.; Johnson, C.C.; Lamerato, L.; Isaacs, C.; Reding, D.J.; Greenlee, R.T.; Yokochi, L.A.; Kessel, B.; et al. Effect of screenning on ovarian cancer mortality: The Prostate, Lung, and Ovarian (PLCO) Cancer Screening randomized controlled trial. *J. Am. Med. Assoc.* **2011**, *305*, 2295–2303. [CrossRef] [PubMed]
12. Jacobs, I.J.; Menon, U.; Ryan, A.; Gentry-Maharaj, A.; Burnell, M.; Kalsi, J.K.; Amso, N.N.; Apostolidou, E.B.; Cruickshank, D.; Crump, D.N.; et al. Ovarian cancer screening and mortality in the UK Collaborative Trial of Ovarian Cancer Screening (UKCTOS): A randomised controlled trial. *Lancet* **2016**, *387*, 945–956. [CrossRef]
13. Menon, U.; Griffin, M.; Gentry-Maharaj, A. Ovarian cancer screening—Current status, future directions. *Gynecol. Oncol.* **2014**, *132*, 490–495. [CrossRef] [PubMed]
14. Reade, C.J.; Riva, J.J.; Busse, J.W.; Goldsmith, C.H.; Elit, L. Risks and benefits of screening asymptomatic women for ovarian cancer: A systematic review and meta-analysis. *Gynecol. Oncol.* **2013**, *130*, 674–681. [CrossRef] [PubMed]
15. Schorge, J.O.; Modesitt, S.C.; Coleman, R.L.; Cohn, D.E.; Kauff, N.D.; Duska, L.R.; Herzog, T.J. SGO white paper on ovarian cancer: Etiology, screening and surveillance. *Gynecol. Oncol.* **2010**, *119*, 7–17. [CrossRef] [PubMed]
16. Van Nagell, J.R., Jr.; Pavlik, E.J. Ovarian cancer screening. *Clin. Obstet. Gynecol.* **2012**, *55*, 43–51. [CrossRef] [PubMed]
17. Moyer, V.A. U.S. Preventive Services Task Force. Screening for ovarian cancer: U.S. Preventive Services Task Force reaffirmation recommendation statement. *Ann. Intern. Med.* **2012**, *157*, 900–904. [CrossRef] [PubMed]
18. Baldwin, L.-M.; Trivers, K.F.; Matthews, B.; Andrilla, C.H.A.; Miller, J.W.; Berry, D.L.; Lishner, D.M.; Goff, B.A. Vignette-based study of ovarian cancer screening: Do U.S. physicians report adhering to evidence-based recommendations. *Ann. Intern. Med.* **2012**, *156*, 182–194. [CrossRef] [PubMed]
19. Pavlik, E.J.; Ueland, F.R.; Miller, R.V.V.; Ubellacker, J.M.; DeSimone, C.P.; Hoff, J.; Baldwin, R.J.; Kryscio, R.J.; van Nagell, J.R., Jr. Frequency and disposition of ovarian abnormalities followed with serial transvaginal sonography. *Obstet. Gynecol.* **2013**, *122*, 210–217. [CrossRef] [PubMed]
20. Andersen, M.R.; Drescher, C.W.; Zheng, Y.; Bowen, D.J.; Wilson, S.; Young, A.; McIntosh, M.; Mahony, B.S.; Lowe, K.A.; Urban, N. Changes in cancer worry associated with participation in ovarian cancer screening. *Psychooncology* **2007**, *16*, 814–820. [CrossRef] [PubMed]
21. Barrett, J.; Jenkins, V.; Farewell, V.; Menon, U.; Jacobs, I.; Kilkerr, J.; Ryan, A.; Langridge, C.; Fallowfield, L.; UKCTOCS Trialists. Psychological morbidity associated with ovarian cancer screening: Results from more than 23,000 women in the randomised trial of ovarian cancer screening (UKCTOCS). *BJOG* **2014**, *121*, 1071–1079. [CrossRef] [PubMed]
22. Andrykowski, M.A.; Boerner, L.M.; Salsman, J.M.; Pavlik, E. Psychological response to test results in an ovarian cancer screening program: A prospective, longitudinal study. *Health Psychol.* **2004**, *23*, 622–630. [CrossRef] [PubMed]
23. Brain, K.E.; Lifford, K.J.; Fraser, L.; Rosenthal, A.N.; Rogers, M.T.; Lancastle, D.; Phelps, C.; Watson, E.K.; Clements, A.; Menon, U. Psychological outcomes of familial ovarian cancer screening: No evidence of long-term harm. *Gynecol. Oncol.* **2012**, *127*, 556–563. [CrossRef] [PubMed]

24. Floyd, A.; Steffens, R.F.; Pavlik, E.; Andrykowski, M.A. Receipt of a false positive test result during routine screening for ovarian cancer: A teachable moment? *J. Clin. Psychol. Med. Settings* **2011**, *18*, 70–77. [CrossRef] [PubMed]
25. Kauff, N.D.; Hurley, K.E.; Hensley, M.L.; Robson, M.E.; Lev, G.; Goldfrank, D.; Castiel, M.; Brown, C.L.; Ostroff, J.S.; Hann, L.E.; et al. Ovarian carcinoma screening in women at intermediate risk: Impact on quality of life and need for invasive follow-up. *Cancer* **2005**, *104*, 314–320. [CrossRef] [PubMed]
26. Portnoy, D.B.; Loud, J.T.; Han, P.K.J.; Mai, P.L.; Greene, M.H. Effects of false-positive cancer screenings and cancer worry on risk-reducing surgery among BRCA1/2 carriers. *Health Psychol.* **2015**, *34*, 709–717. [CrossRef] [PubMed]
27. Wardle, J.; Collins, W.; Pernet, A.L.; Whitehead, M.I.; Bourne, T.H.; Campbell, S. Psychological impact of screening for familial ovarian cancer. *J. Natl. Cancer Inst.* **1993**, *85*, 653–657. [CrossRef] [PubMed]
28. Wardle, J.; Pernet, A.; Collins, W.; Bourne, T. False positive results in ovarian cancer screening: One year follow-up of psychological status. *Psychol. Health* **1994**, *10*, 33–40. [CrossRef]
29. Wiggins, A.; Pavlik, E.J.; Andrykowski, M.A. Affective, cognitive, and behavioral outcomes associated with a false positive screening test for ovarian cancer. *J. Behav. Med.* **2017**, in press.
30. Weller, D.P.; Campbell, C. Uptake in cancer screening programmes: A priority in cancer control. *Br. J. Cancer* **2009**, *101* (Suppl. 2), S55–S59. [CrossRef] [PubMed]
31. McBride, C.M.; Emmons, K.M.; Lipkus, I.M. Understanding the potential of teachable moments: The case of smoking cessation. *Health Educ. Res.* **2003**, *18*, 156–170. [CrossRef] [PubMed]
32. Andolf, E.; Jorgensen, C.; Uddenberg, N.; Ursing, I. Psychological effects of ultrasound screening for ovarian carcinoma. *J. Psychosom. Obstet. Gynaecol.* **1990**, *11*, 155–162. [CrossRef]
33. Gaugler, J.E.; Pavlik, E.; Salsman, J.M.; Andrykowski, M.A. Psychological and behavioral impact of receipt of a "normal" ovarian cancer screening test. *Prev. Med.* **2006**, *42*, 463–470. [CrossRef] [PubMed]
34. Slomski, A. Screening women for ovarian cancer still does more harm than good. *J. Am. Med. Assoc.* **2012**, *307*, 2474–2475. [CrossRef] [PubMed]

8

PSA and PSA Kinetics Thresholds for the Presence of ^{68}Ga-PSMA-11 PET/CT-Detectable Lesions in Patients with Biochemical Recurrent Prostate Cancer

Manuela Andrea Hoffmann [1,2,*], Hans-Georg Buchholz [2], Helmut J. Wieler [3], Matthias Miederer [2], Florian Rosar [2,4], Nicolas Fischer [5], Jonas Müller-Hübenthal [6], Ludwin Trampert [7], Stefanie Pektor [2] and Mathias Schreckenberger [2]

1 Department of Occupational Health & Safety, Federal Ministry of Defense, 53123 Bonn, Germany
2 Clinic of Nuclear Medicine, Johannes Gutenberg-University, 55101 Mainz, Germany; hans-georg.buchholz@unimedizin-mainz.de (H.-G.B.); matthias.miederer@unimedizin-mainz.de (M.M.); florian.rosar@uks.eu (F.R.); stefanie.pektor@unimedizin-mainz.de (S.P.); mathias.schreckenberger@unimedizin-mainz.de (M.S.)
3 Clinic of Nuclear Medicine, Bundeswehr Central Hospital, 56072 Koblenz, Germany; helmut.wieler@web.de
4 Department of Nuclear Medicine, Saarland University Medical Center, 66421 Homburg, Germany
5 Department of Urology, Helios Kliniken Krefeld, 47805 Krefeld, Germany; simplissimus@gmx.de
6 Practice of Radiology and Nuclear Medicine, Praxis im KölnTriangle, 50679 Köln, Germany; jmh@praxis-im-koelntriangle.de
7 Clinic of Nuclear Medicine, Klinikum Mutterhaus der Borromäerinnen, 54290 Trier, Germany; ludwin.trampert@mutterhaus.de
* Correspondence: manuhoffmann@web.de

Abstract: ^{68}Ga-PSMA-11 positron-emission tomography/computed tomography (PET/CT) is commonly used for restaging recurrent prostate cancer (PC) in European clinical practice. The goal of this study is to determine the optimum time for performing these PET/CT scans in a large cohort of patients by identifying the prostate-specific-antigen (PSA) and PSA kinetics thresholds for detecting and localizing recurrent PC. This retrospective analysis includes 581 patients with biochemical recurrence (BC) by definition. The performance of ^{68}Ga-PSMA-11 PET/CT in relation to the PSA value at the scan time as well as PSA kinetics was assessed by the receiver-operating-characteristic-curve (ROC) generated by plotting sensitivity versus 1-specificity. Malignant prostatic lesions were identified in 77%. For patients that were treated with radical prostatectomy (RP) a PSA value of 1.24 ng/mL was found to be the optimal cutoff level for predicting positive and negative scans, while for patients previously treated with radiotherapy (RT) it was 5.75 ng/mL. In RP-patients with PSA value <1.24 ng/mL, 52% scans were positive, whereas patients with PSA ≥1.24 ng/mL had positive scan results in 87%. RT-patients with PSA <5.75 ng/mL had positive scans in 86% and for those with PSA ≥5.75 ng/mL 94% had positive scans. This study identifies the PSA and PSA kinetics threshold levels for the presence of ^{68}Ga-PSMA-11 PET/CT-detectable PC-lesions in BC patients.

Keywords: ^{68}Gallium-PSMA PET/CT; prostate-specific-antigen; prostate cancer; PSA kinetics thresholds; biochemical recurrence; optimal cutoff level

---

1. Introduction

Prostate cancer (PC) is the second most common type of malignant cancers and it accounts for 55% of global cancer incidence, together with lung, stomach, and breast cancer [1]. The global incidence of PC in 2012 is 1.1 million per year and accounts for approximately 7% of deaths in men [2]. PC incidence has increased to 95–116 per 10,000 persons and the incidence of death related to PC is 2 per 10,000 per person years since the introduction of prostate-specific-antigen (PSA)-screening [3].

Most patients with BC of PC are diagnosed at an early tumor stage with local disease. The primary treatment of choice for localized PC is radical prostatectomy (RP) or radiation therapy (RT). In recent years, several alternative treatment options have been approved, especially for the therapy of aggressive PC and/or metastatic spread [4,5]. BC occurs in about 30% of the patients treated, in spite of radical therapy [5,6]. BC is defined as a PSA is > 0.2 ng/mL after radical prostatectomy (RP) or > 2 ng/mL above the nadir following radiotherapy (RT) [7]. The shorter the time between primary treatment and BC is, the greater the risk for metastatic recurrence and clinical progression will be. In comparison, the longer the timeline, the higher the association of localized recurrence [4]. In this setting, PSA and PSA kinetics (i.e., PSA doubling time (PSAdt)—"which measures the exponential increase in serum PSA over time" [8] and PSA velocity (PSAvel)—an indication of the "absolute annual increase in serum PSA (ng/mL/year)" [8]) are valuable for the forecast of recurrent PC [4,9]. However the PSA alone does not indicate the localization of malignant lesions.

Cornford et al. shows imaging guidelines and salvage therapy protocols after primary treatment [7]. In patients with presumptive cancer after initial curative treatment, diagnostic imaging is challenging in the evaluation of patients with recurrent PC and/or distant metastases. Current standard imaging techniques for restaging include transrectal ultrasonography (TRUS), ^{99m}Tc-diphosphonate bone scintigraphy, computed tomography (CT), and magnetic resonance imaging (MRI). Morphological imaging modalities, such as CT and MRI, often fail to visualize cancer lesions. Therefore, their accuracy is limited, especially for the detection of lymph node metastases (LNM). Other diagnostic methods, such as positron-emission tomography (PET) (with various tracers) or MR spectroscopy, which show metabolic activity, will be used, in order to minimize this limitation [10].

Hybrid PET/CT has been favored for several years and has been applied according to international guidelines to improve the diagnostic accuracy [8,11]. ^{68}Gallium (Ga)-prostate specific membrane antigen (PSMA) is currently one of the most successful tracers for PC imaging due to its clinical specificity [12,13]. PSMA is a transmembrane protein that is overexpressed in 95% of PC cells, especially in higher grade PC, recurrent PC and metastatic disease [14]. In benign prostate tissue, it is only weakly or not expressed. PSMA provides an optimal target for the diagnosis of PC as well as the treatment of PC [15]. Different ^{68}Ga-labelled PSMA inhibitors have been studied regarding their sensitivity and specificity to diagnose recurrence of PC such as HBED-CC, which is an efficient ^{68}Ga-chelator [13,16]. A German group has developed Glu-NH-CO-NH-Lys(Ahx)-{^{68}Ga-(N,N′-bis-[2-hydroxy-5-(carboxyethyl)benzyl]ethylen-ediamine-N,N′ -diacetic acid)}(^{68}Ga-HBED-CC-PSMA or ^{68}Ga-PSMA-11), a small-molecule inhibitor for PSMA [6,16]. The HBED-CC ligand has a fast blood and organ clearance and little of the ligand is taken up into the liver. ^{68}Ga-PSMA-11 PET/CT is a favorable diagnostic tool due to its excellent contrast-to-noise ratio and the improved detection of lesions. The HBED-CC conjugated PSMA inhibitor ^{68}Ga-PSMA-11 precisely binds to PSMA-positive cells and it is more specifically internalized into PSMA expressing tumor cells and PSMA-positive metastatic lesion cells of PC [13,16,17]. In recent years, several other PSMA ligands have been developed for labelling with ^{68}Ga and ^{18}F. In particular, the ^{18}F-labelled PSMA ligands continue to be researched [6,18,19]. To date, thousands of patients have been scanned with ^{68}Ga-PSMA, while ^{18}F-PSMA has only been used in a few hundred patients.

The current research is directed toward the development of more sensitive PET molecules for detection of BC at low PSA levels to allow for a personalized treatment planning at an early stage of recurrent disease. PSA kinetics has been proposed to supplement other diagnostic modalities in patient selection, especially with low PSA [9].

The goal of this study is to determine the best time for performing ^{68}Ga-PSMA-11 PET/CT scans in patients with BC by calculating PSA and PSA kinetics thresholds for the detection and localization of recurrent PC.

2. Results

2.1. Clinical Characteristics

Table 1 summarizes the clinical and pathological characteristics of the 581 study patients. At the time of the scan, the median PSA levels were 2.98 ng/mL, range (0.2–2000). Gleason Score (GS, the grading system for determining the aggressiveness of PC) [8] was for GS ≤ 6 in 37 patients. 303 patients had GS 7 (7a + 7b), 104 patients had GS 8, and 139 patients GS > 8. 36% of the patients were treated with systemic androgen deprivation therapy (ADT). The primary treatment of most patients (493) was radical prostatectomy (85%). 88 patients (15%) were primarily treated with radiotherapy (Table 1).

Table 1. Patient characteristics.

Characteristics (*n*)	**Parameters**
Number of patients	581
Age (y) (581)	
Median	71
Range	49–88
Mean ± SD	71.3 ± 7.5
Gleason Score (581)	
≤ 6 (low risk + grade group 1)	37
7 (intermediate risk + grade group 2+3)	303
8 (high risk + grade group 4)	104
> 8 (high risk + grade group 5)	139
PSA (ng/mL) (581)	
Median	2.98
Range	0.2–2000
Mean ± SD	18.21 ± 101.91
PSAvel (ng/mL/y) (196)	
Median	1.24
Range	0–620.1
Mean ± SD	10.89 ± 54.25
PSAdt (months) (581)	
Median	10.35
Range	0–628.2
Mean ± SD	22.1 ± 48.8
Prior treatment of primary tumor (581)	
Surgery (radical prostatectomy)	493
Radiotherapy and other	88
Further treatment	
Anti-androgen therapy	209
Positivity rate	
Total/PET/CT positive patients	450/581

Abbreviations: PSA, prostate-specific-antigen; vel, velocity; dt, doubling time; SD, standard deviation; n, number of patients; y, year.

2.2. *Overall Positivity Rate of ^{68}Ga-PSMA-11 PET/CT*

^{68}Ga-PSMA-11 PET/CT showed a positivity rate in 450 out of 581 patients (77%) (mean PSA 18.21 ± 101.91 ng/mL). The discrimination of the PSA values between patients with a PSMA-positive scan and those with a PSMA-negative scan was statistically significant ($p < 0.001$). The mean PSA levels of patients with positive scans were significantly higher than those of patients with negative scan results (22.94 ± 115.38 ng/mL versus 1.95 ± 3.28 ng/mL, $p < 0.001$, Mann-Whitney-U test) (Table 2).

Table 2. ^{68}Ga-PSMA-11 positron-emission tomography/computed tomography (PET/CT)-11 positive and negative scan results in relation to prostate-specific-antigen (PSA).

PET/CT Results	PSA (ng/mL)		
	Mean ± SD	Median (range)	*p* Value
Positive (450/581)	22.94 ± 115.38	4.01 (0.2-2000)	
Negative (131/581)	1.95 ± 3.28	0.8 (0.2–25.67)	
Total	18.21 ± 101.91	2.98 (0.2–2000)	$p < 0.001$ *

* Mann-Whitney-U test. Abbreviations: PSA, prostate-specific-antigen; SD, standard deviation; $p < 0.05$ is considered significant.

This retrospective analysis includes 581 patients with a BC. We looked at the two groups of patients with different BC by definition (patient-group RP and patient-group RT) separately to ensure proper statistics and a homogeneous patient collective.

2.3. *Positivity Rate of ^{68}Ga-PSMA-11 PET/CT in Detecting Clinical Recurrence Post-Prostatectomy*

^{68}Ga-PSMA-11 PET/CT revealed malignant prostatic lesions in 370 of 493 patients (75%). A statistically significant demarcation in PSA values was shown ($p < 0.001$) between patients with a positive (3.20 ng/mL) and a negative (0.70 ng/mL) ^{68}Ga-PSMA-11 PET/CT scan.

The detection efficacy of ^{68}Ga-PSMA-11 PET/CT for post-prostatectomy (patient-group RP) was 40% (27) for PSA levels of 0.2 to < 0.5 ng/mL and 62% (48), 70% (61), 84% (99), 94% (135) for PSA levels of 0.5 to < 1 ng/mL, 1 to < 2 ng/mL, 2 to < 5 ng/mL, and ≥ 5 ng/mL, respectively ($p < 0.001$) (Table 3A).

Table 3A shows the sites of lesions that were detected by ^{68}Ga-PSMA-11 PET/CT scans in patient-group RP. Local recurrence was evident in 29% (109/370) of the patients with a positive scan. Out of all patients with positive scans, 85% showed metastases. 54% of these patients exhibited local metastases and 23% distant metastases. Multiple metastases were observed in 66% of these patients. Lymph node (LN) metastases (LNM) were evident in 78% of the patients, 75% of which were local, 8% distant LNM, and 18% were local and distant LNM. Bone metastases were revealed in 43% of the patients with positive ^{68}Ga-PSMA-11 PET/CT scans. Visceral metastases rarely occurred in 7% (Table 3A). Single metastases were detected in 28% of the patients ($n = 105$) with positive ^{68}Ga-PSMA-11 PET/CT results and 56% of the patients ($n = 208$) showed multiple PC metastases (Table 4).

Table 3. (**A**) Prostate cancer (PC) recurrence (patient-group radical prostatectomy (RP)) location related to different PSA values. (**B**) PC recurrence (patient-group RT) location related to different PSA values.

(A) Prostate cancer (PC) recurrence (patient-group radical prostatectomy (RP)) location related to different PSA values.

PSA (ng/mL)	0.2–<0.5	0.5–<1.0	1.0–<2.0	2.0–<5.0	≥5.0	Chi^2, p
Number (x/493) patient-group RP	67	78	87	118	143	
PET/CT positive	27	48	61	99	135	$r = 0.413$; $p < 0.001$
Positivity rate	40.3%	61.5%	70.1%	83.9%	94.4%	
Androgen deprivation therapy	15	13	21	31	77	$r = 0.252$; $p < 0.001$
Regions:						
Local recurrence	6	14	19	29	41	$r = 0.149$; $p = 0.02$
Metastases	22	39	49	80	123	$r = 0.365$; $p < 0.001$
Site of metastases:						$r = 0.402$; $p < 0.001$
Local metastases	16	28	32	43	50	
Distant metastases	3	7	12	18	31	
Local + distant metastases	3	4	5	19	42	
Number of metastases:						$r = 0.397$; $p < 0.001$
Single metastases	14	14	23	25	29	
Multiple metastases	8	25	26	55	94	
Lymph node metastases (LNM)	19	30	38	61	97	$r = 0.266$; $p < 0.001$
Site of LNM:						$r = 0.344$; $p < 0.001$
Local LNM	18	28	34	51	52	
Distant LNM	0	0	2	4	13	
Local + distant LNM	1	2	2	6	32	
Bone metastases	8	11	12	33	72	$r = 0.315$; $p < 0.001$
Visceral metastases	1	1	2	5	12	$r = 0.128$; $p = 0.075$ *

(B) PC recurrence (patient-group RT) location related to different PSA values.

PSA (ng/mL)	2.0–<5.0	≥5.0	Chi^2, p
Number (x/88) patient-group RT	33	55	
PET/CT positive	29	51	$r = 0.08$; $p = 0.44$
Positivity rate	87.9%	92.7%	
Androgen deprivation therapy	11	41	$r = 0.406$; $p = 0.001$
Regions:			
Local recurrence	21	29	$r = -0.107$; $p = 0.317$
Metastases	14	37	$r = 0.244$; $p = 0.022$
Site of metastases:			$r = 0.306$; $p = 0.011$
Local metastases	10	12	
Distant metastases	1	13	
Local + distant metastases	3	12	
Number of metastases:			$r = 0.289$; $p = 0.022$

Table 3. *Cont.*

Single metastases	6	7	
Multiple metastases	8	30	
Lymph node metastases (LNM)	12	23	$r = 0.054$; n.s.
Site of LNM:			$r = 0.076$; n.s.
Local LNM	9	17	
Distant LNM	2	1	
Local + distant LNM	1	5	
Bone metastases	5	22	$r = -0.261$; $p = 0.014$
Visceral metastases	2	1	$r = -0.113$; *n.s.*

* Fisher exact test. Abbreviations: PSA, prostate-specific-antigen; LNM, lymph node metastases; $p < 0.05$ is considered significant; r, Pearson correlation coefficient.

Table 4. Tumor location and positivity rate of detected lesions.

Tumor Location	*n* (493)	% (370)	*n* (88)	% (80)
PET/CT positive patients	370		80	
Local recurrence	109	29.5%	50	62.5%
Metastases	313	84.6%	51	63.8%
local	169	45.7%	22	27.5%
distant	71	19.2%	14	17.5%
local and distant	73	19.7%	15	18.8%
single	105	28.4%	13	16.3%
multiple	208	56.2%	38	47.5%
Lymph node metastases	245	66.2%	35	43.8%
Local/regional	183	49.6%	26	32.5%
Distant	19	5.1%	3	3.8%
Local and distant	43	11.6%	6	7.5%
Bone metastases	136	36.8%	27	33.8%
Visceral metastases (lung, liver, adrenals, soft tissue, spleen, thyroid)	21	5.7%	3	7.5%

Abbreviation: *n*, number of patients.

2.4. *Positivity Rate of ^{68}Ga-PSMA-11 PET/CT in Detecting Clinical Recurrence Post-Radiotherapy*

Overall, 80 of 88 patients had a positive ^{68}Ga-PSMA-11 PET/CT scan (91%). The discrimination in PSA values between the patients with a positive (7.15 ng/mL) and a negative (5.25 ng/mL) scan was not statistically significant ($p = 0.384$).

For patients that were treated with RT, the detection efficacy of ^{68}Ga-PSMA-11 PET/CT was 88% (29) for PSA levels of 2 to < 5 ng/mL and 93% (51) for PSA levels of ≥ 5 ng/mL, respectively ($p = 0.44$) (Table 3B).

Table 3B shows the sites of lesions that were detected by ^{68}Ga-PSMA-11 PET/CT scans in patient-group RT. In 63% (50/80) of the patients with a positive scan, local recurrence was detected. Of the positive scans, 64% showed metastases and 43% of these patients exhibited local metastases, whereas 27% showed at least one distant finding (extra pelvic LN and/or bone and/or visceral metastases). Multiple metastases were demonstrated in 75% of these patients. A total of 69% of the patients showed LNM (74% of them local, 9% distant, and 17% local and distant LNM). Bone metastases were revealed in 34% of the patients with positive ^{68}Ga-PSMA-11 PET/CT scans. Visceral metastases were detected in only 4% of the positive scans (Table 3B). Multimetastatic disease was shown in 48% of the PSMA-positive patients ($n = 38$), whereas in 16% of the patients ($n = 13$) single PC metastases were detected (Table 4).

2.5. PSA and PSA Kinetics Threshold Levels

The performance of ^{68}Ga-PSMA-11 PET/CT in relation to the PSA value at the time of the scans, as well as PSA kinetics, were assessed by receiver-operating-characteristic-curve (ROC) generated by plotting sensitivity versus 1-specificity. A PSA value of 1.24 ng/mL was found to be the optimal cutoff level for predicting positive and negative scans by means of ROC analysis (AUC = 0.788; 95% CI 0.746–0.831) in all the patients primarily treated with RP and with RT (the cohort of 581 patients).

2.6. PSA and PSA Kinetics Threshold Levels Post-Prostatectomy

The optimal cutoff level was also 1.24 ng/mL for patients that were treated with radical prostatectomy (370/493 patient-group RP) (AUC = 0.784; 95% CI 0.740–0.828) (Figure 1).

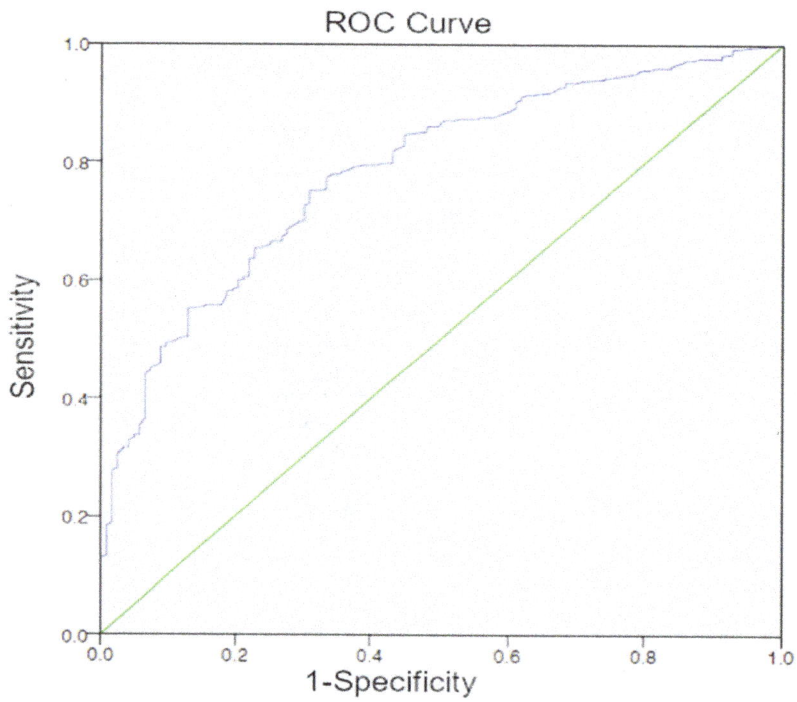

Figure 1. Receiver-operating-characteristic-curve (ROC) curve for PSA (patient-group RP) with an optimal cutoff level of 1.24 ng/mL.

In patients with a PSA value <1.24 ng/mL, 52% (92/177) ^{68}Ga-PSMA-11 PET/CT scans were positive, whereas patients with a PSA ≥1.24 ng/mL exhibited positive scan results in 87% (278/316) ($p < 0.001$). Local recurrence in the prostate bed was noted in 13% vs. 27% of the patients with PSA levels below and above the cutoff. Multimetastatic disease was determined in 21% of the patients with PSA values that were below cutoff level vs. 79% of patients with PSA above cutoff ($p < 0.001$, r 0.315) (Table 5A). The local and distant metastases were determined in 6% (11/177) of patients with PSA values below the cutoff level vs. 20% (62/316) of patients with PSA above cutoff ($p < 0.001$) (Table 5A).

Local metastases were detected in 51 patients (29%) below and in 118 patients (37%) above cutoff PSA values ($p < 0.001$). Distant lesions were identified in 9% below vs. 18% above cutoff levels, respectively ($p < 0.001$; Table 5A). As compared to patients with PSA values that were below the optimal cutoff level, patients with PSA levels ≥ 1.24 more frequently exhibited LNM (25% vs. 75%, $p < 0.001$, r 0.228) and bone metastases (18% vs. 82%, $p < 0.001$, r 0.235).

Table 5. (**A**) ^{68}Ga-PSMA-11 PET/CT positivity rate (RP) of different subgroups related to PSA levels. (**B**) 68Ga-PSMA-11 PET/CT positivity rate (RT) of different subgroups that were related to PSA levels.

(A) ^{68}Ga-PSMA-11 PET/CT positivity rate (RP) of different subgroups related to PSA levels.						
PSA Range (ng/mL)	**Overall Positivity**	***p*/*r* Value**	**Single Metastases**	**Multiple Metastases**		***p*/*r* Value**
0.2 to <1 (145)	75 (51.7%)		28 (19.3%)	33 (22.8%)		
<1.24 (177)	92 (52%)		33 (31%)	44 (21%)		
≥1.24 (316)	278 (87.4%)		72 (69%)	164 (79%)		
Total (493)	370 (75%)	$p < 0.001$: r 0.400	105	208		$p < 0.001$: r 0.315
PSA Range (ng/mL)	**Local Recur-Rence**	***p*/*r* Value**	**Local Metastases**	**Distant Metastases**	**Local + Distant Metastases**	***p*/*r* Value**
0.2 to <1 (145)	20 (13.8%)		44 (30.3%)	10 (6.9%)	7 (4.8%)	
<1.24 (177)	23 (13%)		51 (28.8%)	15 (8.5%)	11 (6.2%)	
≥1.24 (316)	86 (27.2%)		118 (37.3%)	56 (17.7%)	62 (19.6%)	
Total (493)	109	$p < 0.001$; r 0.164	169	71	73	$p < 0.001$; r 0.308
(B) ^{68}Ga-PSMA-11 PET/CT positivity rate (RT) of different subgroups that were related to PSA levels.						
PSA Range (ng/mL)	**Overall Positivity**	***p*/*r* Value**	**Single Metastases**	**Multiple Metastases**		***p*/*r* Value**
<5.75 (36)	31 (86.1%)		15 (41.7%)	19 (52.8%)		
≥5.75 (52)	49 (94.2%)		7 (13.5%)	29 (55.8%)		
Total (88)	80 (91%)	$p = 0.19$; r 0.139	22	48		$p = 0.008$; r 0.255
PSA Range (ng/mL)	**Local Recur-Rence**	***p*/*r* Value**	**Local Metastases**	**Distant Metastases**	**Local + Distant Metastases**	***p*/*r* Value**
<5.75 (36)	22 (61.1%)		11 (30.6%)	1 (2.8%)	4 (11.1%)	
≥5.75 (52)	28 (53.8%)		11 (21.2%)	13 (25%)	11 (21.2%)	
Total (88)	50	$p = 0.5$; r −0.07	22	14	15	$p = 0.01$; r 0.286

Abbreviations: PSA, prostate-specific-antigen; $p < 0.05$ is considered significant; r, Pearson correlation coefficient.

The optimal PSAvel threshold from ROC analysis for the detection of recurrent PC-lesions (patient-group RP) was 1.32 ng/mL/year (AUC = 0.777; 95% CI 0.709–0.845) (Figure 2), which showed significant differences between the PET-positive and PET-negative scans ($p < 0.001$).

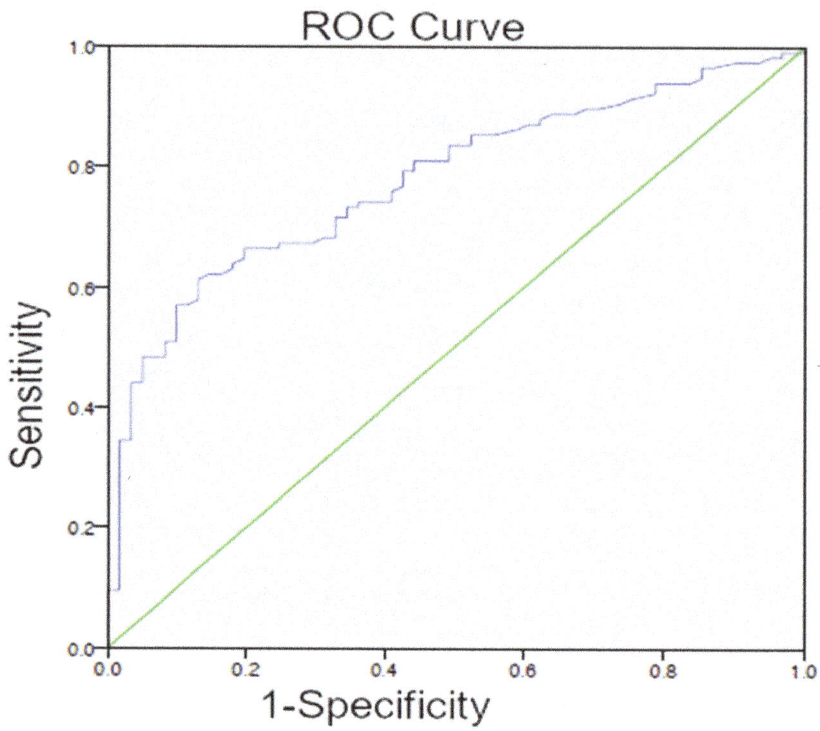

Figure 2. ROC curve for PSAvel (patient-group RP) with an optimal cutoff level of 1.32 ng/mL/year.

The ROC curve analysis showed that PSAdt was not useful in distinguishing between patients with positive and negative ^{68}Ga-PSMA-11 PET/CT scan results with an AUC of 0.450.

2.7. PSA and PSA Kinetics Threshold Levels Post-Radiotherapy

The optimal cutoff level for patients that were previously been treated with RT (80/88 patient-group RT) was 5.75 ng/mL (AUC = 0.594; 95% CI 0.400–0.788) (Figure 3). In patients with a PSA value <5.75 ng/mL, 86% (31/36) ^{68}Ga-PSMA-11 PET/CT scans were positive, whereas patients with a PSA ≥5.75 ng/mL exhibited positive scan results in 94% (49/52) ($p = 0.19$, r 0.139). Local recurrence in the prostate appeared in 61% vs. 54% of the patients with PSA levels that were below and above cutoff, respectively. Multimetastatic disease was determined in 53% of the patients with PSA values that were below cutoff level vs. 56% of patients with PSA above cutoff ($p = 0.008$, r 0.255) (Table 5B). Local and distant metastases were found in 11% (4/36) of patients with PSA values below cutoff level vs. 21% (11/52) of patients with PSA above cutoff ($p = 0.01$, r 0.286) (Table 5B). Patients with PSA levels ≥ 5.75 more frequently exhibited LNM (33% vs. 41%, $p = 0.393$, r 0.076) and bone metastases (26% vs. 41%, $p = 0.089$, r 0.152) as compared to patients with PSA values below the optimal cutoff level.

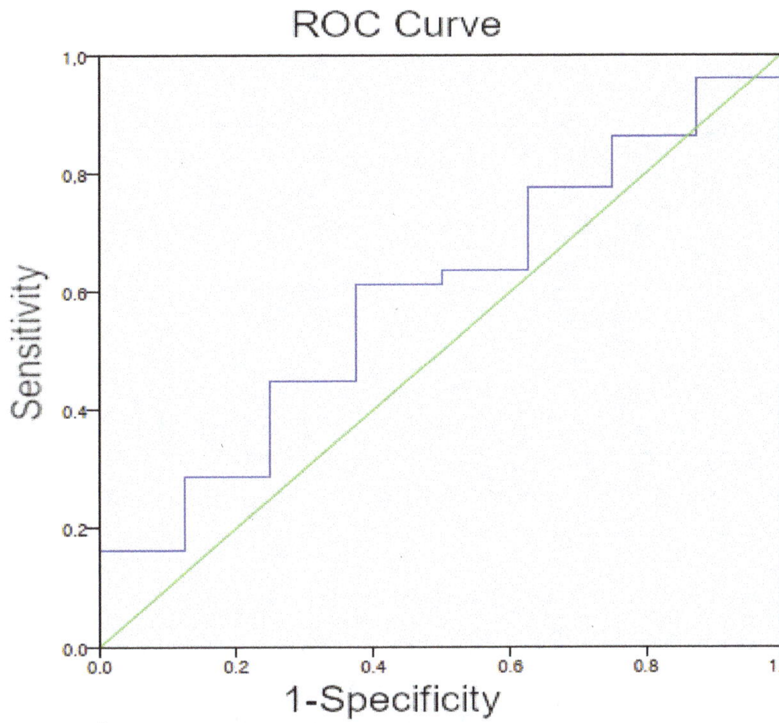

Figure 3. ROC curve for PSA (patient-group RT) with an optimal cutoff level of.5.75 ng/mL.

An optimal PSAvel threshold from ROC analysis for the detection of recurrent PC-lesions (patient-group RT) could not be ascertained, since only 19 patient data sets were available for the calculation of the value, of which a positive scan result was obtained in 18 patients.

ROC curve analysis revealed a PSAdt threshold of 10.6 months (AUC = 0.600; 95% Cl 0.366–0.834) to distinguish patients with positive and negative ^{68}Ga-PSMA-11 PET/CT, but without significance ($p = 0.353$).

2.8. Maximum Standardized Uptake Value (SUV_{max})

As evidenced by the Kolmogorov-Smirnov-Test, the SUV_{max} of the detected sites of malignant lesions were not normally distributed. SUV_{max} was the highest in bone metastases (mean and standard deviation/SD: 22.14 ± 22.98, median: 15) and lowest in lung metastases (mean and SD: 9.84 ± 9.31, median: 6). SUV_{max} of LNM and visceral metastases showed values in between.

2.9. GS

4% of patients with a positive ^{68}Ga-PSMA-11 PET/CT scan were categorized as being low risk PC (International Society of Urological Pathology (ISUP) grade 1; GS < 7), whereas 12% of PSMA-positive patients were categorized GS 7a (ISUP grade 2; intermediate risk), 35% GS 7b (ISUP grade 3; intermediate risk), 22% GS 8 (ISUP grade 4; high risk), and 26% GS > 8 (ISUP grade 5; high risk) [8] (Table 6). High risk (GS 8, GS > 8) as compared to low risk patients (GS < 7) showed a high frequency of positive scan results ($p < 0.001$) and metastases (52% vs. 2%) ($p < 0.001$). When considering local recurrence, the results are similar, but not statistically significant. With regard to the subgroups (GS 7a vs. GS 7b), there is an important distinction between patients with intermediate risk and grade group 2 (GS 7a also called 7 (3 + 4)) (10%) when compared to patients with intermediate risk and grade group 3 (GS 7b also called 7 (4 + 3)) (36%) for PSMA-positive metastases ($p < 0.001$) (Table 6).

Table 6. Gleason Score in relation to ^{68}Ga-PSMA-11 PET/CT-11 positive scan results.

n = 581	GS < 7 (37)	GS 7a (97)	GS 7b (204)	GS 8(104)	GS > 8(139)	Chi^2 r, p Value
PET/CT positive (450/581)	16	52	158	97	117	0.288; $p < 0.001$
Local recurrence (159/581)	9	24	56	32	38	0.027; n.s.
Metastases (364/581)	8	36	132	83	105	0.324; $p < 0.001$

Abbreviations: GS, Gleason Score; n, number of patients; $p < 0.05$ is considered significant; r, Pearson correlation coefficient.

2.10. ADT

ADT was significantly associated with increased probability of a positive ^{68}Ga-PSMA-11 PET/CT scan ($p < 0.001$). 37% of PSMA PET/CT-positive and 18% of PSMA PET/CT-negative patients were treated with ADT ($p < 0.001$, r 0.173) in the patient-group RP. For the patient-group RT, 59% of the patients with a positive PSMA scan and 63% with a negative scan were treated with androgens ($p = 0.837$, r = ™0.022).

2.11. Alkaline Phosphatase (AP)

AP has been described as an efficient and functional biomarker for the prognosis of PC (43). We wanted to verify whether AP is a predictor for bone involvement of PC. In our study, AP levels of patients with positive ^{68}Ga-PSMA-11 PET/CT scan results were higher than those of patients with negative scans (93 ± 53 IU/L vs. 74 ± 24 IU/L, $p < 0.001$, Mann-Whitney-U test). Patients exhibiting bone metastases showed higher AP than patients without bone metastases (108 ± 70 IU/L vs. 76 ± 23 IU/L; $p < 0.001$).

2.12. Subpopulation

EAU guidelines suggest PSMA PET/CT for restaging PC in the case of patients that were treated with RP, if the PSA level is > 0.2 ng/mL and if the results would influence subsequent treatment decisions [8]. In the event that PSMA PET/CT is not available and the PSA level is ≥ 1 ng/mL, PET/CT with other tracers (Fluciclovine or Choline) has been suggested, if the results could influence subsequent treatment decisions [8]. For PSA recurrence after RT, EAU guidelines recommend performing PSMA PET/CT (if available) or fluciclovine PET/CT or choline PET/CT in patients that qualified for curative salvage treatment [8]. Therefore, we analyzed the PSA range from 0.2 ng/mL to < 1 ng/mL for post-prostatectomy patients. We did not form a separate subgroup for the irradiated patients, as no PSA threshold was stated in the EAU guidelines with regard to them.

All of the prostatectomized patients, 29% (145/493) exhibited PSA levels between 0.2 and < 1 ng/mL and 52% of these patients showed positive PET/CT scans (positive: 0.2 to < 0.5 ng/mL 40% and 0.5 to < 1 ng/mL 62%; $p < 0.001$, r 0.413) (Table 3A). In this subpopulation (overall positivity rate in scans and PSA levels between 0.2 ng/mL and < 1 ng/mL), ^{68}Ga-PSMA-11 PET/CT showed the presence of local recurrence in the prostate bed in 27% (20 of 75), of local metastases in 59% (44 of 75), of distant metastases in 13% (10 of 75), and of local and distant metastases in 9% (7 of 75). Multimetastatic carcinoma was detected in 44% (33 of 75) (Table 3A). The absolute PSA value at the time of the ^{68}Ga-PSMA-11 scan was associated with an increased probability of a positive scan result ($p < 0.001$).

3. Discussion

We evaluated ^{68}Ga-PSMA-11 PET/CT scans in 581 BC patients after primary curative PC therapy (RP as well as RT) in this retrospective study. A high positivity rate of 77% (450/581 patients) for the detection of malignant prostatic lesions was shown (Figure 4A,B)). Our data reflects the positive results of several other studies and confirms that ^{68}Ga-PSMA-11 PET/CT is a promising method for diagnosing PC [12,20–24]. For restaging prostatectomized BC patients by PSMA PET/CT, the EAU guidelines recommend a PSA level of > 0.2 ng/mL [8]. Patients with low cancer burdens have the best chance of a salvage RT to be curative. For this reason, imaging with subsequent therapy planning at an early stage of recurrent disease makes sense, from the point at which carcinoma foci are detectable, even with low PSA [25]. The EAU guidelines report that salvage RT in BC patients after RP was correlated with a tripling in PC-specific survival when compared to the patients who did not get salvage therapy [8]. The purpose of our study was to determine the best time for performing ^{68}Ga-PSMA-11 PET/CT scans in BC patients. For that reason, we calculated the PSA and PSA kinetics thresholds for the detection and localization of recurrent PC. The PSA levels and PSA kinetics were assessed by ROC generated by plotting sensitivity versus 1-specificity.

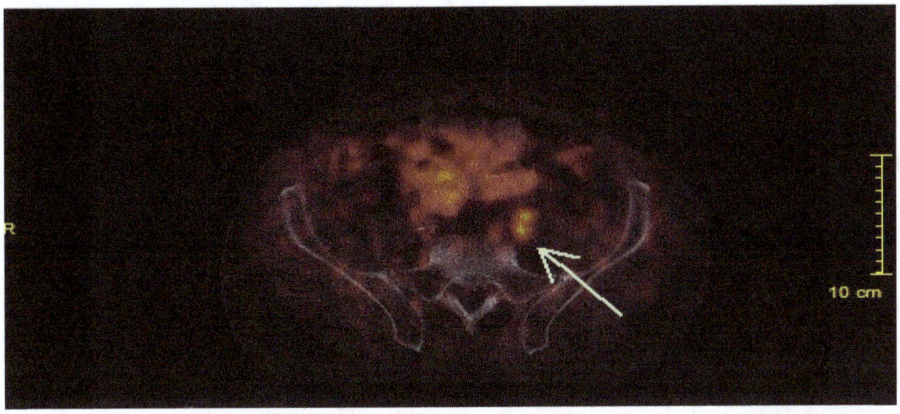

(A)

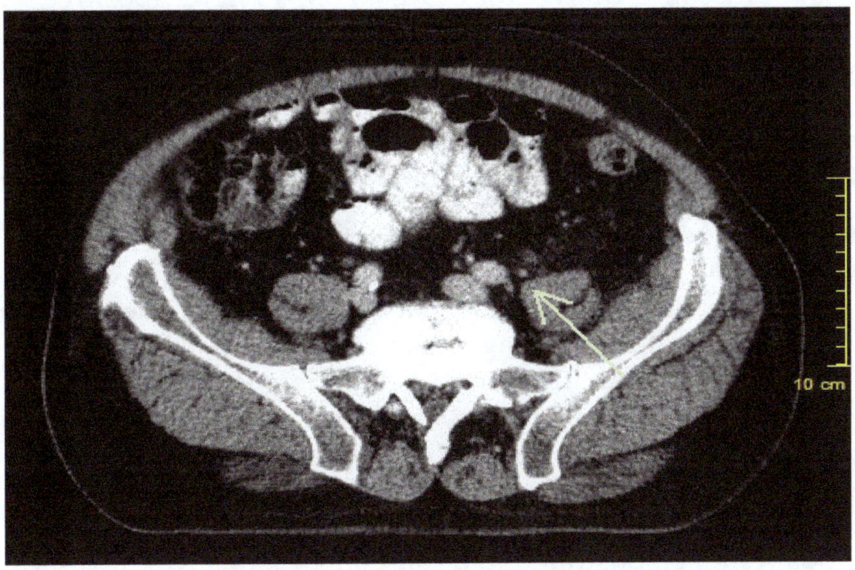

(B)

Figure 4. (**A**) History of a patient with prostate cancer followed by radical prostatectomy and lymphadenectomy (pT3, pN0, cM0, G3) in 2012. PSA doubles within three months. ^{68}Ga-PSMA-11 PET/CT scan shows two lymph node metastases with high prostate specific membrane antigen (PSMA)-avidity. (**B**) The two small lymph node metastases are detectable on CT alone, but not suspect of malignancy.

3.1. Overall Positivity Rate

The positivity rate of ^{68}Ga-PSMA-11 PET/CT of the present study was 77% over all patients (mean PSA 22.94 ± 115.38 ng/mL), thereby confirming the results of previous studies where detection rates of 74% to 83% were reported for restaging PET/CT [6,12,26]. There was a statistically significant ability to discriminate PSA values between PSMA-positive and PSMA-negative scans ($p < 0.001$). The overall patient group was divided into the group of patients who were primarily treated with prostatectomy (patient-group RP) and the group of patients who were primarily treated with RT (patient-group RT) to ensure clean statistics.

3.2. Positivity Rate (RP)

In the group of prostatectomized patients, the positivity rate was 75% (370/493 patients) (see Table 3A). Therefore, a clinically relevant percentage of patients with low PSA levels (< 0.5 ng/mL) could be diagnosed with the recurrence of PC, being comparable to the results of other studies [6,12,23,26]. In recent studies of restaging by ^{68}Ga-PSMA PET/CT, the detection rate was 50% at PSA levels of 0.2 to 0.49 ng/mL [6] and, in another study, 57.9% of the patients were ^{68}Ga-PSMA PET/CT-positive at PSA levels from 0.2 to < 0.5 ng/mL [20]. The results from the present study emphasize that ^{68}Ga-PSMA PET/CT is a sensitive tool for restaging PC, even at low PSA values [23]. After early salvage RT (PSA ≤ 0.5 ng/mL), an undetectable PSA level can be reached in 60% of the patients, being associated with a chance of 80% for a progression free five-year survival. This is indicated as second line therapy with curative intent [8,25]. Salvage RT is usually indicated after a persistent increase in PSA after RP, when systemic metastases are not found during staging imaging. If conventional imaging does not show any malignant foci (local and/or distant metastases), only the prostate bed is typically irradiated by Radiation Oncologists. Eiber et al. described that the detection of malignant lesions by PET was extremely important for the final diagnosis in over 50%. They showed lesions that were not detected by computed tomography (CT) [20,23]. Another study demonstrated that, in patients with BC after RP while using the standard procedure, nearly 20% of ^{68}Ga-PSMA PET/CT-positive lesions—suspicious of malignancy—would not have been included in the radiation field. All of these patients belonged to the crucial collective with PSA of < 1 ng/mL. ^{68}Ga-PSMA-11 PET/CT hybrid imaging opens up the possibility of changing the therapy [23,27]. Based on the data, both radiation therapists and urologists should have a more accurate road map for directing therapy. In the end, the radiation therapist should point where to direct his device. If a LN is resectable, a urologist might also resect it.

In comparison to other radiopharmaceuticals (e. g. ^{11}C- and ^{18}F-choline), detection rates of ^{68}Ga-PSMA at low PSA levels were higher [28,29]. PSA levels and ^{11}C-choline scans with positive results were linearily correlated [30–32]. The positivity rate of ^{11}C-choline scans for restaging was 73% at PSA levels of ≥ 3 ng/mL, but at PSA < 1 ng/mL the rate decreased dramatically to 19–36% [4,28]. However, a recent study showed that the second-generation of labelling of PSMA tracers with ^{18}F (e.g., ^{18}F-DCFPyL-PSMA) was superior to ^{68}Ga-PSMA for restaging at PSA levels of 0.5 to 3.5 μg/L with a sensitivity of 88% (15 of 17 patients) vs. 66% (23 of 35 patients). But at PSA values < 0.5 and > 3.5 μg/L, the sensitivity of both methods was comparable. Nevertheless, in 36% of the patients with positive scans, additional lesions were found, while using ^{18}F-PSMA vs. ^{68}Ga-PSMA [18]. Overall, the results of both methods were demonstrated to be similar [18]; this was also shown in a recent study, which compared ^{68}Ga-PSMA-11 and ^{18}F-PSMA-1007 in the case of staging PC [33].

3.3. Positivity Rate (RT)

The positivity rate of RT patients was 91%, but no statistically significant differences could be shown in the distinction of PSA levels between patients with positive and negative scans ($p = 0.384$) (see Table 3B). The EAU Guidelines recommend that PSMA PET/CT can be crucial for PC detection in the setting of BC after RT. However, they suggest that further studies be conducted [8].

3.4. PSA and PSA Kinetics Threshold Levels

We assessed the performance of ^{68}Ga-PSMA-11 PET/CT regarding pre-scan PSA levels by ROC curve separating the two patient-groups RP and RT. Based on the results of previous studies [4,9], which emphasized the importance of PSA kinetics for patient selection and detection, we also calculated PSAvel and PSAdt (see introduction), as they are valuable parameters for the prediction of clinical progression. However, it should also be borne in mind that there are non-PSA-producing tumor masses in metastatic and fully treated PCs.

3.5. PSA and PSA Kinetics Threshold Levels (RP)

In our study, a PSA of 1.24 ng/mL was the optimal cutoff level for distinguishing between positive and negative ^{68}Ga-PSMA-11 PET/CT scans. ^{68}Ga-PSMA-11 PET/CT showed the presence of multimetastatic PC in 21% of the positive lesions in patients with PSA levels below the cutoff value and in 79% in patients with PSA above the cutoff (Table 5A). Thus, we conclude that the cutoff by hybrid imaging with ^{68}Ga-PSMA-11 can be used for patient selection for restaging and also fits well into clinical practice. If you convert 1.24 ng/mL to tumor mass, it might be a small LNM or tissue volume of less than one cubic milliliter.

Significant differences between PET-positive and PET-negative patients were calculated with corresponding optimal PSAvel threshold of 1.32 ng/mL/year ($p < 0.001$). Similarly to other studies, our data show higher positivity rates corresponding to a higher PSAvel, which was also seen in studies with ^{18}F-choline. Like other authors, we propose that in addition to the PSA level, PSAvel could be taken into account in patient selection [9,20,32,34]. On the other hand, a recent study, which assessed a large cohort of patients, did not show significant correlation between ^{68}Ga-PSMA-11 PET/CT positivity and PSAvel [35].

In this study, PSAdt was not significantly associated with ^{68}Ga-PSMA-11 PET/CT positivity. For distinguishing between the positive and negative PSMA-PET findings, no optimal PSAdt cutoff could be determined by ROC analysis (AUC = 0.450). The value of PSA in patient selection is controversial [9]. Verburg et al. recommended combining serum PSA with PSAdt in order to achieve the best PSMA-positive scan result or the detection of distant LNM; in which they emphasized the importance of PSA over that of PSAdt [26]. Ceci et al. demonstrated PSAdt as a valuable predictor of positive ^{68}Ga-PSMA PET/CT scans and pointed out that patients with a short PSAdt and low PSA values showed positive PSMA scans in 85% [36]. Corresponding to the EAU guidelines, these patients were ideal candidates for salvage RT, as salvage RT has been described to be mostly efficient in patients with short PSAdt [8,36]. In contrast, in the same study, 18.7% of patients had low PSA values, but long PSAdt, and also showed positive PSMA-PET/CT findings [36].

3.6. PSA and PSA Kinetics Threshold Levels (RT)

In our study, we calculated an optimal PSA cutoff level from ROC curve of 5.75 ng/mL (Table 5B). We were not able to determine an optimal PSAvel threshold for the irradiated patient-group based on the available data. ROC analysis revealed a PSAdt cutoff of 10.6 months for the identification of RT patients with positive and negative scans, which did not find significance ($p = 0.353$).

At the present time, our cutoff results cannot be compared with the results of other studies in terms of thresholds, since they consider both (the prostatectomized and the irradiated patients) in one common patient group. Otherwise, only the RP-group is analyzed. Radiation groups are rarely examined alone for calculating cutoff levels.

3.7. Subpopulations

The performance of ^{68}Ga-PSMA-11 PET/CT has to be appraised for a therapeutic approach. In particular, the detection of local LNM should be considered, which could lead to a changed therapeutic approach (salvage RP plus LNM dissection or salvage RT with extended radiation field).

We took a closer look at PSA range between 0.2 ng/mL to < 1 ng/mL for post-prostatectomized patients based on the EAU guidelines for performing PSMA PET/CT in different initial situations [8]. The guidelines do not specify a threshold after primary radiation, so we have not formed a subgroup for these patients [8]. In the RP-group, 29% of patients showed PSA values that were between 0.2 and < 1 ng/mL with a PSMA-positivity rate of 52%. There was a significant association between the pre-scan PSA and an increased likelihood of a positive PSMA-scan was proven ($p < 0.001$). In comparison, Eiber et al. demonstrated positive scans in 57.9% for PSA values of 0.2 to < 0.5 ng/mL and even 72.7% at 0.5 to < 1 ng/mL [20]. A published study by Graziani et al. showed that only about 45% of the scans were positive while using hybrid imaging with ^{11}C-choline PET/CT in patients, even with PSA levels between 1 and 2 ng/mL. Multimetastatic disease was detected in 38% of all scans and distant lesions in 19% of the patients with PSA levels between 1–2 ng/mL [37]. In the present study, ^{68}Ga-PSMA-11 PET/CT revealed local metastases in 59%, multimetastatic disease in 44%, and distant lesions were shown in 13% of the subpopulation patients. A clinically relevant number of patients can be selected for salvage therapy due to the effectiveness of ^{68}Ga-PSMA-11 PET/CT for the detection of metastases, which is apparently higher than that of ^{11}C-choline, possibly even for metastatic-directed treatment, which might justify salvage LN dissection rather than systemic therapeutic path, thereby help to avoid unnecessary procedures and complications and also improve the chance of a clinical recurrence-free survival [38,39].

3.8. GS

Histopathological GS was significantly associated with positive ^{68}Ga-PSMA-11 PET/CT results ($p < 0.001$). Patients with GS of 7b (intermediate risk and grade group 3) and > 7 (high risk and grade group 4 or 5) showed an increased incidence of positive ^{68}Ga-PSMA-11 PET/CT scans ($p < 0.001$). Between patients with PSMA-positive scans corresponding to GS 7a (intermediate risk and grade group 2) and PSMA-positive scans corresponding to GS 7b, there was a significant demarcation ($p < 0.001$). Regarding the clinically important, highly significant differentiation between GS 7a (3 + 4) and 7b (4 + 3), patients with GS 7b exhibited more frequent pathologic ^{68}Ga-PSMA-11 PET/CT scans and metastases [8,40]. Therefore, the findings of hybrid imaging with ^{68}Ga-PSMA-11 agree in many cases with higher risk relapses on the basis of histology (frequency and detection of metastases). Our results are in line with other studies, which could possibly be due to the fact that the PSMA expression is usually more intense in higher-grade GS lesions than in lesions with a lower-grade GS [8,12,23,41]. Our results correspond to the immunohistochemical results of PSMA expression in PC [20].

3.9. ADT

The positivity rate of ^{68}Ga-PSMA-11 PET/CT was significantly correlated with accompanying ADT in this study. This is in line with the results of a study, in which the ADT-treated patients revealed positive PET/CT results more often and that was believed to be due to the frequent use of ADT in patients with advanced disease [20]. The same phenomenon has also been described when using ^{11}C-choline [37]. Furthermore, there have been reports of higher PSMA-expression of PC tumor cells as part of ADT [42]. Overall, the scientific knowledge on this issue remains unclear and further studies are needed [12,20].

3.10. AP

In our study, patients with PSMA-positive lesions showed higher AP levels than patients with negative PSMA scans ($p < 0.001$). Additionally, the detection of bone metastases was significantly associated with high AP. Our results corroborate the findings of other studies where serum AP was found to be a predictor for bone involvement of PC and to be an efficient and reliable biomarker for the prognosis of PC [43]. The AP levels were higher in patients with positive ^{68}Ga-PSMA-11 PET/CT scan results, with higher PSA levels, in patients receiving ADT and in patients exhibiting bone metastases in our study. Li et al. suggest that high AP is significantly related to poor overall survival and poor progression-free survival in PC, but there is no apparent association to cancer specific survival [43]. Skeletal AP is prognostic for bone metastases for M-staging of PC, and it is a dependable marker of osteoblastic activity. Another study demonstrated that AP levels were more closely associated with pathological bone scans than with PSA values and that the amount of AP was positively related to bone metastases [44]. From this, we conclude that the term "bone-specific AP" can reasonably be used.

4. Materials and Methods

4.1. Patient Characteristics

581 BC patients that had previously been treated with RP or RT, underwent ^{68}Ga-PSMA-11 (Glu-urea-Lys(Ahx)-HBED-CC) PET/CT between 2015 and 2019 and were retrospectively evaluated. The inclusion criteria for the performance of a ^{68}Ga-PSMA-11 PET/CT scan were: (a) histopathologically proven primary PC; (b) treatment with RP or RT (with or without ADT); and, (c) proven BC by definition (BC is defined as an elevation of the PSA value after primary treatment to > 0.2 ng/mL after RP or > 2 ng/mL above nadir following RT). The data on some of the patients included were already considered in another study with different aim. The PSA levels were available at the time of surgery as well as nadir, interim, and PET/CT scans (BC). Mean relapse PSA levels were 18.21 ng/mL ± 101.91 ng/mL (median 2.98, range 0.2–2000). 209 patients were treated with anti-androgens (Table 1). The patient data were collected from four Nuclear Medicine Institutions (a–d) in Germany. We have classified the patients into the following groups: (1) To obtain a clean statistic, we looked at the patient-group after RP and the patient group after RT separately, as, by definition, they have a different BC. (2) The subgroup of RP-patients was divided into five groups: 0.2 to < 0.5 ng/mL, 0.5 to < 1 ng/mL, 1 to < 2 ng/mL, 2 to < 5 ng/mL, and 5 ng/mL, and above. (3) The RT-patients were divided into two groups: 2 to < 5 ng/mL and 5 ng/mL and above. Additionally, patients were assigned to five-tiered GS groups: < 7, 7a and 7b, 8 and > 8, respectively. The following parameters were evaluated: ^{68}Ga-PSMA PET/CT scan results, PSA values, PSA kinetics, SUV_{max} of the malignant lesions, GS, ADT, AP and local/distant/single/multiple metastases, regional and/or distant LNM, bone metastases, and visceral metastases (e.g., lung). The main limitation of this retrospective study as compared to many other retrospective studies is that most of the patients did not have histopathological confirmation of the lesions. As a result, we use the term positivity rate instead of detection rate in this study. In addition to the histopathological findings (when available), we used a significant increase in PSA or a decrease in PSA after subsequent therapy (e.g. salvage RT) or a confirmation of the pathological focus in follow-up imaging or an increase and/or enlargement of the lesions in follow-up imaging, as indicators. We evaluated the optimal cutoff level by calculating PSA and PSA kinetics thresholds while using the ROC curve to determine the best time to perform ^{68}Ga-PSMA-11 PET/CT scans in patients with BC. The present study was in accordance with the Helsinki Declaration and the German Medicinal Products Act, AMG §13.2b. The retrospective study was conducted in accordance with the Declaration of Helsinki, and the Ethics Committee of Laek Rlp (2018-13390, approval date: 29 October 2018) and Aek No (41/2019, approval date: 22 February 2019) approved the protocol. All of the patients gave their written informed consent for the examination and for inclusion in the study.

4.2. Radiopharmaceuticals

The ^{68}Ga-labelled PSMA ligand, Glu-urea-Lys(Ahx)-HBED-CC (^{68}Ga-PSMA-11), was synthesized while using modification of a method described in 2012 [16]. In short, ^{68}Ga was achieved from a ^{68}Ge/^{68}Ga radionuclide generator (Garching, Germany) to be used to label the PSMA ligand. The labelled tracer without carrier additive was cleaned using a reverse phase cartridge (Sep-Pak C18 Plus Light cartridge, 130 mg Sorbent; Waters) and formulated in 10 mL phosphate-buffered saline with 5% by volume ETOH. Confirmation by radio thin-layer chromatography (TLC) and high-performance liquid chromatography (HPLC) was able to show a radiochemical purification yield of over 98%. ^{68}Ga-PSMA-11 was obtained from the Clinic of Nuclear Medicine of the Medical Center of the University Johannes Gutenberg (Mainz, Germany; b, c), from Advanced Accelerator Applications (Bonn, Germany; b, c), from Eckert & Ziegler (Bonn, Germany; d) or was produced in house (Mainz, Germany; a), depending on the availability.

4.3. Imaging Protocol

Each patient received an intravenous injection of ^{68}Ga-PSMA-11 (mean and SD: 199 ± 61 MBq, median activity: 200 MBq, range: 50–390 MBq). The PET data of tracer distribution were acquired 60 ± 10 min. (whole body) after injection of ^{68}Ga-PSMA-11. The patients were imaged on a PET/CT scanner named Gemini TF16 (Philips Medical Systems, Best, The Netherlands) (a, c) or a PET/CT scanner, named Biograph 64/Z64, R4 (HD and time of flight)/Biograph 64 TruePoint (True V HD; Siemens, Erlangen, Germany) (b, d). Either a mid-inspiratory low-dose CT scan (120 kV, 20–60 mAs, CT transverse scan field 50 cm, 70 cm extended field of view, high contrast resolution 1.0 s, 0.6 mm) without contrast enhancement or a maximum inspiratory venous-phase diagnostic contrast enhanced (Ultravist 300; Bayer AG, Berlin, Germany) CT scan (140 kV, 100–400 mAs, dose modulation) from the head to the upper-thigh was used for anatomical correlation and for attenuation corrections. PET was performed while using a standard technique on a dedicated three-dimensional (3D) system (a, c: matrix 144 × 144; d: 400 × 400; b: 168 × 168), with an acquisition time of 3 min. per bed position (axial field of view d: 13.3 cm; b: 21.8 cm; c: 19 cm; a: 18 cm). Random, scatter, and decay correction were applied to the emission data. Ordered-subsets expectation maximization method (OSEM) (a: three iterations, 33 subsets, Gaussian filtering, 4.3 mm full-width at half-maximum; b, c: two iterations, 14 subsets, Gaussian filtering, 5 mm (c) or 4.2 mm (b) transaxial resolution, full-width at half-maximum; d: three iterations, 24 subsets, Gaussian filtering, 5 mm transaxial resolution, full-width at half-maximum) was used for PET image reconstruction. The CT data were converted to attenuation coefficients at 511 keV and applied for attenuation corrections of the PET images.

4.4. Imaging Analysis

The PET/CT images were first visually assessed by individual specialists (nuclear medicine physician, radiologist) while applying coronal, transaxial, and sagittal layers. Subsequently, all of the images were interpreted in consensus by at least one experienced nuclear medicine physician, and two experienced radiologists, each of them board-certified and with PET/CT experience of more than five years as well as rich experience in interpretation of hybrid imaging with ^{68}Ga-PSMA-11. The final diagnosis was reached by consensus. Any PSMA-avid lesion with a morphological substrate on CT and an uptake above the background (but not correlated with physiological tracer uptake) was considered as being suggestive of PC. The SUV_{max} was measured for all lesions, suspicious of malignancy. PSMA-PET-avid lesions as described above were classified as suspected local recurrence in the prostate or prostate bed, as local/regional LN in the pelvis (iliac and/or pararectal) or as distant/extrapelvic LN (retroperitoneal and/or above the iliac bifurcation), as well as bone metastases and visceral metastases (lung, liver, adrenals, soft tissue, spleen, thyroid). When conflicting interpretations were identified, they were discussed and solved by the panel and consensus was passed between the reviewing physicians.

4.5. Statistical Analysis

Statistical analyses were performed while using SPSS version 24.0 (IBM Corporation, Ehningen, Germany). For continuous metric normally distributed variables, Students t-test was performed to determine differences between two groups. Multivariate variance analysis was used for comparison of more than two groups. We analyzed non-normally distributed continuous variables by Mann-Whitney-U test. The Wilcoxon signed rank test was calculated for determining the changes of PSA levels. For further analysis, we subdivided the metric values (e.g., PSAvel and PSAdt) into categories. We analyzed these nominal and ordinal parameters with Chi-square test and Pearson correlation. The performance of ^{68}Ga-PSMA-11 PET/CT was assessed in relation to these parameters by

ROC curves in order to determine the optimal cutoff of PSA levels and of PSA kinetics to differentiate between positive and negative scan results. The data are presented as mean, SD, and/or median and range. $p < 0.05$ was considered to be significant.

5. Conclusions

This study identifies the PSA and PSA kinetics thresholds for the presence of ^{68}Ga-PSMA-11 PET/CT-detectable PC-lesions in patients with BC. Pre-scan PSA was the main predictor of a positive scan with an optimal cutoff level of 1.24 ng/mL for patients that were primarily treated with RP. In this subgroup, kinetics analysis of PSA calculated a threshold velocity of 1.32 ng/mL/year.

We conclude that the PSA levels and kinetics (PSAvel) are suitable risk markers for optimizing the selection of patients who may benefit from ^{68}Ga-PSMA-11 PET/CT, especially in the subgroup of prostatectomized patients. ^{68}Ga-PSMA-11 PET/CT has a great impact on selecting patients with primary RP for salvage RT with curative intent.

Author Contributions: Conceptualization, M.A.H., H.-G.B., H.J.W., M.M. and M.S.; methodology, M.A.H., H.-G.B., H.J.W., M.M., F.R. and M.S.; software, M.A.H., H.-G.B., N.F., J.M.-H. and L.T.; validation, M.A.H., H.-G.B., H.J.W., M.M., F.R., N.F. and M.S.; formal analysis, M.A.H., H.-G.B., H.J.W., M.M., F.R., N.F. and S.P.; investigation, M.A.H., H.J.W., M.M., J.M.-H., L.T. and S.P.; resources, M.A.H., H.-G.B., H.J.W. and M.M.; data curation, H.J.W., M.M., J.M.-H., L.T. and M.S.; writing—original draft preparation, M.A.H., H.-G.B., H.J.W., M.M. and M.S.; writing—review and editing, H.J.W., M.M., F.R., N.F., S.P. and M.S.; visualization, M.A.H., H.-G.B., S.P., and M.S.; supervision, M.M. and M.S.; project administration, H.J.W., M.M. and M.S. All authors have read and agreed to the published version of the manuscript.

Acknowledgments: The authors thank Ed Michaelson, MD, Fort Lauderdale, Florida, for language revision and Jennifer Steffens, Germany, for technical assistance.

References

1. Pilleron, S.; Sarfati, D.; Janssen-Heijnen, M.; Vignat, J.; Ferlay, J.; Bray, F.; Soerjomataram, I. Global Cancer Incidence in Older Adults, 2012 and 2035: A population-based study. *Int. J. Cancer* **2019**, *144*, 49–58. [CrossRef]
2. World Health Organization. Healthy Ageing. In *World Report an Ageing and Health*; WHO Press: Geneva, Switzerland, 2015; Available online: https://apps.who.int/iris/bitstream/handle/10665/186463/9789240694811_eng.pdf?sequence=1 (accessed on 15 November 2019).
3. Andriole, G.L.; Crawford, E.D.; Grubb, R.L., 3rd; Buys, S.S.; Chia, D.; Church, T.R.; Fouad, M.N.; Gelmann, E.P.; Kvale, P.A.; Reding, D.J.; et al. Mortality results from a randomized prostate-cancer screening trial. *N. Engl. J. Med.* **2009**, *360*, 1310–1319. [CrossRef] [PubMed]
4. Castellucci, P.; Picchio, M. 11C-choline PET/CT and PSA kinetics. *Eur. J. Nucl. Med. Mol. Imaging* **2013**, *40*, 36–40. [CrossRef] [PubMed]
5. Darwish, O.M.; Raj, G.V. Management of biochemical recurrence after primary localized therapy for prostate cancer. *Front. Oncol.* **2012**, *2*, 48. [CrossRef]
6. Von Eyben, F.E.; Picchio, M.; Von Eyben, R.; Rhee, H.; Bauman, G. ^{68}Ga-Labeled Prostate-specific Membrane Antigen Ligand Positron Emission Tomography/Computed Tomography for Prostate Cancer: A Systematic Review and Meta-analysis. *Eur. Urol. Focus* **2018**, *4*, 686–693. [CrossRef]
7. Cornford, P.; Bellmunt, J.; Bolla, M.; Briers, E.; De Santis, M.; Gross, T.; Henry, A.M.; Joniau, S.; Lam, T.B.; Mason, M.D.; et al. EAU-ESTRO-SIOG Guidelines on Prostate Cancer. Part II: Treatment of Relapsing, Metastatic, and Castration-Resistant Prostate Cancer. *Eur. Urol.* **2017**, *71*, 630–642. [CrossRef]
8. Mottet, N.; Bellmunt, J.; Briers, E.; Bolla, M.; Bourke, L.; Cornford, P.; De Santis, M.; Henry, A.; Joniau, S.; Lam, T. Members of the EAU-ESTRO-ESUR-SIOG Prostate Cancer Guidelines Panel. EAU-ESTRO-ESUR-SIOG Guidelines on Prostate Cancer. Available online: https://uroweb.org/guideline/prostate-cancer/ (accessed on 19 March 2019).
9. Chiaravalloti, A.; Di Biagio, D.; Tavolozza, M.; Calabria, F.; Schillaci, O. PET/CT with (18)F-choline after radical prostatectomy in patients with PSA. *Eur. J. Nucl. Med. Mol. Imaging* **2016**, *43*, 1418–1424. [CrossRef] [PubMed]

10. Pijoan, J.M. Diagnostic methodology for the biochemical recurrence of prostate cancer after radiotherapy. *Arch. Españoles Urol.* **2006**, *59*, 1053–1062.
11. Wayant, C.; Cooper, C.; Turner, D.; Vassar, M. Evaluation of the NCCN guidelines using the RIGHT Statement and AGREE II instrument: A cross-sectional review. *BMJ Evid.-Based Med.* **2019**, *24*, 219–226. [CrossRef] [PubMed]
12. Afshar-Oromieh, A.; Avtzi, E.; Giesel, F.L.; Holland-Letz, T.; Linhart, H.G.; Eder, M.; Eisenhut, M.; Boxler, S.; Hadaschik, B.A.; Kratochwil, C.; et al. The diagnostic value of PET/CT imaging with the $^{(68)}$Ga-labelled PSMA ligand HBED-CC in the diagnosis of recurrent prostate cancer. *Eur. J. Nucl. Med. Mol. Imaging* **2015**, *42*, 197–209. [CrossRef]
13. Banerjee, S.R.; Pullambhatla, M.; Byun, Y.; Nimmagadda, S.; Green, G.; Fox, J.J.; Horti, A.; Mease, R.C.; Pomper, M.G. ^{68}Ga-labeled inhibitors of prostate-specific membrane antigen (PSMA) for imaging prostate cancer. *J. Med. Chem.* **2010**, *53*, 5333–5341. [CrossRef]
14. Mestre, R.P.; Treglia, G.; Ferrari, M.; Pascale, M.; Mazzara, C.; Azinwi, N.C.; Llado', A.; Stathis, A.; Giovanella, L.; Roggero, E. Correlation between PSA kinetics and PSMA-PET in prostate cancer restaging: A meta-analysis. *Eur. J. Clin. Investig.* **2019**, *49*, e13063. [CrossRef]
15. Eder, M.; Neels, O.; Müller, M.; Bauder-Wüst, U.; Remde, Y.; Schäfer, M.; Hennrich, U.; Eisenhut, M.; Afshar-Oromieh, A.; Haberkorn, U.; et al. Novel Preclinical and Radiopharma-ceutical Aspects of [68Ga]Ga-PSMA-HBED-CC: A new PET tracer for imaging of prostate cancer. *Pharmaceuticals* **2014**, *7*, 779–796. [CrossRef]
16. Eder, M.; Schäfer, M.; Bauder-Wüst, U.; Hull, W.-E.; Wängler, C.; Mier, W.; Haberkorn, U.; Eisenhut, M. ^{68}Ga-Complex Lipophilicity and the Targeting Property of a Urea-Based PSMA Inhibitor for PET Imaging. *Bioconjugate Chem.* **2012**, *23*, 688–697. [CrossRef]
17. Mottet, N.; Bellmunt, J.; Bolla, M.; Briers, E.; Cumberbatch, M.G.; De Santis, M.; Fossati, N.; Gross, T.; Henri, A.M.; Henry, A.M.; et al. EAU-ESTRO-SIOG Guidelines on Prostate Cancer. Part I: Screening, Diagnosis, and Local Treatment with Curative Intent. *Eur. Urol.* **2017**, *71*, 618–629. [CrossRef] [PubMed]
18. Dietlein, F.; Kobe, C.; Neubauer, S.; Schmidt, M.; Stockter, S.; Fischer, T.; Schomäcker, K.; Heidenreich, A.; Zlatopolskiy, B.D.; Neumaier, B.; et al. PSA-Stratified Performance of (18)F- and (68)Ga-PSMA PET in Patients with Biochemical Recurrence of Prostate Cancer. *J. Nucl. Med.* **2017**, *58*, 947–952. [CrossRef] [PubMed]
19. Giesel, F.L.; Hadaschik, B.; Cardinale, J.; Radtke, J.; Vinsensia, M.; Lehnert, W.; Kesch, C.; Tolstov, Y.; Singer, S.; Grabe, N.; et al. F-18 labelled PSMA-1007: Biodistribution, radiation dosimetry and histopathological validation of tumor lesions in prostate cancer patients. *Eur. J. Nucl. Med. Mol. Imaging* **2017**, *44*, 678–688. [CrossRef] [PubMed]
20. Eiber, M.; Maurer, T.; Souvatzoglou, M.; Beer, A.J.; Ruffani, A.; Haller, B.; Graner, F.-P.; Kübler, H.; Haberhorn, U.; Eisenhut, M.; et al. Evaluation of Hybrid 68Ga-PSMA Ligand PET/CT in 248 Patients with Biochemical Recurrence After Radical Prostatectomy. *J. Nucl. Med.* **2015**, *56*, 668–674. [CrossRef]
21. Fanti, S.; Oyen, W.; Lalumera, E. Consensus Procedures in Oncological Imaging: The Case of Prostate Cancer. *Cancers* **2019**, *11*, 1788. [CrossRef]
22. Zhao, Z.; Weickmann, S.; Jung, M.; Lein, M.; Kilic, E.; Stephan, C.; Erbersdobler, A.; Fendler, A.; Jung, K. A Novel Predictor Tool of Biochemical Recurrence after Radical Prostatectomy Based on a Five-MicroRNA Tissue Signature. *Cancers* **2019**, *11*, 1603. [CrossRef]
23. Hoffmann, M.A.; Wieler, H.J.; Baues, C.; Kuntz, N.J.; Richardsen, I.; Schreckenberger, M. The impact of ^{68}Ga-PSMA PET/CT and PET/MRT on the management of prostate cancer. *Urology* **2019**, *130*, 1–12. [CrossRef] [PubMed]
24. Hoffmann, M.A.; Miederer, M.; Wieler, H.J.; Ruf, C.; Jakobs, F.M.; Schreckenberger, M. Diagnostic performance of ^{68}Gallium-PSMA-11 PET/CT to detect significant prostate cancer and comparison with 18FEC PET/CT. *Oncotarget* **2017**, *8*, 111073–111083. [CrossRef] [PubMed]
25. Stephenson, A.J.; Scardino, P.T.; Kattan, M.W.; Pisansky, T.M.; Slawin, K.M.; Klein, E.A.; Anscher, M.S.; Michalski, J.M.; Sandler, H.M.; Lin, D.W.; et al. Predicting the Outcome of Salvage Radiation Therapy for Recurrent Prostate Cancer After Radical Prostatectomy. *J. Clin. Oncol.* **2007**, *25*, 2035–2041. [CrossRef]
26. Verburg, F.A.; Pfister, D.; Heidenreich, A.; Vogg, A.; Drude, N.I.; Vöö, S.; Mottaghy, F.M.; Behrendt, F.F. Extent of disease in recurrent prostate cancer determined by [(68)Ga]PSMA-HBED-CC PET/CT in relation to PSA levels, PSA doubling time and Gleason score. *Eur. J. Nucl. Med. Mol. Imaging* **2016**, *43*, 397–403. [CrossRef]

27. Calais, J.; Czernin, J.; Cao, M.; Kishan, A.U.; Hegde, J.V.; Shaverdian, N.; Sandler, K.; Chu, F.I.; King, C.R.; Steinberg, M.L.; et al. ^{68}Ga-PSMA-11 PET/CT mapping of prostate cancer biochemical recurrence after radical prostatectomy in 270 patients with a PSA level of less than 1.0 ng/mL: Impact on salvage radiotherapy planning. *J. Nucl. Med.* **2018**, *59*, 230–237. [CrossRef] [PubMed]
28. Mapelli, P.; Incerti, E.; Ceci, F.; Castellucci, P.; Fanti, S.; Picchio, M. 11C- or 18F-Choline PET/CT for Imaging Evaluation of Biochemical Recurrence of Prostate Cancer. *J. Nucl. Med.* **2016**, *57*, 43–48. [CrossRef] [PubMed]
29. Afshar-Oromieh, A.; Zechmann, C.M.; Malcher, A.; Eder, M.; Eisenhut, M.; Linhart, H.G.; Holland-Letz, T.; Hadaschik, B.A.; Giesel, F.L.; Debus, J.; et al. Comparison of PET imaging with a (68)Ga-labelled PSMA ligand and (18)F-choline-based PET/CT for the diagnosis of recurrent prostate cancer. *Eur. J. Nucl. Med. Mol. Imaging* **2014**, *41*, 11–20. [CrossRef]
30. Krause, B.J.; Souvatzoglou, M.; Treiber, U. Imaging of prostate cancer with PET/CT and radioactively labeled choline derivates. *Urol. Oncol. Semin. Orig. Investig.* **2013**, *31*, 427–435. [CrossRef]
31. Kitajima, K.; Murphy, R.C.; Nathan, M.A. Choline PET/CT for imaging prostate cancer: An update. *Ann. Nucl. Med.* **2013**, *27*, 581–591. [CrossRef]
32. Graute, V.; Jansen, N.; Ubleis, C.; Seitz, M.; Hartenbach, M.; Scherr, M.K.; Thieme, S.; Cumming, P.; Klanke, K.; Tiling, R.; et al. Relationship between PSA kinetics and [18F]fluorocholine PET/CT detection rates of recurrence in patients with prostate cancer after total prostatectomy. *Eur. J. Nucl. Med. Mol. Imaging* **2012**, *39*, 271–282. [CrossRef]
33. Kuten, J.; Fahoum, I.; Savin, Z.; Shamni, O.; Gitstein, G.; Hershkovitz, V.; Mabjeesh, N.J.; Yossepowitch, O.; Mishani, E.; Even-Sapir, E. Head- to head Comparison of 68Ga-PSMA-11 with 18F-PSMA-1007 PET/CT in Staging Prostate Cancer Using Histopathology and Immunohistochemical Analysis as Reference-Standard. *J. Nucl. Med.* **2019**. [CrossRef] [PubMed]
34. Schillaci, O.; Calabria, F.; Tavolozza, M.; Caracciolo, C.R.; Agrò, E.F.; Miano, R.; Orlacchio, A.; Danieli, R.; Simonetti, G. Influence of PSA, PSA velocity and PSA doubling time on contrast-enhanced 18F-choline PET/CT detection rate in patients with rising PSA after radical prostatectomy. *Eur. J. Nucl. Med. Mol. Imaging* **2012**, *39*, 589–596. [CrossRef] [PubMed]
35. Afshar-Oromieh, A.; Holland-Letz, T.; Giesel, F.L.; Kratochwil, C.; Mier, W.; Haufe, S.; Debus, N.; Eder, M.; Eisenhut, M.; Schäfer, M.; et al. Diagnostic performance of 68Ga-PSMA-11 (HBED-CC) PET/CT in patients with recurrent prostate cancer: Evaluation in 1007 patients. *Eur. J. Nucl. Med. Mol. Imaging* **2017**, *44*, 1258–1268. [CrossRef] [PubMed]
36. Ceci, F.; Uprimny, C.; Nilica, B.; Geraldo, L.; Kendler, D.; Kroiss, A.; Bektic, J.; Horninger, W.; Lukas, P.; Decristoforo, C.; et al. ^{68}Ga-PSMA PET/CT for restaging recurrent prostate cancer: Which factors are associated with PET/CT detection rate? *Eur. J. Nucl. Med. Mol. Imaging* **2015**, *42*, 1284–1294. [CrossRef]
37. Graziani, T.; Ceci, F.; Castellucci, P.; Polverari, G.; Lima, G.M.; Lodi, F.; Morganti, A.G.; Ardizzoni, A.; Schiavina, R.; Fanti, S. 11C-Choline PET/CT for restaging prostate cancer. Results from 4,426 scans in a single-centre patient series. *Eur. J. Nucl. Med. Mol. Imaging* **2016**, *43*, 1971–1979. [CrossRef]
38. Suardi, N.; Gandaglia, G.; Gallina, A.; Di Trapani, E.; Scattoni, V.; Vizziello, D.; Cucchiara, V.; Bertini, R.; Colombo, R.; Picchio, M.; et al. Long-term Outcomes of Salvage Lymph Node Dissection for Clinically Recurrent Prostate Cancer: Results of a Single-institution Series with a Minimum Follow-up of 5 Years. *Eur. Urol.* **2015**, *67*, 299–309. [CrossRef]
39. Ost, P.; Bossi, A.; Decaestecker, K.; De Meerleer, G.; Giannarini, G.; Karnes, R.J.; Roach, M.; Briganti, A. Metastasis-directed Therapy of Regional and Distant Recurrences After Curative Treatment of Prostate Cancer: A Systematic Review of the Literature. *Eur. Urol.* **2015**, *67*, 852–863. [CrossRef]
40. Kane, C.J.; Eggener, S.E.; Shindel, A.W.; Andriole, G.L. Variability in Outcomes for Patients with Intermediate-risk Prostate Cancer (Gleason Score 7, International Society of Urological Pathology Gleason Group 2–3) and Implications for Risk Stratification: A Systematic Review. *Eur. Urol. Focus* **2017**, *3*, 487–497. [CrossRef]
41. Kasperzyk, J.L.; Finn, S.P.; Flavin, R.; Fiorentino, M.; Lis, R.; Hendrickson, W.K.; Clinton, S.K.; Sesso, H.D.; Giovannucci, E.L.; Stampfer, M.J.; et al. Prostate-specific membrane antigen protein expression in tumor tissue and risk of lethal prostate cancer. *Cancer Epidemiol. Biomark. Prev.* **2013**, *22*, 2354–2363. [CrossRef]
42. Mostaghel, E.A.; Page, S.T.; Lin, D.W.; Fazli, L.; Coleman, I.M.; True, L.D.; Knudsen, B.; Hess, D.L.; Nelson, C.C.; Matsumoto, A.M.; et al. Intraprostatic Androgens and Androgen-Regulated Gene Expression

Persist after Testosterone Suppression: Therapeutic Implications for Castration-Resistant Prostate Cancer. *Cancer Res.* **2007**, *67*, 5033–5041. [CrossRef]

43. Li, N.; Lv, H.; Hao, X.; Hu, B.; Song, Y. Prognostic value of serum alkaline phosphatase in the survival of prostate cancer: Evidence from a meta-analysis. *Cancer Manag. Res.* **2018**, *10*, 3125–3139. [CrossRef] [PubMed]
44. Wymenga, L.; Boomsma, J.; Groenier, K.; Piers, D.; Mensink, H. Routine bone scans in patients with prostate cancer related to serum prostate-specific antigen and alkaline phosphatase. *BJU Int.* **2001**, *88*, 226–230. [CrossRef] [PubMed]

9

Diffusion-Weighted Imaging Can Differentiate between Malignant and Benign Pleural Diseases

Katsuo Usuda [1,*], Shun Iwai [1], Aika Funasaki [1], Atsushi Sekimura [1], Nozomu Motono [1], Munetaka Matoba [2], Mariko Doai [2], Sohsuke Yamada [3], Yoshimichi Ueda [4] and Hidetaka Uramoto [1]

1 Department of Thoracic Surgery, Kanazawa Medical University, Ishikawa 920-0293, Japan; mhg1214@kanazawa-med.ac.jp (S.I.); aicarby@kanazawa-med.ac.jp (A.F.); a24seki@kanazawa-med.ac.jp (A.S.); motono@kanazawa-med.ac.jp (N.M.); hidetaka@kanazawa-med.ac.jp (H.U.)

2 Department of Radiology, Kanazawa Medical University, Ishikawa 920-0293, Japan; m-matoba@kanazawa-med.ac.jp (M.M.); doaimari@kanazawa-med.ac.jp (M.D.)

3 Department of Pathology and Laboratory Medicine, Kanazawa Medical University, Ishikawa 920-0293, Japan; sohsuke@kanazawa-med.ac.jp

4 Department of Pathophysiological and Experimental Pathology, Kanazawa Medical University, Ishikawa 920-0293, Japan; z-ueda@kanazawa-med.ac.jp

* Correspondence: usuda@kanazawa-med.ac.jp

Abstract: It is not clear whether magnetic resonance imaging (MRI) is useful for the assessment of pleural diseases. The aim of this study is to determine whether diffusion-weighted magnetic resonance imaging (DWI) can differentiate malignant pleural mesothelioma (MPM) from pleural dissemination of lung cancer, empyema or pleural effusion. The DWI was calibrated with the b value of 0 and 800 s/mm^2. There were 11 MPMs (8 epithelioid and 3 biphasic), 10 pleural disseminations of lung cancer, 10 empyemas, and 12 pleural effusions. The apparent diffusion coefficient (ADC) of the pleural diseases was $1.22 \pm 0.25 \times 10^{-3}$ mm^2/s in the MPMs, $1.31 \pm 0.49 \times 10^{-3}$ mm^2/s in the pleural disseminations, $2.01 \pm 0.45 \times 10^{-3}$ mm^2/s in the empyemas and $3.76 \pm 0.62 \times 10^{-3}$ mm^2/s in the pleural effusions. The ADC of the MPMs and the pleural disseminations were significantly lower than the ADC of the empyemas and the pleural effusions. Concerning the diffusion pattern of DWI, all 11 MPMs showed strong continuous diffusion, 9 of 10 pleural disseminations showed strong scattered diffusion and 1 pleural dissemination showed strong continuous diffusion, all 10 empyemas showed weak continuous diffusion, and all 12 pleural effusions showed no decreased diffusion. DWI can evaluate pleural diseases morphologically and qualitatively, and thus differentiate between malignant and benign pleural diseases.

Keywords: magnetic resonance imaging; diffusion-weighted imaging; malignant pleural mesothelioma; pleural dissemination; empyema; pleural effusion

---

1. Introduction

Malignant pleural mesothelioma (MPM) is a highly lethal disease with limited therapeutic options that are difficult for patients to endure. Computed tomography (CT) is the primary imaging modality used to evaluate MPM and accurately track the spread of the primary tumor, the intrathoracic lymphadenopathy, as well as the extrathoracic spread. Early diagnosis of MPM is usually difficult in the modality of a chest CT, because pleural thickness or pleural effusion due to MPM can resemble a benign disease on a CT scan image. Additional imaging modalities, such as magnetic resonance imaging (MRI) and fluoro-2-deoxy-glucose positron emission tomography/computed tomography (FDG-PET/CT), have emerged in recent years and are complementary to CT for disease staging and evaluation of patients with MPM [1]. There have been several recent research papers that have shown that MRI is the best modality for the assessment of the pleural interface, characterization of complex pleural effusion, and identification of exudate and hemorrhages, and staging accuracy [2]. MRI is more accurate than CT in staging evaluation of local invasions in the endothoracic fascia or single chest wall focus (68% vs. 46%) and the diaphragm (82% vs. 55%) [3]. Diffusion-weighted magnetic resonance imaging (DWI) has reportedly been useful in differentiating malignant pleural diseases from benign alterations [4]. DWI utilizes the random, translational motion, or so-called Brownian movement, of water molecules in biologic tissue [5]. DWI has been used for brain imaging, mainly for the assessment of acute ischemic strokes, intracranial tumors and demyelinating diseases [6].

The purpose of this study was to determine whether DWI can differentiate MPM from pleural dissemination of lung cancer, empyema, or pleural effusion.

2. Results

Below is shown typical radiological imaging of an MPM (Figure 1), a pleural dissemination of lung cancer (Figure 2), an empyema (Figure 3) and a pleural effusion (Figure 4).

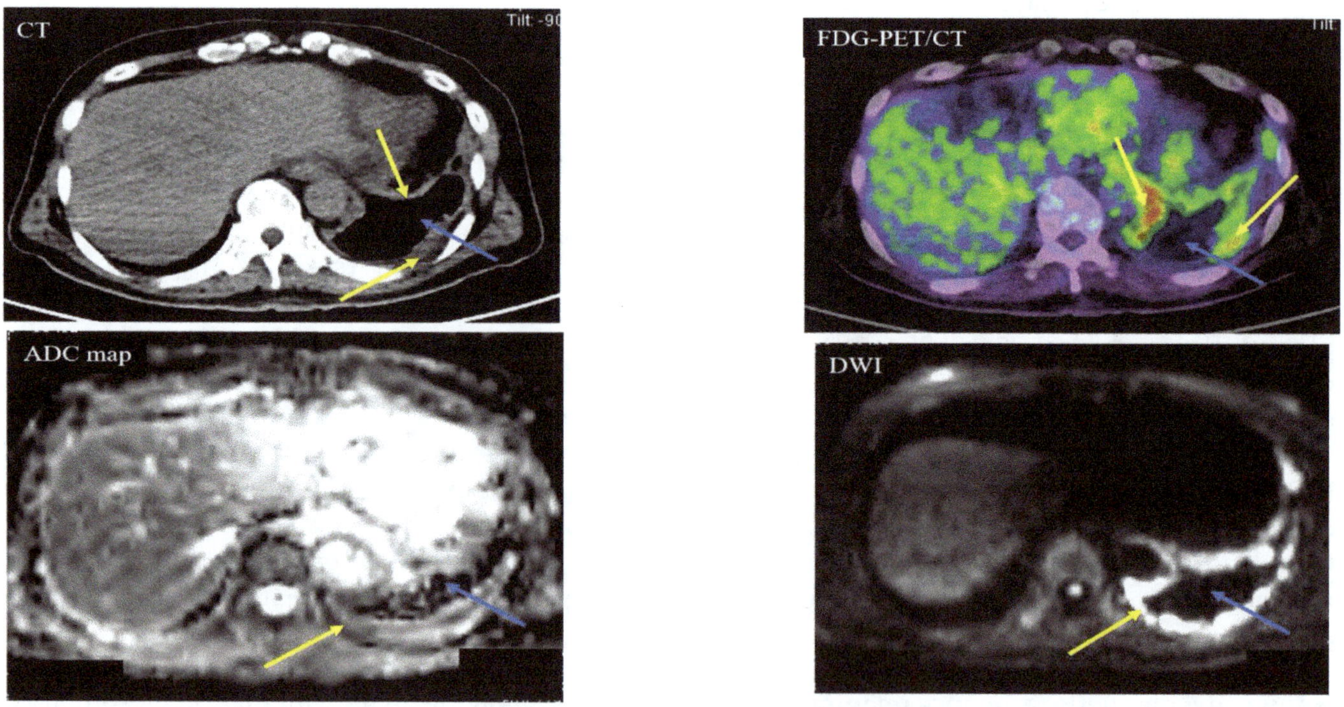

Figure 1. Case 1—Malignant Pleural Mesothelioma (MPM). A 64-year-old male with MPM (cT4N2M0). The yellow arrows indicate the MPM. The blue arrows indicate pleural effusion. Computed tomography (CT) showed left pleural thickness of the MPM. The apparent diffusion coefficient (ADC) of the MPM was 0.84×10^{-3} mm^2/s (positive) and the ADC of the pleural fluid was 3.95×10^{-3} mm^2/s (negative). Fluorodeoxyglucose (FDG)-position emission tomography (PET)/CT showed partial accumulation (standardized uptake value (SUV)max: 12.39) of FDG on the MPM.

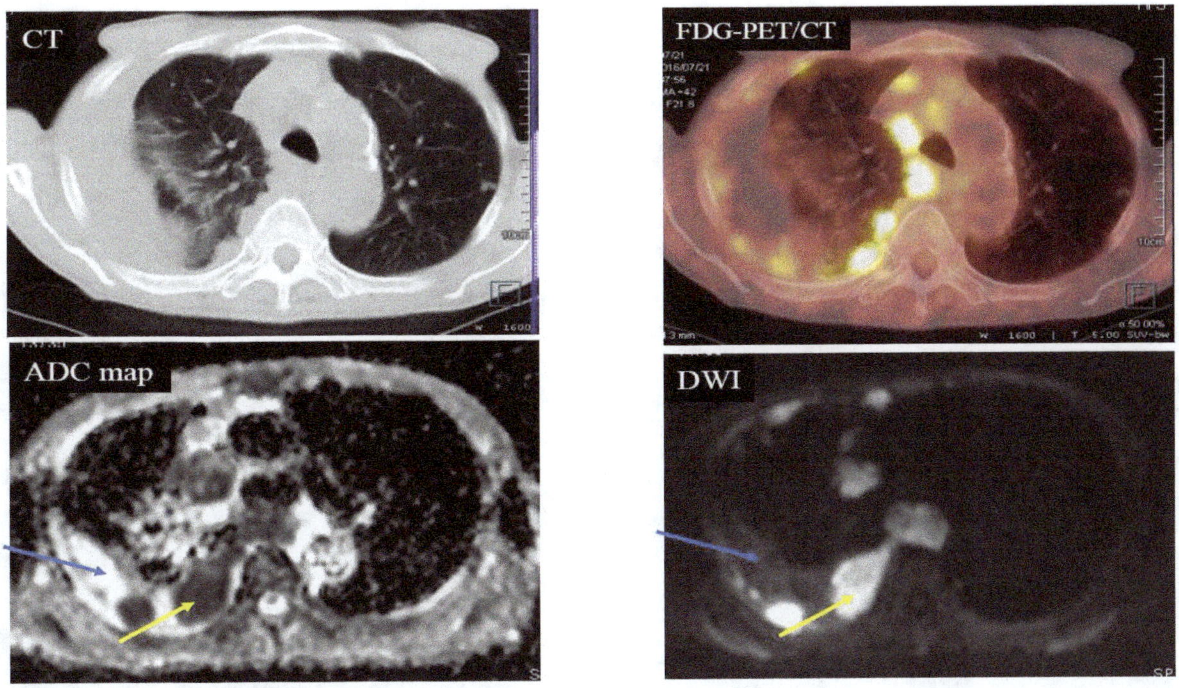

Figure 2. Case 2—Pleural dissemination of lung cancer. An 81-year-old male with pleural dissemination of a large cell neuroendocrine carcinoma. The yellow arrows indicate pleural dissemination. The blue arrows indicate pleural fluid. The apparent diffusion coefficient (ADC) of the pleural dissemination was 0.67×10^{-3} mm^2/s (positive) and the ADC of the pleural fluid was 3.03×10^{-3} mm^2/s (negative). Fluorodeoxyglucose-position emission tomography/computed tomography (FDG-PET/CT) showed scattered accumulation (standardized uptake value (SUVmax): 14.7) of the FDG on the pleural dissemination.

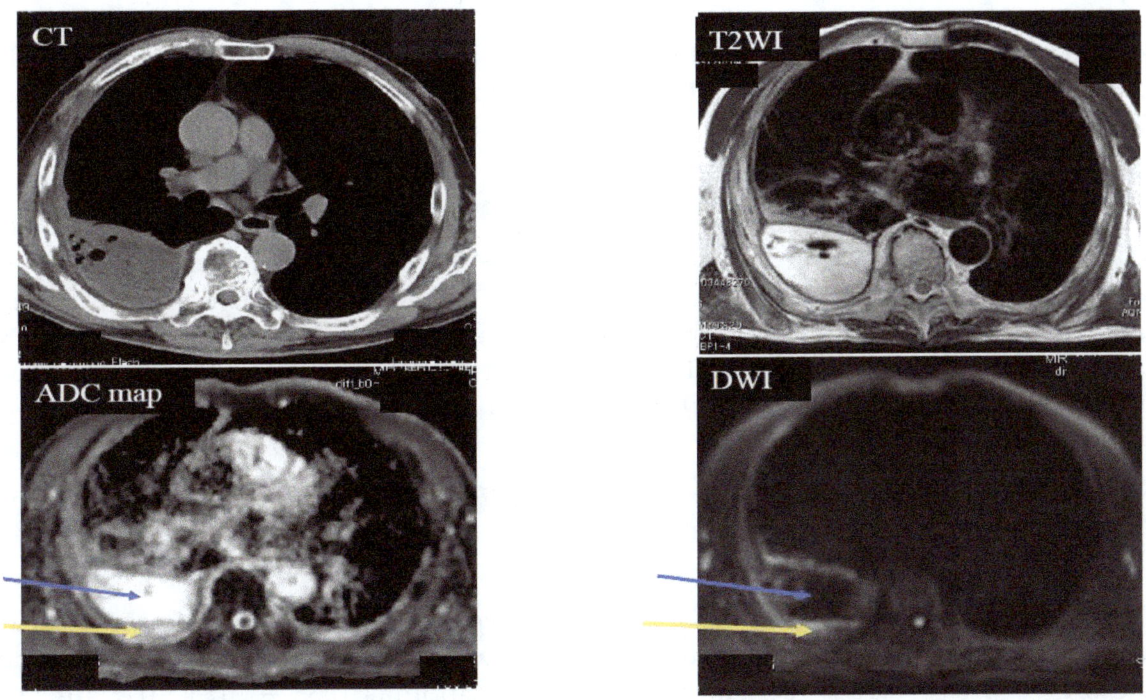

Figure 3. Case 3—Empyema. A 70-year-old male with right empyema. The yellow arrows indicate pleural thickness. The blue arrows indicate pleural fluid. The apparent diffusion coefficient (ADC) of the pleural thickness was 1.82×10^{-3} mm^2/s (negative) and the ADC of the pleural fluid was 3.95×10^{-3} mm^2/s (negative).

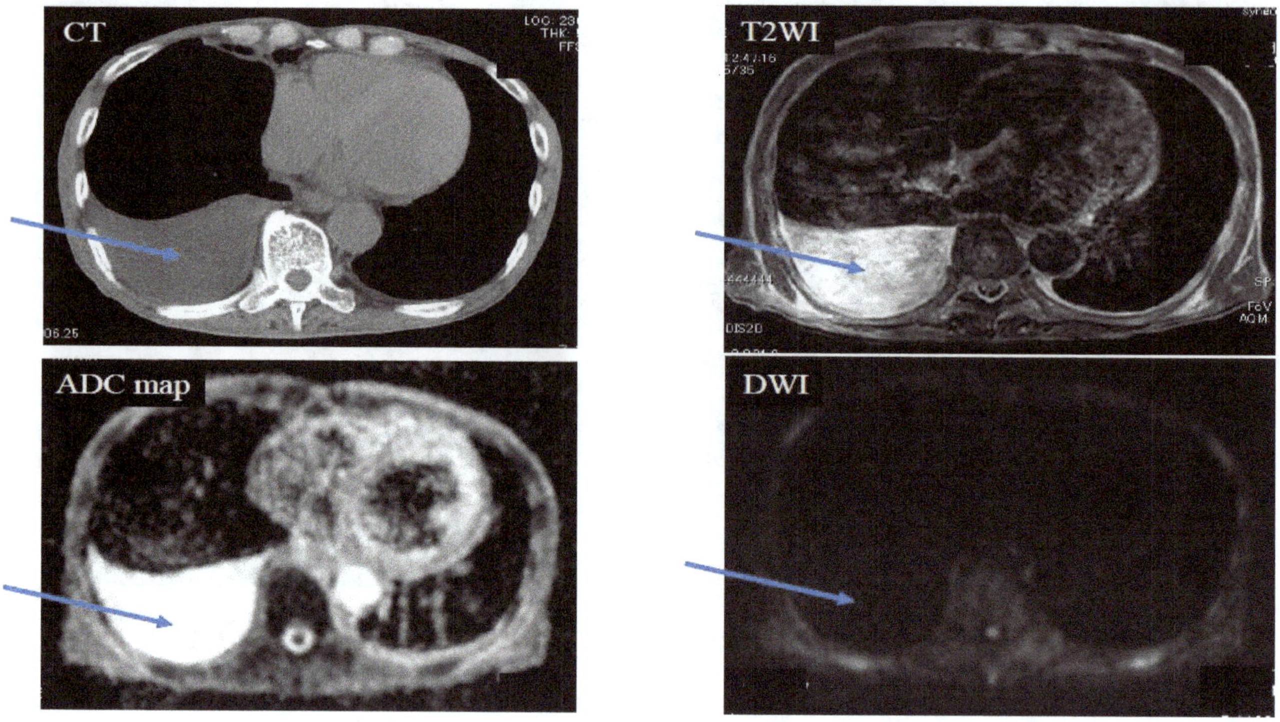

Figure 4. Case 4—Pleural effusion due to exudative pleurisy in a 79-year-old male, who suffered from right pneumonia. The blue arrows indicate pleural fluid. Pleural effusion was not seen in diffusion weighted magnetic resonance imaging (DWI). The apparent diffusion coefficient (ADC) of pleural fluid was 4.02×10^{-3} mm^2/s (negative).

Diffusion patterns based on pleural lesions are shown in Table 1. All 11 cases of MPM showed strong continuous diffusion. Nine of the 10 pleural disseminations showed strong scattered diffusion, and one pleural dissemination showed strong continuous diffusion. All 10 empyemas showed weak continuous diffusion. All 12 pleural effusions showed no decreased diffusion.

The ADC values of the pleural diseases were $1.22 \pm 0.25 \times 10^{-3}$ mm^2/s in the MPMs, $1.31 \pm 0.49 \times 10^{-3}$ mm^2/s in the pleural disseminations, $2.01 \pm 0.45 \times 10^{-3}$ mm^2/s in the empyemas and $3.76 \pm 0.62 \times 10^{-3}$ mm^2/s in the pleural effusions (Figure 5). The ADC of the MPMs was significantly lower than that of the empyemas ($P = 0.0007$) and the pleural effusions ($P < 0.0001$). The ADC values of the pleural disseminations were significantly lower than that of the empyemas ($P = 0.0086$) and the pleural effusions ($P < 0.0001$). The ADC of the MPM was not significantly different from that of pleural dissemination.

There were eight epithelioid and three biphasic MPMs. The ADC ($1.23 \pm 0.26 \times 10^{-3}$ mm^2/s) of the epithelioid MPMs was not significantly higher than the ADC ($1.17 \pm 0.21 \times 10^{-3}$ mm^2/s) of the biphasic MPMs ($P = 0.73$).

Of the 10 pleural disseminations of lung cancer, seven were adenocarcinomas, two were small cell carcinomas, and one was large cell neuroendocrine carcinoma (LCNEC). The ADC of the pleural dissemination was $1.63 \pm 0.13 \times 10^{-3}$ mm^2/s in adenocarcinomas, $0.68 \pm 0.18 \times 10^{-3}$ mm^2/s in small cell carcinomas, and 0.67×10^{-3} mm^2/s in a LCNEC. The ADC of adenocarcinomas was significantly higher than that of small cell carcinomas ($P = 0.0002$).

Six of the pleural effusions were exudative, two were caused by atelectasis, two were caused by malignant uterus tumors, one was caused by trauma, and one was caused by asbestosis. Because the two patients with malignant uterus tumors had negative results of pleural cytology and did not have pleural dissemination, the causes of pleural effusion in the malignant uterus tumors were not clear.

Table 1. Diffusion patterns of DWI for pleural lesions.

Diffusion Pattern		Strong Continuous	Strong Scattered	Weak Continuous	No Decreased	No. of Cases
Diagnosis	MPM	11	0	0	0	11
	Pleural dissemination	1	9	0	0	10
	Empyema	0	0	10	0	10
	Pleural effusion	0	0	0	12	12
No. of cases		12	9	10	12	43

MPM: Malignant Pleural Mesothelioma.

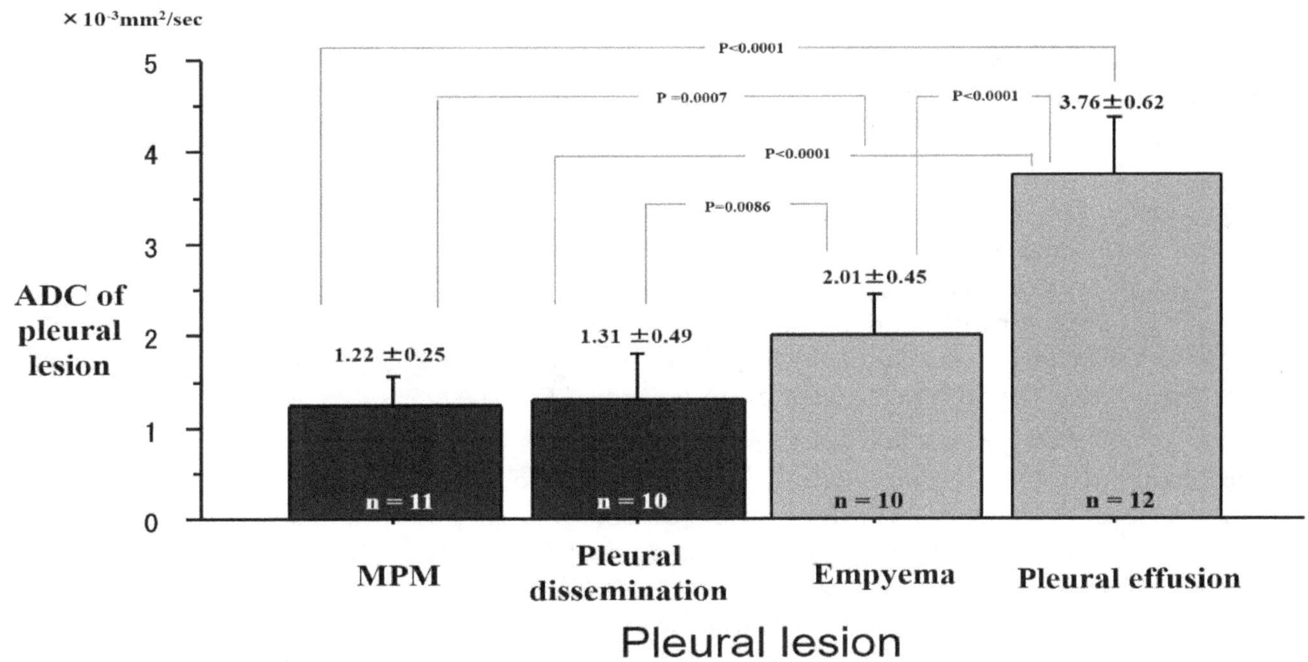

Figure 5. Differences of apparent diffusion coefficient (ADC) of pleural lesions. Mean ADCs were $1.22 \pm 0.25 \times 10^{-3}$ mm^2/s in Malignant Pleural Mesothelioma (MPM), $1.31 \pm 0.49 \times 10^{-3}$ mm^2/s in pleural dissemination, $2.01 \pm 0.45 \times 10^{-3}$ mm^2/s in empyema, and $3.76 \pm 0.62 \times 10^{-3}$ mm^2/s on pleural effusion. The ADC of the MPM was significantly lower than that of empyema ($P = 0.0007$) or pleural effusion ($P < 0.0001$). The ADC of pleural dissemination was significantly lower than that of empyema ($P = 0.0086$) or pleural effusion ($P < 0.0001$).

The ADC values of the pleural fluid were $3.87 \pm 0.29 \times 10^{-3}$ mm^2/s in MPMs, $3.59 \pm 0.57 \times 10^{-3}$ mm^2/s in the pleural disseminations, $2.40 \pm 1.26 \times 10^{-3}$ mm^2/s in the empyemas, and $3.94 \pm 0.27 \times 10^{-3}$ mm^2/s in the pleural effusions (Figure 6). The ADC of pleural fluid was significantly lower in the empyemas than in the MPMs ($P = 0.0023$), the pleural disseminations ($P = 0.0286$) and the pleural effusions ($P = 0.0009$). No significant differences in pleural fluid were found in MPMs, pleural disseminations, and pleural effusions.

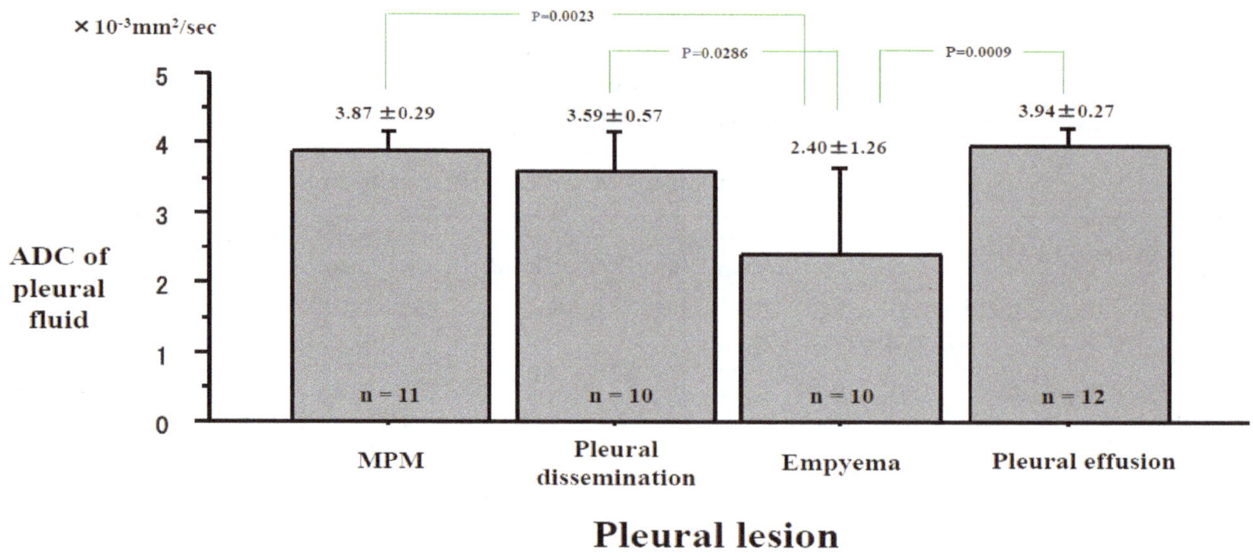

Figure 6. Differences in the apparent diffusion coefficient (ADC) of the pleural effusion inside the pleural lesions. The ADCs of pleural fluid were $3.87 \pm 0.29 \times 10^{-3}$ mm^2/s in Malignant Pleural Mesothelioma (MPM), $3.59 \pm 0.57 \times 10^{-3}$ mm^2/s in the pleural dissemination, $2.40 \pm 1.26 \times 10^{-3}$ mm^2/s in the empyema, and $3.94 \pm 0.27 \times 10^{-3}$ mm^2/s in the pleural effusion.

3. Discussion

DWI can be used to detect the restricted diffusion of water molecules in the body. Evidence has shown the advantage of DWI for functional information of neoplasm [7]. It has been reported that DWI has the potential for differential diagnosis of pulmonary nodules and masses, and evaluation of N factor/M factor/stage of lung cancer [8–11]. Two reports of meta-analysis concluded that DWI was an accurate modality to evaluate N factor of lung cancer [12,13].

Diagnosing MPM correctly in its early phases is very difficult with CT because of fewer symptoms, less pleural thickness or pleural effusion. At this stage, a chest CT would be performed to assess the pleural disease, but the MPM might not be detected. MRI is an important adjunctive imaging examination in thoracic oncologic imaging that is applied as a problem-solving tool to evaluate chest wall invasion, intraspinal extension, and cardiac/vascular invasion [14]. Moreover, functional MR imaging modality, such as DWI and dynamic contrast material–enhanced MR imaging modality, have already proven effective in differentiating malignant from benign pleural diseases and assessing chest wall and diaphragmatic involvement [15–19]. As this research has shown, DWI can diagnose an MPM as a malignant tumor with strong continuous diffusion over the entire circumference of the pleural with an ADC of less than 1.70×10^{-3} mm^2/s. The MPMs present marked restricted diffusion of the pleural tumor in DWI [20].

Coolen et al. [4] reported that visual evaluation of pleural pointillism was denoted by the presence of multiple, hyperintense pleural spots on high-b-value DWI. It is useful to differentiate MPM from benign alterations, which perform substantially better than mediastinal pleural thickness and shrinking lung. Pleural pointillism could be used to provide guidance for biopsies and thoracoscopic evaluations. In our article, one MPM also had hyperintense pleural diffusion on DWI, which we expressed as "strong continuous diffusion". Strong continuous diffusion and pleural pointillism can be seen in DWI of MPMs. Although pleural pointillism on high-*b*-value DWI had better sensitivity and accuracy than pleural thickness and lung shrinkage, the specificity was not significantly better, which suggests that the three parameters should complement, rather than substitute, one another. Gill et al. [19] also reported that the ADC value ($1.31 \pm 0.15 \times 10^{-3}$ mm^2/s) of the epithelioid MPMs was statistically higher than that ($1.01 \pm 0.11 \times 10^{-3}$ mm^2/s) of the biphasic MPMs (P = 0.00024). In our study, we could not repeat the results from Gill's article due to small sample size.

MRI has advantages over FDG-PET/CT due to its excellent soft tissue contrast and absence of ionizing radiation [7]. Uptake of FDG in FDG-PET/CT is not always tumor specific, as seen in benign inflammatory lesions, which can make accurate staging of MPMs difficult [21]. Although FDG-PET/CT is more effective than CT for differentiating malignant from benign pleural diseases [22], its utility is limited to assessing the primary tumor extension and the nodal status of MPM [23]. In general, FDG-PET/CT can detect thicker parts of MPMs, but not thinner parts of MPMs.

DWI could diagnose pleural dissemination from lung cancer as a malignant tumor with strong scattered diffusion along the pleura when the ADC was less than 1.70×10^{-3} mm^2/s. Pleural metastasis from breast cancer can be detected with DWI [24]. Moreover, DWI can evaluate pleural lesions morphologically and qualitatively, while also differentiating between malignant pleural diseases and benign pleural diseases. We have also shown that DWI can differentiate MPM from pleural dissemination.

In our cases of empyema, The ADC of the pleural effusion decreased due to pus. The ADC of pleural fluid in empyemas was significantly lower than the ADC of the MPMs, the pleural disseminations, and the pleural effusions. Abscesses and thrombi impede the diffusivity of water molecules due to their hyperviscous nature [7,25]. Therefore, the ADC value of empyema was significantly lower without a significant decreased diffusion of the pleura. To diagnose empyema, the ADC value of pleura and pleural cavity must be carefully evaluated.

MRI has proven superior to CT in the characterization of pleural fluid [26]. Pleural fluid is typically hypointense on T1-weighted imaging and hyperintense on T2-weighted imaging [2]. As shown in this article, when a patient with pleural fluid shows no decreased diffusion in DWI, and when the ADC of the pleural fluid is higher, the pleural disease can be identified as benign.

MRIs have several advantages. They do not involve contrast agents and examinations take less time. Furthermore, MRIs do not have the downside of radiation exposure and are suitable for children with negative reactions to radiation [27]. On the other hand, an MRI is not a viable option for people with devices, such as pacemakers, or tattoos. In addition, MRI examinations are loud, and can cause some patients anxiety.

Limitations

There are two important limitations in this study. First, this study was performed at a single institution and dealt with a small number of patients, which unavoidably introduced selection bias. Second, we could not acquire consent forms from all the patients who developed pleural lesions in the period from March 2015 to February 2019. Due to these limitations, our sample size was small. Our ADC measurements were repeated three times and the minimum ADC value was recorded. Thus, this ADC may not fully represent the whole tumor. There is no overwhelming agreement in the literature concerning optimal DWI techniques and image analysis procedures, including region of interest (ROI) size and placement.

Nevertheless, DWI has two limitations. First, some of the more common benign diseases which present decreased diffusion and lower ADC values in DWI are pulmonary abscesses and empyemas with histopathological necrosis. Second, mucinous adenocarcinomas were usually hypointense in DWI and showed higher ADC values, which could be misjudged as benign lesions in DWI [28]. Since mucinous adenocarcinomas had lower cellularity than tubular adenocarcinomas, it had lower DWI signal intensity and higher ADC values than tubular adenocarcinoma in the ano-rectal region [29].

4. Patients and Methods

4.1. Eligibility

The study protocol for evaluating pleural lesions with CT and MRI with DWI was approved by the ethical committee of Kanazawa Medical University (the approval number: No.189, the approval date:

25th January 2012). After discussing the risks and benefits of the examinations with their surgeons, we obtained written informed consents for CT and MRI from each patient.

4.2. Patients

A total of 43 patients with pleural diseases or pleural effusions underwent CT scans and MRI examinations and were enrolled in this study in the period from March 2015 to February 2019. Exclusion criteria were unwillingness to undergo an MRI examination, and the general issues that exclude most patients from getting an MRI (e.g., incompatible implanted medical devices, claustrophobia, and tattoos).

The diagnosis of MPM and pleural dissemination of lung cancers were confirmed histopathologically by biopsy or surgical procedure. The diagnosis of empyema was confirmed by positive culture of pleural effusion or by purulent pleural effusion. The diagnosis of pleural effusion was confirmed by negative cytology and negative culture of pleural effusion.

There were 11 MPMs, 10 pleural disseminations of lung cancers, 10 empyemas and 12 pleural effusions.

4.3. Magnetic Resonance Imaging (MRI)

The 1.5 T superconducting magnetic scanner (Magnetom Avanto; Siemens, Erlangen, Germany) with two anterior six-channel body phased-array coils and two posterior spinal clusters (six-channels each) was used for MRI examinations. The conventional MRI consisted of a coronal T1-weighted spin-echo sequence and coronal and axial T2-weighted fast spin-echo sequences. DWI using a single-shot echo-planar technique were performed under SPAIR (spectral attenuated inversion recovery) with respiratory triggered scan with the following parameter: b value = 0 and 800 s/mm^2; TR/TE/flip angle, 3000–4500/65/90; diffusion gradient encoding in three orthogonal directions; receiver bandwidth, 2442 Hz/Px; voxel size, 2.7 × 2.7 × 6.0 mm; field of view, 350 mm; matrix size, 128 × 128; number of excitations, 5; section thickness, 6 mm and section gap, 0 mm. After image reconstruction, a 2-dimensional (2D) round or elliptical ROI was marked on the lesion which was detected visually on the ADC map with reference to T1-weighted or CT image by a radiologist (M.D.) with 26 years of MRI experience who was unaware of the patients' clinical data. The procedure was done three times and we recorded the minimum apparent diffusion coefficient (ADC) value. A consensus was reached if there were any differences of opinion. The optical cutoff value (OCV) of ADC for diagnosing malignancy in DWI was determined to be 1.70×10^{-3} mm^2/s using the receiver operating characteristics (ROC) curve, as previously described [8]. Pleural lesions with an ADC value of the same or less than the OCV were classified as positive. Pleural lesions with ADC value of more than the OCV or those that could not be detected on DWI were classified as negative. Diffusion pattern of DWI were divided into 4 categories: ① strong continuous diffusion, ② strong scattered diffusion, ③ weak continuous diffusion and ④ no decreased diffusion.

FDG-PET/CTs were also used for the evaluation. FDG-PET/CTs were done with a dedicated PET camera (SIEMENS Biograph Sensation 16, Erlangen Germany). All patients fasted for 6 hours before the scans. The OCV of maximum standardized uptake value (SUVmax) for diagnosing malignancy in FDG-PET/CT was determined to be 4.45 using the ROC curve, as previously described [8].

4.4. Statistical Analysis

Using StatView for Windows (Version 5.0; SAS Institute Inc. Cary, NC, USA), statistical analysis was performed. The data is presented as the mean ± standard deviation. A two-tailed Student t test was used for comparison of ADC values of various pleural lesions. A p-value of <0.05 was deemed statistically significant.

5. Conclusions

DWI can evaluate pleural diseases morphologically and qualitatively, while also differentiating between malignant pleural diseases and benign pleural diseases. DWI has the ability to differentiate MPM from pleural dissemination.

Author Contributions: Conceptualization, K.U.; methodology, M.M. and M.D.; formal analysis, S.Y.; investigation, Y.U.; resources, S.I. and A.F.; data curation, A.S. and N.M.; writing—original draft preparation, K.U.; writing—review and editing, K.U.; supervision, H.U.

Acknowledgments: We are grateful to Keiya Hirata of the MRI Center, Kanazawa Medical University, for technical assistance. We are grateful to Dustin Keeling for proofreading this paper.

References

1. Nickell, L.T., Jr.; Lichtenberger, J.P., 3rd; Khorashadi, L.; Abbott, G.F.; Carter, B.W. Multimodality imaging for characterization, classification, and staging of malignant pleural mesothelioma. *Radiographics* **2014**, *34*, 1692–1706. [CrossRef] [PubMed]
2. Pessôa, F.M.; de Melo, A.S.; Souza, A.S.; de Souza, L.S.; Hochhegger, B.; Zanetti, G.; Marchiori, E. Applications of magnetic resonance imaging of the thorax in pleural diseases: A state-of-the-art review. *Lung* **2016**, *194*, 501–509. [CrossRef] [PubMed]
3. Heelan, R.T. Staging of malignant pleural mesothelioma: Comparison of CT and MR imaging. *Am. J. Roentgenol* **1999**, *172*, 1039–1047. [CrossRef] [PubMed]
4. Coolen, J.; De Keyzer, F.; Nafteux, P.; De Wever, W.; Dooms, C.; Vansteenkiste, J.; Derweduwen, A.; Roebben, I.; Verbeken, E.; De Leyn, P.; et al. Malignant pleural mesothelioma: Visual assessment by using pleural pointillism at diffusion-weighted MR imaging. *Radiology* **2015**, *274*, 576–584. [CrossRef] [PubMed]
5. Le Bihan, D.; Breton, E.; Lallemand, D.; Aubin, M.L.; Vignaud, J.; Laval-Jeantet, M. Separation of diffusion and perfusion in intravoxel incoherent motion MR imaging. *Radiology* **1988**, *168*, 497–505. [CrossRef] [PubMed]
6. Tien, R.D.; Felsberg, G.J.; Friedman, H.; Brown, M.; MacFall, J. MR imaging of high-grade cerebral gliomas: Value of diffusion-weighted echoplanar plus sequences. *Am. J. Roentgenol.* **1994**, *162*, 671–676. [CrossRef] [PubMed]
7. Kwee, T.C.; Takahara, T.; Ochiai, R.; Koh, D.M.; Ohno, Y.; Nakanishi, K.; Niwa, T.; Chenevert, T.L.; Luijten, P.R.; Alavi, A. Complementary roles of whole-body diffusion-weighted MRI and 18F-FDG PET: The state of the art and potential applications. *J. Nucl. Med.* **2010**, *51*, 1549–1558. [CrossRef] [PubMed]
8. Usuda, K.; Sagawa, M.; Motono, N.; Ueno, M.; Tanaka, M.; Machida, Y.; Matoba, M.; Kuginuki, Y.; Taniguchi, M.; Ueda, Y.; et al. Advantages of diffusion-weighted imaging over positron emission tomography-computed tomography in assessment of hilar and mediastinal lymph node in lung cancer. *Ann. Surg. Oncol.* **2013**, *20*, 1676–1683. [CrossRef]
9. Li, B.; Li, Q.; Chen, C.; Guan, Y.; Liu, S. A systematic review and meta-analysis of the accuracy of diffusion-weighted MRI in the detection of malignant pulmonary nodules and masses. *Acad. Radiol.* **2014**, *21*, 21–29. [CrossRef] [PubMed]
10. Shen, G.; Jia, Z.; Deng, H. Apparent diffusion coefficient values of diffusion-weighted imaging for distinguishing focal pulmonary lesions and characterizing the subtype of lung cancer: A meta-analysis. *Eur. Radiol.* **2016**, *26*, 556–566. [CrossRef]
11. Usuda, K.; Zhao, X.T.; Sagawa, M.; Matoba, M.; Kuginuki, Y.; Ueda, Y.; Sakuma, T. Diffusion-weighted imaging is superior to positron emission tomography in the detection and nodal assessment of lung cancers. *Ann. Thorac. Surg.* **2011**, *91*, 1689–1695. [CrossRef] [PubMed]
12. Peerlings, J.; Troost, E.G.; Nelemans, P.J.; Cobben, D.C.; de Boer, J.C.; Hoffmann, A.L.; Beets-Tan, R.G. The diagnostic value of MR Imaging in determining the lymph node status of patients with non-small cell lung cancer: A meta-analysis. *Radiology* **2016**, *281*, 86–98. [CrossRef] [PubMed]
13. Shen, G.; Hu, S.; Deng, H.; Kuang, A. Performance of DWI in the nodal characterization and assessment of lung cancer: A meta-analysis. *Am. J. Roentgenol.* **2016**, *206*, 283–290. [CrossRef] [PubMed]
14. Hayes, S.A.; Plodkowski, A.J.; Ginsberg, M.S. Imaging of Thoracic Cavity Tumors. *Surgical Oncology Clinics* **2014**, *23*, 709–733. [CrossRef] [PubMed]

15. Hierholzer, J.; Luo, L.; Bittner, R.C.; Stroszczynski, C.; Schröder, R.J.; Schoenfeld, N.; Dorow, P.; Loddenkemper, R.; Grassot, A. MRI and CT in the differential diagnosis of disease. *Chest* **2000**, *118*, 604–609. [CrossRef] [PubMed]
16. Luo, L.; Hierholzer, J.; Bittner, R.C.; Chen, J.; Huang, L. Magnetic resonance i pleural maging in distinguishing malignant from benign pleural disease. *Chin. Med. J.* **2001**, *114*, 645–649.
17. Luna, A.; Sanchez-Gonzalez, J.; Caro, P. Diffusion weighted imaging of the chest. *Magn. Reason. Imaging Clin. N. Am.* **2011**, *19*, 69–94. [CrossRef] [PubMed]
18. Coolen, J.; De Keyzer, F.; Nafteux, P.; De Wever, W.; Dooms, C.; Vansteenkiste, J.; Roebben, I.; Verbeken, E.; De Leyn, P.; Van Raemdonck, D.; et al. Malignant pleural disease: Diagnosis by using diffusion-weighted and dynamic contrast-enhanced MR imaging-initial experience. *Radiology* **2012**, *263*, 884–892. [CrossRef] [PubMed]
19. Gill, R.R.; Umeoka, S.; Mamata, H.; Tilleman, T.R.; Stanwell, P.; Woodhams, R.; Padera, R.F.; Sugarbaker, D.J.; Hatabu, H. Diffusion-weighted MRI of malignant pleural mesothelioma: Preliminary assessment of apparent diffusion coefficient in histologic subtypes. *Am. J. Roentgenol.* **2010**, *195*, W125–W130. [CrossRef] [PubMed]
20. Bonomi, M.; De Filippis, C.; Lopci, E.; Gianoncelli, L.; Rizzardi, G.; Cerchiaro, E.; Bortolotti, L.; Zanello, A.; Ceresoli, G.L. Clinical staging of malignant pleural mesothelioma: Current perspectives. *Lung Cancer Target Ther.* **2017**, *8*, 127–139. [CrossRef]
21. Jaruskova, M.; Belohlavek, O. Role of FDG-PET and PET/CT in the diagnosis of prolonged febrile states. *Eur. J. Nucl. Med. Mol. Imaging* **2006**, *33*, 913–918. [CrossRef] [PubMed]
22. Flores, R.M.; Akhurst, T.; Gonen, M.; Larson, S.M.; Rusch, V.W. Positron emission tomography defines metastatic disease but not locoregional disease in patients with malignant pleural mesothelioma. *J. Thorac. Cardiovasc. Surg.* **2003**, *126*, 11–16. [CrossRef]
23. Otsuka, H.; Terazawa, K.; Morita, N.; Otomi, Y.; Yamashita, K.; Nishitani, H. Is FDG-PET/CT useful for managing malignant pleural mesothelioma? *J. Med. Investig.* **2009**, *56*, 16–20. [CrossRef] [PubMed]
24. Yang, S.M.; Kim, S.H.; Kang, B.J.; Song, B.J. Extramammary findings on breast MRI: Prevalence and imaging characteristics favoring malignancy detection: A retrospective analysis. *World J. Surg. Oncol.* **2016**, *14*, 119. [CrossRef] [PubMed]
25. Desprechins, B.; Stadnik, T.; Koerts, G.; Shabana, W.; Breucq, C.; Osteaux, M. Use of diffusion-weighted MR imaging in differential diagnosis between intracerebral necrotic tumors and cerebral abscesses. *Am. J. Neuroradiol.* **1999**, *20*, 1252–1257. [PubMed]
26. Qureshi, N.R.; Gleeson, F.V. Imaging of pleural disease. *Clin. Chest Med.* **2006**, *27*, 193–213. [CrossRef] [PubMed]
27. Darge, K.; Jaramillo, D.; Siegel, M.J. Whole-body MRI in children: Current status and future applications. *Eur. J. Radiol.* **2008**, *68*, 289–298. [CrossRef] [PubMed]
28. Usuda, K.; Sagawa, M.; Motono, N.; Ueno, M.; Tanaka, M.; Machida, Y.; Tonami, H. Diagnostic performance of diffusion weighted imaging of malignant and benign pulmonary nodules and masses: Comparison with positron emission tomography. *Asian Pac. J. Cancer Prev.* **2014**, *15*, 4629–4635. [CrossRef] [PubMed]
29. Nasu, K.; Kuroki, Y.; Minami, M. Diffusion-weighted imaging findings of mucinous carcinoma arising in the ano-rectal region. Comparison of apparent diffusion coefficient with that of tubular adenocarcinoma. *Jpn. J. Radiol.* **2012**, *30*, 120–127. [CrossRef] [PubMed]

10

Role of Baseline and Post-Therapy ^{18}F-FDG PET in the Prognostic Stratification of Metastatic Castration-Resistant Prostate Cancer (mCRPC) Patients Treated with Radium-223

Matteo Bauckneht [1,*], Selene Capitanio [1], Maria Isabella Donegani [2], Elisa Zanardi [3,4], Alberto Miceli [2], Roberto Murialdo [5], Stefano Raffa [2], Laura Tomasello [3], Martina Vitti [2], Alessia Cavo [6], Fabio Catalano [7], Manlio Mencoboni [6], Marcello Ceppi [8], Cecilia Marini [2,9], Giuseppe Fornarini [7], Francesco Boccardo [3,4], Gianmario Sambuceti [1,2] and Silvia Morbelli [1,2]

1 Nuclear Medicine Unit, IRCCS Ospedale Policlinico San Martino, 16132 Genoa, Italy; selene.capitanio@hsanmartino.it (S.C.); sambuceti@unige.it (G.S.); silviadaniela.morbelli@hsanmartino.it (S.M.)
2 Department of Health Sciences (DISSAL), University of Genova, 16132 Genoa, Italy; isabella.donegani@gmail.com (M.I.D.); albertomiceli23@gmail.com (A.M.); stefanoraffa@live.com (S.R.); vitti.martina@hotmail.it (M.V.); cecilia.marini@unige.it (C.M.)
3 Academic Unit of Medical Oncology, IRCCS Ospedale Policlinico San Martino, 16132 Genoa, Italy; elisa.zanardi@unige.it (E.Z.); laura.tomasello@hsanmartino.it (L.T.); fboccardo@unige.it (F.B.)
4 Department of Internal Medicine and Medical Specialties (DIMI), University of Genoa, 16132 Genoa, Italy
5 Internal Medicine Unit, IRCCS Ospedale Policlinico San Martino, 16132 Genoa, Italy; roberto.murialdo@hsanmartino.it
6 Oncology Unit, Villa Scassi Hospital, 16149, Genova, Italy; alessia.cavo@asl3.liguria.it (A.C.); manlio.mencoboni@asl3.liguria.it (M.M.)
7 Medical Oncology Unit, IRCCS Ospedale Policlinico San Martino, 16132 Genoa, Italy; catalan.fab@gmail.com (F.C.); giuseppe.fornarini@hsanmartino.it (G.F.)
8 Clinical Epidemiology Unit, IRCCS Ospedale Policlinico San Martino, 16132 Genoa, Italy; marcello.ceppi@hsanmartino.it
9 CNR Institute of Molecular Bioimaging and Physiology (IBFM), 20090 Segrate (MI), Italy
* Correspondence: matteo.bauckneht@hsanmartino.it

Abstract: Radium-223 dichloride (Ra223) represents the unique bone-directed treatment option that shows an improvement in overall survival (OS) in metastatic castrate resistant prostate cancer (mCRPC). However, there is an urgent need for the identification of reliable biomarkers to non-invasively determine its efficacy (possibly improving patients' selection or identifying responders' after therapy completion). 18F-Fluorodeoxyglucose (FDG)-avidity is low in naïve prostate cancer, but it is enhanced in advanced and chemotherapy-refractory mCRPC, providing prognostic insights. Moreover, this tool showed high potential for the evaluation of response in cancer patients with bone involvement. For these reasons, FDG Positron Emission Tomography (FDG-PET) might represent an effective tool that is able to provide prognostic stratification (improving patients selection) at baseline and assessing the treatment response to Ra223. We conducted a retrospective analysis of 28 mCRPC patients that were treated with Ra223 and submitted to bone scan and FDG-PET/CT for prognostic purposes at baseline and within two months after therapy completion. The following parameters were measured: number of bone lesions at bone scan, SUVmax of the hottest bone lesion, metabolic tumor volume (MTV), and total lesion glycolysis (TLG). In patients who underwent post-therapy 18F-Fluorodeoxyglucose Positron Emission Tomography/Computed Tomography (FDG-PET/CT), (20/28), PET Response Criteria in Solid Tumors (PERCIST), and European Organization for Research and Treatment of Cancer (EORTC) criteria were applied to evaluate the metabolic treatment response. The difference between end of therapy and baseline values was also calculated for Metabolic Tumor Volume (MTV),

TLG, prostate-specific antigen (PSA), alkaline phosphatase (AP), and lactate dehydrogenase (LDH) (termed deltaMTV, deltaTLG, deltaPSA, deltaAP and deltaLDH, respectively). Predictive power of baseline and post-therapy PET- and biochemical-derived parameters on OS were assessed by Kaplan–Meier, univariate and multivariate analyses. At baseline, PSA, LDH, and MTV significantly predicted OS. However, MTV (but not PSA nor LDH) was able to identify a subgroup of patients with worse prognosis, even after adjusting for the number of lesions at bone scan (which, in turn, was not an independent predictor of OS). After therapy, PERCIST criteria were able to capture the response to Ra223 by demonstrating longer OS in patients with partial metabolic response. Moreover, the biochemical parameters were outperformed by PERCIST in the post-treatment setting, as their variation after therapy was not informative on long term OS. The present study supports the role of FDG-PET as a tool for patient's selection and response assessment in mCRPC patients undergoing Ra223 administration.

Keywords: Radium-223; positron emission tomography; FDG; castrate resistant prostate cancer

---

1. Introduction

Radium-223 dichloride (Ra223) is a radionuclide that selectively binds to areas of increased bone turnover in bone metastases. The short range of energy delivery that is typical of its apha-emission makes Ra223 an effective therapeutic approach for symptomatic patients with bone metastatic castration-resistant prostate cancer (mCRPC) [1].

Besides documenting its effect on pain palliation, the pivotal phase 3 Alpharadin in Symptomatic Prostate Cancer Patients (ALSYMPCA) trial demonstrated the prognostic benefit that is induced by this radio-metabolic approach that prolonged overall survival (OS) and delayed time to the first symptomatic skeletal event with respect to the placebo arm [1]. However, in the last few years, some retrospective studies suggested that the OS benefit in real-life patients might be lower than that reported in the ALSYMPCA study [2–5]. These evidences might be explained either by the suboptimal sequence of Ra223 use in the castrate-resistant phase or as the result of a suboptimal selection of patients with poorer prognostic clinical characteristics. A similar consideration also applies to the monitoring of therapy effectiveness: a number of limitations hamper the direct evaluation of bone lesion evolution asking for a combined approach while using clinical, biochemical (e.g. prostate-specific antigen (PSA), serum alkaline phosphatase (AP)), and imaging assessments [6]. However, this approach is also hampered by the so-called flare effect: the early and transient rise in the PSA levels or tracer uptake at bone scan, followed by a later decline that is commonly observed in prostate cancer patients treated with chemotherapy, luteinizing hormone-releasing hormone, and even Ra223 [7]. Indeed, the role of imaging for capturing response to Ra223 is still unclear and data regarding the most accurate modality for evaluating treated patients are lacking.

In this framework, while 18F-Fluorodeoxyglucose Positron Emission Tomography/Computed Tomography (FDG-PET/CT) is not indicated in naïve prostate cancer, as they have low FDG-avidity, mCRPC patients, and, even more, chemotherapy-refractory mCRPC are characterized by higher FDG uptake. For this reason, FDG has been proposed as a tool that is able to aggressively identify disease in mCRPC [8–11], and more in general molecular imaging with PET has high potential for the evaluation of response in cancer patients with bone involvement [12]. Based on these considerations, FDG-PET/CT might represent an effective tool for measuring disease burden and aggressiveness at baseline and for assessing the treatment response to Ra223 in mCRPC.

In the present retrospective, single center study, we aimed to evaluate the potential role of FDG-PET/CT in patient's selection and evaluation of response in a cohort of mCRPC treated with Ra223. To this aim, FDG-avid metabolic tumor burden at baseline and post-therapy of patients that were treated with Ra223 was computed and its relationship with biochemical parameters as well as progression-free (PFS) and overall survival (OS) was assessed.

2. Patients and Methods

2.1. Study Protocol

We conducted a retrospective review of mCRPC patients treated with Ra223 and submitted to FDG-PET/CT at baseline and within two months after therapy between September 2016 and November 2018 in our institution. All of the patients with an available baseline FDG-PET/CT scan were included (regardless of the availability of a post-therapy scan). By contrast, patients with an available post-therapy were only included when a baseline scan was available in the 30 days preceding Ra223 administration. Patients were candidate to FDG-PET/CT, in agreement with the evidence reported in national guidelines of the Italian Association of Medical Oncology (AOIM) on the emerging role of FDG-PET/CT in patients with mCRPC or in patients with poorly differentiated prostate cancer (Gleason score ≥ 8) [13,14]. According to our standard procedure, all of the patients signed a written informed consent form, which encompassed the use of anonymized data for retrospective research purposes, before each PET/CT scan.

All of the patients obviously had to fulfill all of the inclusion criteria for Ra223 treatment and they were treated with standard Ra223 regimen encompassing six administrations every four weeks (55 KBq/kg, intravenously). According to the established selection criteria for Ra223 patient's selection [13], in the previous four weeks preceding the first administration, each patient underwent contrast enhanced CT (ceCT) and bone scan, in order to select mCRPC patients with symptomatic bone metastases in the absence of visceral metastases (with the exception for lymph nodes with maximum diameter < 3 cm). Similarly, a bone marrow reserve fulfilling the hematologic criteria necessary for administering Ra223 and Eastern Cooperative Oncology Group (ECOG) performance status of 0–1 (life expectancy greater than six months) were verified [13]. Clinical and biochemical variables at baseline, in course and at the end of therapy, also had to be available at the time of our study. These variables included: ECOG performance status, PSA, AP, and lactate dehydrogenase (LDH). During treatment, the patients were maintained under androgen deprivation therapy.

2.2. Imaging Procedures

Bone scan and FDG-PET/CT were performed according to European Association of Nuclear Medicine (EANM) Guidelines [15,16], as detailed in the Supplementary Materials. Briefly, bone scan was acquired 3 h after the injection of 740 MBq of 99mTc-methilen diphosphonate. A dual-head gamma camera (Millennium; GE Healthcare, Boston, USA) that was equipped with a parallel-hole, low-energy, high-resolution collimator on a 10% energy window centered on the 99mTc photopeak was used to acquire planar whole-body acquisitions, and, if needed, Single Photon Emission Computed Tomography (SPECT) images. FDG-PET/CT was performed while using a 16-slices PET/CT hybrid system (Hirez-Biograph 16, Siemens Medical Solutions, Munich, Germany). After blood glucose levels measurement (to ensure blood glucose levels <160 mg/dL), fasting patients underwent the intravenous injection of 300–400 MBq of FDG. The patients were asked to drink 500 mL of water 1h prior to image acquisition and empty the bladder just before the acquisition start. Imaging started 60 ± 15 minutes after tracer administration. The acquired PET data were reconstructed into a 128 × 128 matrix using an iterative reconstruction algorithm (three iterative steps, eight subsets). Raw images were scatter-corrected and processed while using a three-dimensional (3D) Gaussian filter, while CT was used for attenuation correction. Image quality control documented a spatial resolution of 4.0 mm full width at half-maximum.

2.3. Image Analysis

The bone scan images were qualitatively evaluated, and number of lesions present at baseline and after therapy was recorded. The following semiquantitative parameters were computed on both baseline and post-therapy FDG-PET/CT scans: maximum standard uptake value (SUVmax) of the hottest bone lesion, Metabolic Tumor Volume (MTV) and Total Lesion Glycolysis (TLG). MTV was estimated from the volumes of interest SUV isocontours that were automatically drawn by setting a relative threshold of 40% of the SUVmax [17]. TLG was calculated as SUVmean × MTV. All of the semiquantitative variables were estimated at baseline and after therapy to calculate their difference (termed deltaMTV and deltaTLG, respectively). However, deltaSUVmax was not calculated, as the hottest bone lesion at post-therapy FDG-PET/CT might not correspond to the hottest lesion at baseline. The metabolic response to Ra223 was also evaluated by two independent readers (MB, SM) while using PET Response Criteria in Solid Tumors (PERCIST) and European Organization for Research and Treatment of Cancer (EORTC) criteria [18,19], see also Supplementary Materials for details on PERCIST and EORTC criteria). The PET readers were blinded to ceCT and bone scan results. DeltaPSA, deltaAP, and deltaLDH were also calculated as the difference between post-therapy and baseline levels.

2.4. Statistical Analysis

PFS and OS curves were computed according to Kaplan–Meier with the Log Rank test determining statistical significance. This analysis was performed by dividing the population into tertiles for all tested variables, with the only exception of bone scan lesions whose number was divided in ≤ 6, 6–20, and > 20, as performed in a sub-analysis of the ALSYMPCA study [1]. A binary classification of response to therapy was applied to PERCIST scores due to the small numbers involved, as previously described [20]. In particular, patients showing partial metabolic response (PMR) were considered as "responders", while stable metabolic disease (SMD) and progressive metabolic disease (PMD) were classified as "non-responders". A set of univariate and multivariate Cox proportional hazard models were fitted to the data to assess the predictive value of baseline parameters: in univariate analyses, OS and PFS were modeled as a function of each tested variable. Subsequently, all of the tested variables were tentatively included in a multivariate Cox's model by means of a step-down (backward) procedure, based on the likelihood ratio test: variables with a p value < 0.1 were removed from the model. Proportionality assumptions were assessed, as previously described [21]. Analyses were conducted with IBM-SPSS release 23 (IBM, Armonk, USA).

3. Results

The interrogation of our database identified 28 mCRPC patients who met the inclusion criteria and they were submitted to baseline FDG-PET/CT. Within this cohort, six patients died before treatment completion, while two refused the post-therapy FDG-PET/CT, but were still alive at the time of database interrogation. Accordingly, functional imaging at both time points was available in 20 subjects. The median interval between the two PET/CT scan was 213 days. Table 1 summarizes the overall patient's characteristics. Once completed the treatment protocol, the 20 remaining patients were monitored for twelve months after the post-therapy PET/CT. During this one-year follow-up, further 10/20 (50%) patients died. Figure S1 reports OS in the whole study cohort (since treatment start).

3.1. Prognostic Role of Baseline Parameters

As shown in Figure 1, Kaplan–Meyer analysis revealed that the biochemical parameters PSA, AP, and LDH, as well as the FDG imaging ones MTV and TLG provided a risk stratification power. In fact, the death rate was highest in mCRPC patients' candidates to Ra223 clustered within the highest tertile for each of them ($p < 0.01$, respectively). By contrast, the whole body bone scan was devoid of this prognostic penetrance, since mortality rate was remarkably similar among patients with low, intermediate, or high number of detectable bone lesions [1]. Univariate analysis that reported a significant association between overall survival and PSA, LDH, and MTV confirmed this observation ($p < 0.01$ each, respectively), as shown in Table 2 (see also Table S1 for the univariate analysis including the same variables as categorial). Multivariate Cox Regression analysis reported that each of these variables was characterized an additive predictive capability (Table 2, see also Table S1 for the multivariate analysis, including the same variables as categorial). By contrast, no baseline clinical or imaging variable was able to predict the PFS.

Table 1. Patients characteristics.

	Baseline ($n = 28$)	End of Therapy ($n = 20$)	p
Age	76.71 ± 7.1	-	-
Gleason score at diagnosis	-	-	-
5	1 (3.6%)	-	-
6	6 (21.4%)	-	-
7	9 (32.1%)	-	-
8	9 (32.1%)	-	-
9	2 (7.2%)	-	-
10	1 (3.6%)	-	-
Time evolution of prostate cancer (months)	90.59 ± 156.3	-	-
Time gap from diagnosis to mCRPC (months)	40.22 ± 54.7	-	-
Number of previous systemic therapies for mCRPC	-	-	-
1	8 (28.6%)	-	
2	6 (21.4%)	-	
3	7 (25%)	-	
4	6 (21.4%)	-	
5	1 (3.6%)	-	
ECOG score	-	-	-
0	5 (17%)	3 (15%)	p = ns
1	23 (82%)	17 (85%)	p = ns
Number of Ra223 administered doses	-	5.3 ± 1.1	-
Pain response	-	6 (30%)	-
Lab tests	-	-	
Hemoglobin (g/dL)	12.34 ± 1.6	10.87 ± 1.1	$p < 0.05$
White Blood Cells (x10^9/L)	6.6 ± 2.2	5.5 ± 1.9	$p < 0.05$
Platelets (x10^9/L)	236 ± 72.9	214.7 ± 84.3	p = ns
PSA (ng/mL)	119.25 ± 171.5	347.80 ± 468.1	$p<0.01$
AP (UI/L)	213.3 ± 295.4	133.46 ± 159.1	$p < 0.05$
LDH (UI/L)	265.23 ± 112.1	317.36 ± 241.9	$p < 0.05$
Bone scintigraphy parameters	-	-	-
1–6 lesions	7 (25%)	9 (45%)	p = ns
6-20 lesions	9 (32%)	3 (15%)	p = ns
> 20 lesions	9 (32%)	4 (20%)	p = ns
Superscan	3 (10%)	4 (20%)	p = ns
Extraosseus involvement	-	-	-
Lymph nodes	4 (14.3%)	6 (30%)	
Prostate	2 (7%)	2 (1%)	
FDG PET/CT paramethers	-	-	-
SUVmax of the hottest bone lesion	7.25 ± 3.4	8.04 ± 4.3	ns
MTV (cm3)	352.71 ± 384.3	468.01 ± 489.9	$p < 0.01$
TLG	1358.92 ± 1560.9	1877.69 ± 2179.13	$p < 0.01$

Of note, focusing the survival analysis on the 12 patients showing >20 bone lesions at bone scan, neither PSA, AP, nor LDH serum levels significantly predicted OS, while MTV was able to stratify three different prognostic classes ($p < 0.01$, Figure 2). Again, the multivariate analysis confirmed these data (Cox Regression, backward stepwise, LR; $p < 0.0001$).

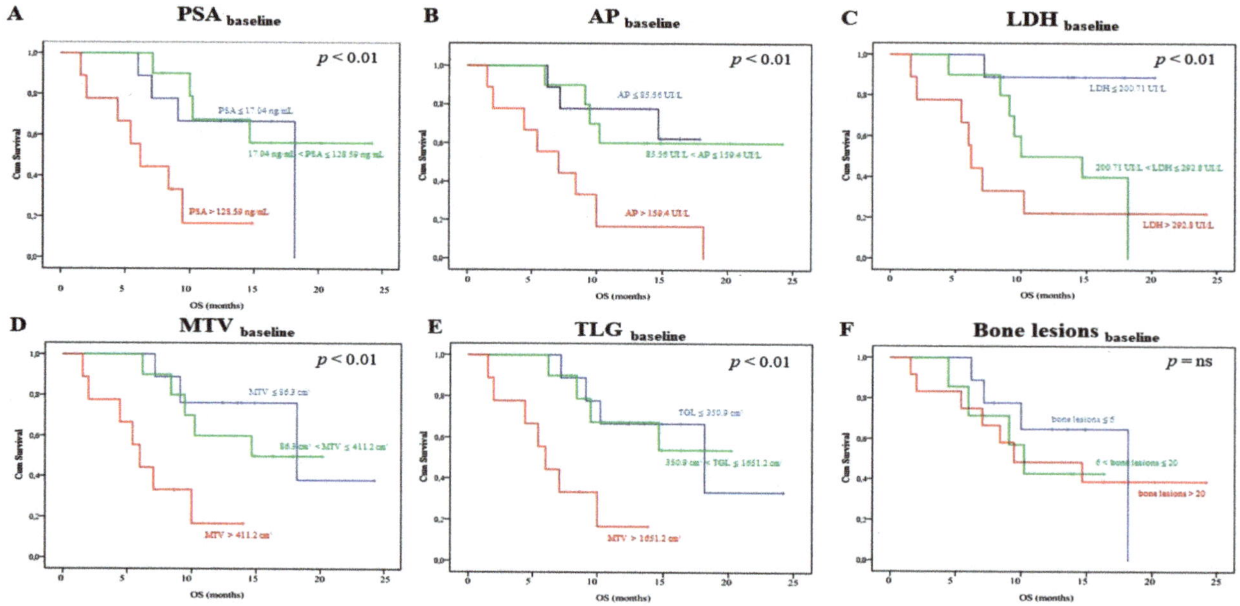

Figure 1. Kaplan–Meyer analysis including baseline biochemical and imaging variables. Each panel show the overall survival (OS) curves depending on baseline prostate-specific antigen (PSA), alkaline phosphatase (AP), lactate dehydrogenase (LDH), metabolic tumor volume (MTV), total lesion glycolysis (TLG), and bone lesions, respectively. In each case, but Panel F, patients were divided in three tertiles (first tertile: blue; second tertile: green; third tertile: orange). Following a subgroup analysis proposed in the ALSYMPCA study, in Panel F, patients were divided in three subgroups according to the number bone lesions at bone scan in < 6 (blue), 6–19 (green), and > 20 (orange) bone metastases, respectively.

Table 2. The prognostic role of baseline parameters: uni- and multivariate analyses.

	Univariate Analysis					Multivariate Analysis				
	df	p	H.R.	95% CI			p	H.R.	95% CI	
PSA	1	0.001	1.007	1.003	-	1.010	0.004	1.007	1.002 -	1.011
AP	1	0.020	1.001	0.000	-	0.001	0.443	*		
LDH	1	0.001	1.009	1.004	-	1.015	0.010	1.009	1.002 -	1.016
Number of bone lesions	1	0.960	1.009	−0.002	-	0.019	0.300	*		
SUVmax	1	0.976	1.001	−0.055	-	0.057	0.204	*		
MTV	1	0.001	1.002	1.001	-	1.003	0.044	1.002	1.000 -	1.003
TLG	1	0.134	5×10^{-005}	0.339	-	0.733	0.411	*		

* = excluded from the final model.

3.2. FDG PET/CT in the Response Evaluation Following Ra223

Table 1 sumamrizes the overall clinical characteristics of the 20 patients who underwent FDG-PET/CT post therapy evaluation. Ra223 administration caused a measurable response in most of the tested variables. In particular, hematopoietic response was confirmed by a decrease in hemoglobin levels and in white blood cells count, while the decrease in platelet number did not reach the statistical significance. AP showed a significant decrease. Nevertheless, the suggested reduction in osteoblastic activity was devoid of any significant risk prediction power, as reported in Supplementary Materials Figure S2, Panel B. The tumor burden indexes showed an opposite response that roughly approached 25% for LDH and almost 300% for PSA. Again, this response was not able to stratify patient's outcome (Figure S2, Panels A and C), which confirmed a relevant interference of the so-called "flair effect" after radiometabolic treatment of bone lesions.

A completely different consideration applied to imaging indexes of treatment effectiveness. PERCIST scores significantly predicted OS (Figure 3, $p < 0.05$), while this prognostic penetrance did not reach statistical significance for EORTC, deltaMTV, and deltaTLG evaluations.

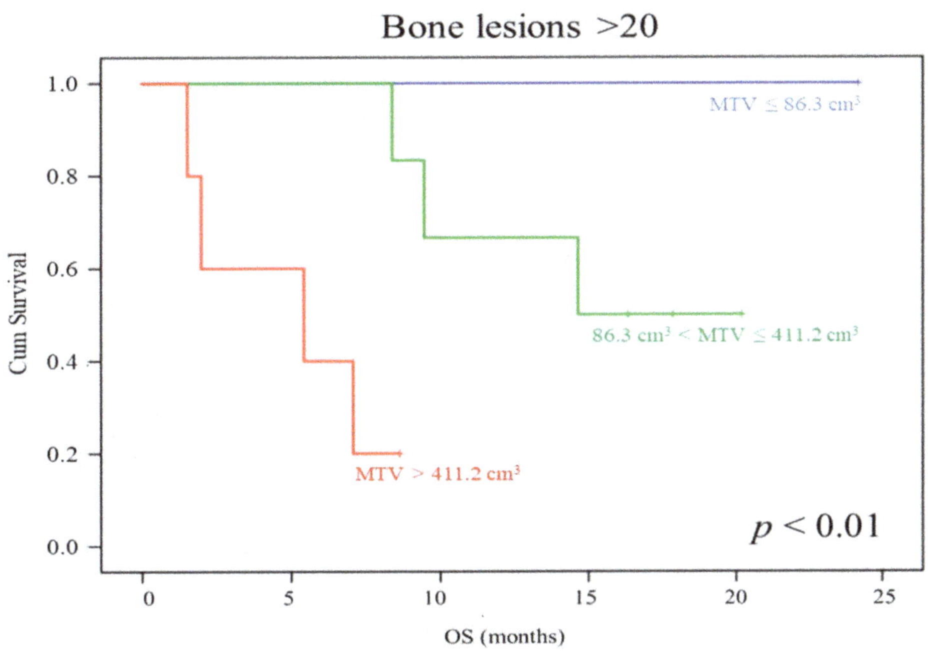

Figure 2. MTV prognostic power in patients showing >20 lesions at bone scan. OS curves depending on baseline MTV (first tertile: blue; second tertile: green; third tertile: orange) in the subgroup of patients showing > 20 bone lesions at bone scan.

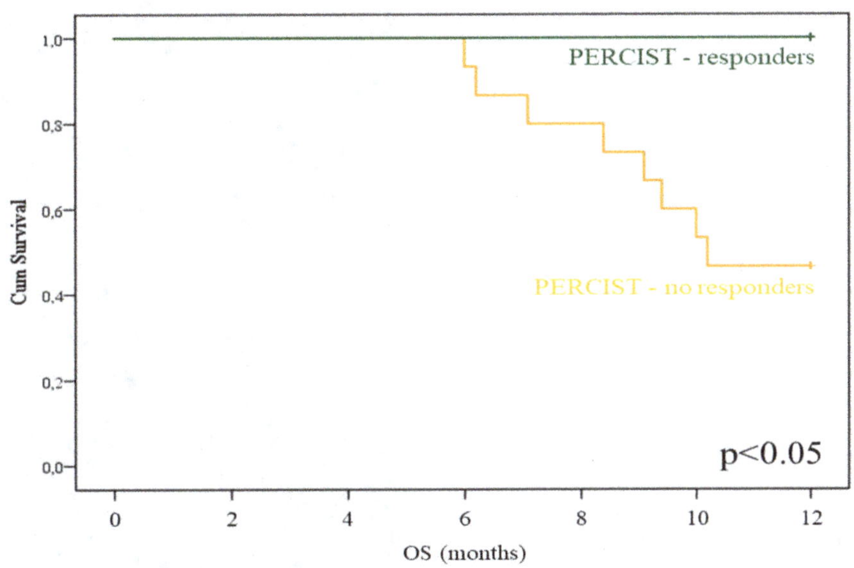

Figure 3. PET Response Criteria in Solid Tumors (PERCIST) prognostic power in Radium-223 treated patients. OS curves depending on PERCIST score (PMR: blue; SMD+PMD: green) in the subgroup of patients submitted to post-therapy 18F-Fluorodeoxyglucose Positron Emission Tomography/Computed Tomography (FDG-PET/CT).

Multivariate Cox analysis, including deltaPSA, deltaAP, deltaLDH, and PERCIST score, confirmed the additive value of PERCIST score with respect to all of the remaining variables (p = 0.012). In agreement with this finding, the imaging index virtually preserved its capability to predict the response to treatment in patients with the highest increase in PSA after Ra223 administration, as suggested by the almost significant p value (p = 0.1 in each subgroup, see also Figure 4) and the emblematic example reported in Figure 5.

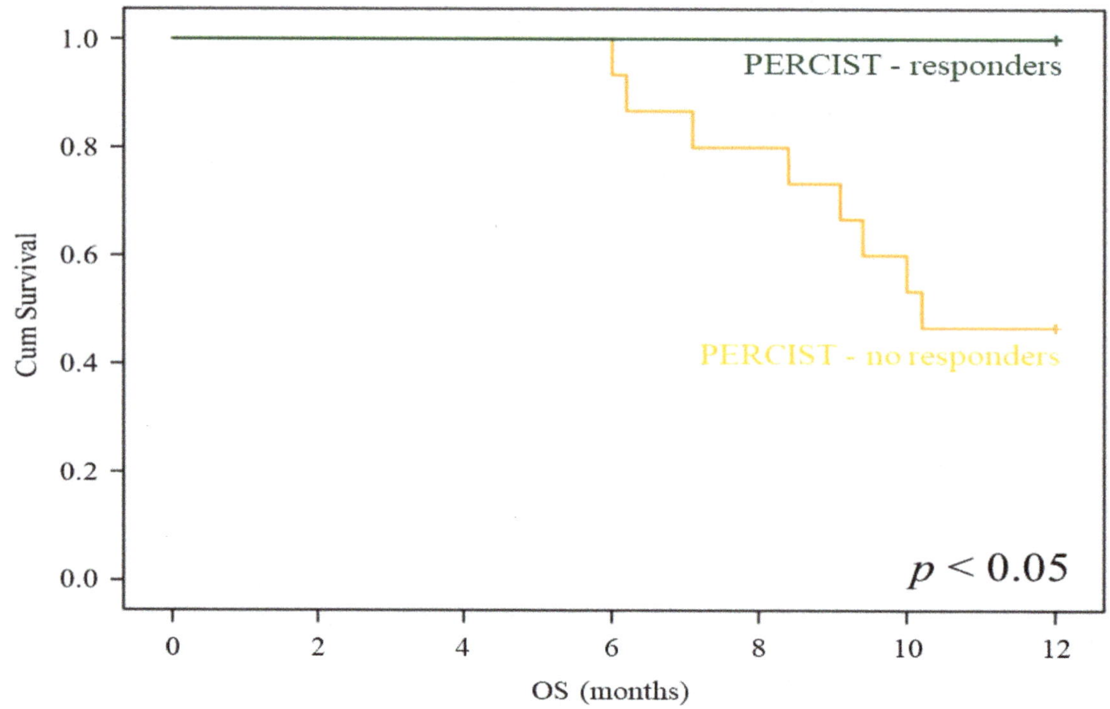

Figure 4. PERCIST prognostic stratification in deltaPSA classes. OS curves depending on PERCIST score (PMR: blue; SMD+PMD: green) in the subgroups of patients submitted to post-therapy FDG-PET/CT classified on the basis of the deltaPSA class.

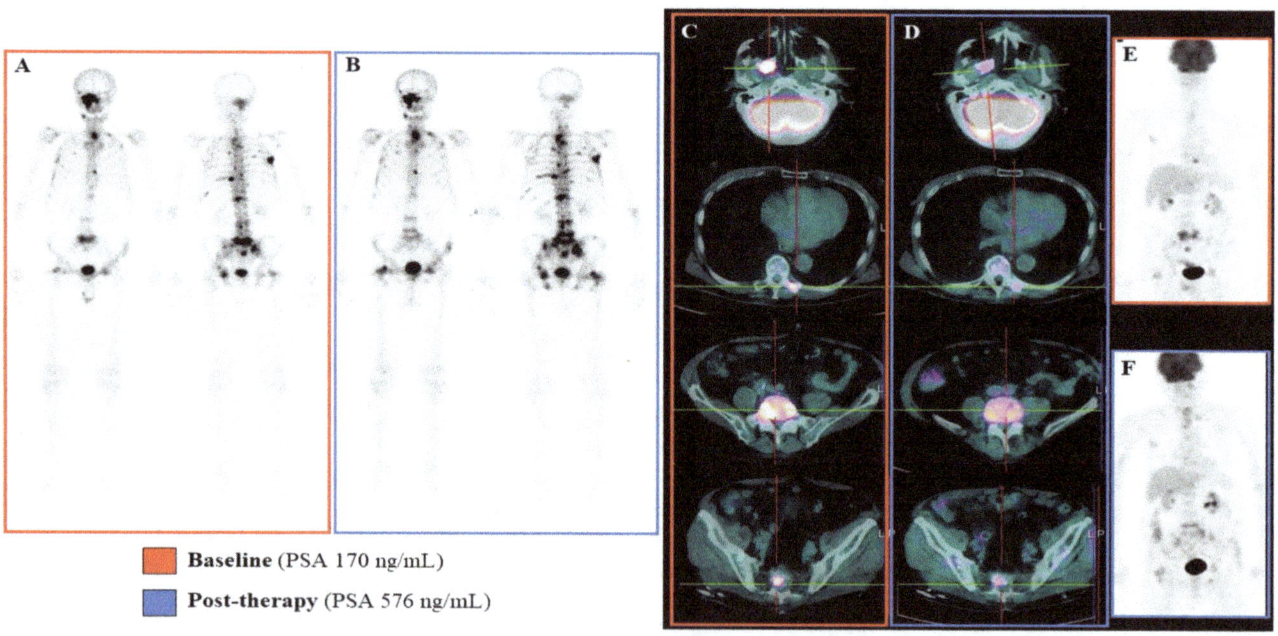

Figure 5. Emblematic example of mismatch between metabolic and biochemical/bone scan response. In this emblematic case a mismatch between metabolic data and biochemical/bone scan results was observed. At baseline the bone scan revealed the presence of several osteoblastic bone lesions (Panel **A**) that were mainly FDG-avid (Panels **C** and **E**). The post-therapy evaluation, performed six weeks after Ra223 protocol completion, showed the persistence of osteoblastic bone lesions that were occasionally more extended and diphosphonate-avid (Panel **B**). This finding was paralleled by increased serum PSA levels (576 vs 170 ng/mL at baseline). However, the post-therapy FDG PET/CT showed a significant reduction in bone lesions FDG uptake, leading to a Partial Metabolic Response according to PERCIST criteria (Panels **D** and **F**).

4. Discussion

The present results support the role of both baseline and post-therapy FDG-PET/CT in mCRPC patients treated with Ra223. In fact, MTV evaluation of baseline metabolically active skeletal disease burden was able to predict OS with an additive independent value, as documented by multivariate Cox regression analysis. By contrast, the number of lesions, as assessed by bone scan, was characterized by a largely less evident prognostic penetrance. Similarly, biochemical biomarkers PSA, AP, and LDH confirmed their predictive value when assessed before Ra223 treatment. However, their response to therapy was virtually devoid of any prognostic penetrance. By contrast, PET-based evaluations and, in particular, PERCIST criteria, were able to predict the response to Ra223 by demonstrating a lower mortality rate in patients with partial metabolic response.

4.1. Patient's Selection for Ra223

Patients' selection is a crucial point when discussing the role of Ra223 in mCRPC patients. In 2018, the European Medicines Agency (EMA) issued a specific note on the indications for treatment with Ra223 in a review of an ongoing phase 3 trial by the EMA's Pharmacovigilance Risk Assessment Committee, basically moving Ra223 to a third-line of treatment of mCRPC patients (EMA/500948/2018; https://www.ema.europa.eu/en/documents/press-release/ema-restricts-use-prostate-cancer-medicine-xofigo_en.pdf). The observation of increased the risk of fractures, in the absence of statistically significant survival benefit in patients with <6 bone lesions enrolled in the ERA-223 study, receiving Ra223 in combination with abiraterone acetate plus prednisone/prednisolone, motivated this action [22]. In fact, patients with lower skeletal disease burden might have a larger proportion of Ra223 homing to healthy bone, as compared to patients with extensive bone metastases. Indeed, sites of bony metastases are known to have a higher bone turnover and the sequestration of administered Ra223 (the so-called "sink-effect"), which might limit Ra223 deposition in the non-diseased skeleton [23,24]. However, besides the mere number of bone lesions, a huge variability in Ra223-avid bone disease can be observed. Preclinical prostate cancer models showed that the short range of alpha particles results in a lower tumor control-rate of large metastatic deposits as compared to near eradication of small lesions [25]. These data suggest the inadequacy of the mere bone lesion number count in the identification of the right candidate to Ra223.

Previous studies showed that the quantification of skeletal tumor burden by means of bone scintigraphy or 18F-NaF PET/CT might predict patients' OS and reflect the risk of hematological toxicity related to Ra223 administration [26,27]. The present study is in keeping with these evidences as also FDG-PET/CT-derived tumor volume and not the mere number of bone lesions predicted patients' prognosis. However, the present findings further extend this evidence by demonstrating the specific weight of metabolic active tumor burden.

Indeed, the higher predictive value of 18F-FDG PET/CT with respect to bone scan might be due to its capability to capture bone marrow involvement, which is obviously underestimated by the simple osteoblastic bone disease detected by bone scan (and even by 18F-NaF-PET/CT) [28]. On the other hand, the detection of FDG-avid de-differentiated and non-osteoblastic bone disease [10,29,30] might mirror greater tumour aggressiveness, also possibly predicting the lower Ra223 accumulation and the consequent low-response rate. Moreover, as the added prognostic value of the extent of metabolic active disease was preserved in patients showing >20 bone lesions at bone scan, FDG-PET/CT might play a role in the selection of patients with larger tumour burden. This finding is of potential clinical relevance, since high-volume bone disease predicts higher degrees of haematological toxicity and the selection of this group of patients for Ra223 should be even more thoughtful [26,31]. Finally, if confirmed in larger studies, the highlighted FDG-PET/CT capability rule out high-risk candidates to Ra223 might be relevant for the cost/effectiveness of Ra223 administration, thus reducing the risk of ineffective treatments in patients with worst prognosis and higher risk of hematological toxicity.

4.2. Post-Therapy Assessment

In the ALSYMPCA trial, Ra223 showed a modest effect on serum PSA levels, which reached a ≥30% reduction in just 16% of treated patients, despite improving OS [1]. Moreover, a minor correlation between OS and PSA changes at week 12 was observed [32] and, especially during the first three months of treatment, possible flare phenomena have been described [33–35]. AP and LDH kinetics under Ra223 administration has been proposed as an alternative approach to the PSA monitoring [1,36]. However, post-hoc analyses from the ALSYMPCA trial showed that these biomarkers did not meet the needed statistical surrogacy requirement for OS [32]. Therefore, the low predictive value of these biochemical biomarkers raises the urgent need for the identification of novel biomarkers, even if the dynamic monitoring of AP and LDH serum levels is still recommended during Ra223 administration.

Even though imaging was not routinely performed in the ALSYMPCA trial, imaging with bone-targeted radiopharmaceuticals has been proposed as a tool for monitoring treatment response when clinically indicated [1]. However, bon flare phenomenon resulting in false-positive tracer uptake, even in responsive cases, has been described [23,37,38], which complicates the evaluation of response at a single patient level. Recently, the 2 + 2 rule has been proposed for overcoming this limitation of osteotropic radiotracers [26,34,39]. However, its reliability in the clinical setting still needs to be validated. On the other hand, ceCT scan can be used in case of suspicious disease progression. However, in prostate cancer metastatic lymph nodes can be normal sized resulting false-negative at anatomic imaging [40,41], profoundly underpowering the accuracy of this tool in the evaluation of response to Ra223. In this scenario, 18F-Fluorocholine or 68Ga-PSMA PET/CT have been recently proposed as promising tools for monitoring the response to Ra223 treatment [31,42–45].

To the best of our knowledge, a case report of mCRPC [46], a small case series [47], and a phase IIa metastatic breast cancer study represent the sole available reports on FDG-PET/CT used for the evaluation of Ra223 response [48]. In the present study, the application of PERCIST criteria to FDG-PET/CT images overpowered bone scan and biochemical parameters in the evaluation of response to Ra223 treatment. Moreover, a trend in the post-treatment prognostic assessment was maintained when the PERCIST classes were analyzed in patients experiencing an increase in PSA levels. This latter finding suggests the potential role for FDG-PET/CT in the identification of the PSA-flare phenomenon. The observed discordance in the bone imaging patterns between bone scan and FDG-PET/CT after Ra223 administration might be related to bone marrow metastases, which cannot be detected by bone scintigraphy. Importantly, these discordances have been observed, not only in case of disease progression, but also in metabolic responders, although the magnitude of this discordance seems to be larger in cases of progression. On one side, this finding fits with the acknowledged limited efficacy of Ra223 in bone marrow metastases, as consistent with its mode of action [34,49–51]. On the other hand, it highlights a need for optimal clinical management of Ra223-treated patients who present with marrow metastases at baseline.

4.3. Limitations

The present study has some drawbacks. First, the relatively small population. However, its monocentric nature represents one of its strengths. Accordingly, all of the enrolled patients were submitted to FDG-PET/CT while using the same PET/CT scanner avoiding the possible influence of inter-scanner variability on PET results. Second, in the multivariate analyses, we did not consider other potential prognostic factors in the cohort able to influence OS and, consequently, the impact of the different response criteria investigated. Finally, bone scan images were qualitatively evaluated, while the application of semi-quantification tools [26,52] might have provided the estimation of the "osteoblastic tumor volume", improving the comparison between bone scan and metabolic parameters that were obtained by FDG-PET/CT.

5. Conclusions

FDG-PET/CT can represent a widely available method for directly measuring active de-differentiated tumor burden in mCRPC patients' candidates to Ra223, providing prognostic information overpowering biochemical and other imaging parameters. After treatment, it can assess tumor load reduction particularly in patients showing increased PSA, helping in the differential diagnosis between progression and pseudoprogression (related to the PSA flare phenomenon).

Author Contributions: Study concept and design M.B., S.M., G.S., S.C.; recruitment and collection data: M.I.D., E.Z., A.M., S.R., L.T., R.M., M.V., A.C., F.C., M.M., G.F., C.M.; quality control of data and algorithm: M.B.; data analysis, statistical analysis and interpretation: M.B., M.C., G.S.; manuscript preparation: M.B., S.C., S.M., G.S.; editing, review, supervision, approval final version of the manuscript, all authors. All authors have read and agreed to the published version of the manuscript.

References

1. Parker, C.; Nilsson, S.; Heinrich, D.; Helle, S.I.; O'Sullivan, J.M.; Fosså, S.D.; Chodacki, A.; Wiechno, P.; Logue, J.; Seke, M.; et al. ALSYMPCA Investigators. Alpha emitter radium-223 and survival in metastatic prostate cancer. *N. Engl. J. Med.* **2013**, *369*, 213–223. [CrossRef] [PubMed]
2. Parikh, S.; Murray, L.; Kenning, L.; Bottomley, D.; Din, O.; Dixit, S.; Ferguson, C.; Handforth, C.; Joseph, L.; Mokhtar, D.; et al. Real-world outcomes and factors predicting survival and completion of radium 223 in metastatic castrate-resistant prostate cancer. *Clin. Oncol.* **2018**, *30*, 548–555. [CrossRef] [PubMed]
3. Wong, W.W.; Anderson, E.M.; Mohammadi, H.; Daniels, T.B.; Schild, S.E.; Keole, S.R.; Choo, C.R.; Tzou, K.S.; Bryce, A.H.; Ho, T.H.; et al. Factors associated with survival following radium-223 treatment for metastatic castration-resistant prostate cancer. *Clin. Genitourin. Cancer* **2017**, *15*, e969–e975. [CrossRef] [PubMed]
4. Frantellizzi, V.; Farcomeni, A.; Follacchio, G.A.; Pacilio, M.; Pellegrini, R.; Pani, R.; De Vincentis, G. A 3-variable prognostic score (3-PS) for overall survival prediction in metastatic castration-resistant prostate cancer treated with 223Radium-dichloride. *Ann. Nucl. Med.* **2018**, *32*, 142–148. [CrossRef]
5. Saad, F.; Carles, J.; Gillessen, S.; Heidenreich, A.; Heinrich, D.; Gratt, J.; Lévy, J.; Miller, K.; Nilsson, S.; Petrenciuc, O.; et al. Radium-223 International Early Access Program Investigators. Radium-223 and concomitant therapies in patients with metastatic castration-resistant prostate cancer: An international, early access, open-label, single-arm phase 3b trial. *Lancet Oncol.* **2016**, *17*, 1306–1316. [CrossRef]
6. Clamp, A.; Danson, S.; Nguyen, H.; Cole, D.; Clemons, M. Assessment of therapeutic response in patients with metastatic bone disease. *Lancet Oncol.* **2004**, *5*, 607–616. [CrossRef]
7. Castello, A.; Macapinlac, H.A.; Lopci, E.; Santos, E.B. Prostate-specific antigen flare induced by 223RaCl2 in patients with metastatic castration-resistant prostate cancer. *Eur. J. Nucl. Med. Mol. Imaging* **2018**, *45*, 2256–2263. [CrossRef]
8. Oyama, N.; Akino, H.; Suzuki, Y.; Kanamaru, H.; Miwa, Y.; Tsuka, H.; Sadato, N.; Yonekura, Y.; Okada, K. Prognostic value of 2-deoxy-2-[F-18]fluoro-D-glucose positron emission tomography imaging for patients with prostate cancer. *Mol. Imaging Biol.* **2002**, *4*, 99–104. [CrossRef]
9. Meirelles, G.S.; Schöder, H.; Ravizzini, G.C.; Gönen, M.; Fox, J.J.; Humm, J.; Morris, M.J.; Scher, H.I.; Larson, S.M. Prognostic value of baseline [18F] fluorodeoxyglucose positron emission tomography and 99mTc-MDP bone scan in progressing metastatic prostate cancer. *Clin. Cancer Res.* **2010**, *16*, 6093–6096. [CrossRef]
10. Jadvar, H.; Desai, B.; Ji, L.; Conti, P.S.; Dorff, T.B.; Groshen, S.G.; Pinski, J.K.; Quinn, D.I. Baseline 18F FDG PET/CT parameters as imaging biomarkers of overall survival in castrate-resistant metastatic prostate cancer. *J. Nucl. Med.* **2013**, *54*, 1195–1201. [CrossRef]
11. Vargas, H.A.; Wassberg, C.; Fox, J.J.; Wibmer, A.; Goldman, D.A.; Kuk, D.; Gonen, M.; Larson, S.M.; Morris, M.J.; Scher, H.I.; et al. Bone metastases in castration-resistant prostate cancer: Associations between morphologic CT patterns, Glycolytic activity, and androgen receptor expression on PET and overall survival. *Radiology* **2014**, *271*, 220–229. [CrossRef] [PubMed]
12. Capitanio, S.; Bongioanni, F.; Piccardo, A.; Campus, C.; Gonella, R.; Tixi, L.; Naseri, M.; Pennone, M.; Altrinetti, V.; Buschiazzo, A.; et al. Comparisons between glucose analogue 2-deoxy-2-((18)F)fluoro-D-glucose

and (18)F-sodium fluoride positron emission tomography/computed tomography in breast cancer patients with bone lesions. *World J. Radiol.* **2016**, *8*, 200–209. [CrossRef] [PubMed]
13. AIOM 2019 Prostate Cancer Guidelines. Available online: https://www.aiom.it/linee-guida-aiom-carcinoma-della-prostata-2019/14 (accessed on 23 November 2019).
14. Jadvar, H. Prostate cancer: PET with 18F-FDG, 18F- or 11C-acetate, and 18F- or 11C-choline. *J. Nucl. Med.* **2011**, *52*, 81–89. [CrossRef]
15. Boellaard, R.; Delgado-Bolton, R.; Oyen, W.J.; Giammarile, F.; Tatsch, K.; Eschner, W.; Verzijlbergen, F.J.; Barrington, S.F.; Pike, L.C.; Weber, W.A.; et al. European Association of Nuclear Medicine (EANM). FDG PET/CT: EANM procedure guidelines for tumour imaging: Version 2.0. *Eur. J. Nucl. Med. Mol. Imaging* **2015**, *42*, 328–354. [CrossRef] [PubMed]
16. Van den Wyngaert, T.; Strobel, K.; Kampen, W.U.; Kuwert, T.; van der Bruggen, W.; Mohan, H.K.; Gnanasegaran, G.; Delgado-Bolton, R.; Weber, W.A.; Beheshti, M.; et al. The EANM practice guidelines for bone scintigraphy. *Eur. J. Nucl. Med. Mol. Imaging* **2016**, *43*, 1723–1738. [CrossRef] [PubMed]
17. Kruse, V.; Mees, G.; Maes, A.; D'Asseler, Y.; Borms, M.; Cocquyt, V.; Van De Wiele, C. Reproducibility of FDG PET based metabolic tumor volume measurements and of their FDG distribution within. *Q. J. Nucl. Med. Mol. Imaging* **2015**, *59*, 462–468. [PubMed]
18. Young, H.; Baum, R.; Cremerius, U.; Herholz, K.; Hoekstra, O.; Lammertsma, A.A.; Pruim, J.; Price, P. Measurement of clinical and subclinical tumour response using [18F]-fluorodeoxyglucose and positron emission tomography: Review and 1999 EORTC recommendations. European Organization for Research and Treatment of Cancer (EORTC) PET Study Group. *Eur. J. Cancer* **1999**, *35*, 1773–1782. [CrossRef]
19. Wahl, R.L.; Jacene, H.; Kasamon, Y.; Lodge, M.A. From RECIST to PERCIST: Evolving Considerations for PET response criteria in solid tumors. *J. Nucl. Med.* **2009**, *50*, 122S–150S. [CrossRef]
20. Rossi, G.; Bauckneht, M.; Genova, C.; Rijavec, E.; Biello, F.; Mennella, S.; Dal Bello, M.G.; Cittadini, G.; Bruzzi, P.; Piva, R.; et al. Comparison between 18F-FDG-PET- and CT-based criteria in non-small cell lung cancer (NSCLC) patients treated with Nivolumab. *J. Nucl. Med.* **2019**. [CrossRef]
21. Grambsch, P.M.; Therneau, T.M. Proportional hazards tests and diagnostics based on weighted residuals. *Biometrika* **1994**, *81*, 515–526. [CrossRef]
22. Smith, M.; Parker, C.; Saad, F.; Miller, K.; Tombal, B.; Ng, Q.S.; Boegemann, M.; Matveev, V.; Piulats, J.M.; Zucca, L.E.; et al. Addition of radium-223 to abiraterone acetate and prednisone or prednisolone in patients with castration-resistant prostate cancer and bone metastases (ERA 223): A randomised, double-blind, placebo-controlled, phase 3 trial. *Lancet Oncol.* **2019**, *20*, 408–419. [CrossRef]
23. Nilsson, S.; Larsen, R.H.; Fosså, S.D.; Balteskard, L.; Borch, K.W.; Westlin, J.E.; Salberg, G.; Bruland, O.S. First clinical experience with alpha-emitting radium-223 in the treatment of skeletal metastases. *Clin. Cancer Res.* **2005**, *11*, 4451–4459. [CrossRef] [PubMed]
24. Beauregard, J.M.; Hofman, M.S.; Kong, G.; Hicks, R.J. The tumour sink effect on the biodistribution of 68Ga-DOTA-octreotate: Implications for peptide receptor radionuclide therapy. *Eur. J. Nucl. Med. Mol. Imaging* **2012**, *39*, 50–56. [CrossRef] [PubMed]
25. Dondossola, E.; Casarin, S.; Paindelli, C.; De-Juan-Pardo, E.M.; Hutmacher, D.W.; Logothetis, C.J.; Friedl, P. Radium 223-Mediated Zonal Cytotoxicity of Prostate Cancer in Bone. *J. Natl. Cancer Inst.* **2019**, *111*, 1042–1050. [CrossRef]
26. Føsbol, M.O.; Petersen, P.M.; Kjaer, A.; Mortensen, J. 223Ra Therapy of Advanced Metastatic Castration-Resistant Prostate Cancer: Quantitative Assessment of Skeletal Tumor Burden for Prognostication of Clinical Outcome and Hematologic Toxicity. *J. Nucl. Med.* **2018**, *59*, 596–602. [CrossRef]
27. Etchebehere, E.C.; Araujo, J.C.; Fox, P.S.; Swanston, N.M.; Macapinlac, H.A.; Rohren, E.M. Prognostic factors in patients treated with 223ra: The role of skeletal tumor burden on baseline 18F-fluoride PET/CT in predicting overall survival. *J. Nucl. Med.* **2015**, *56*, 1177–1184. [CrossRef]
28. Raynor, W.Y.; Al-Zaghal, A.; Zadeh, M.Z.; Seraj, S.M.; Alavi, A. Metastatic Seeding Attacks Bone Marrow, Not Bone: Rectifying Ongoing Misconceptions. *PET Clin.* **2019**, *14*, 135–144. [CrossRef]
29. Jadvar, H. Is There Use for FDG-PET in Prostate Cancer? *Semin. Nucl. Med.* **2016**, *46*, 502–506. [CrossRef]
30. Fox, J.J.; Gavane, S.C.; Blanc-Autran, E.; Nehmeh, S.; Gönen, M.; Beattie, B.; Vargas, H.A.; Schöder, H.; Humm, J.L.; Fine, S.W.; et al. Positron Emission Tomography/Computed Tomography-Based Assessments of Androgen Receptor Expression and Glycolytic Activity as a Prognostic Biomarker for Metastatic Castration-Resistant Prostate Cancer. *JAMA Oncol.* **2018**, *4*, 217–224. [CrossRef]

31. Etchebehere, E.C.; Araujo, J.C.; Milton, D.R.; Erwin, W.D.; Wendt, R.E., 3rd; Swanston, N.M.; Fox, P.; Macapinlac, H.A.; Rohren, E.M. Skeletal tumor burden on baseline 18F-fluoride PET/CT predicts bone marrow failure after 223Ra therapy. *Clin. Nucl. Med.* **2016**, *41*, 268–273. [CrossRef]
32. Sartor, O.; Coleman, R.E.; Nilsson, S.; Heinrich, D.; Helle, S.I.; O'Sullivan, J.M.; Vogelzang, N.J.; Bruland, Ø.; Kobina, S.; Wilhelm, S.; et al. An exploratory analysis of alkaline phosphatase, lactate dehydrogenase, and prostate-specific antigen dynamics in the phase 3 ALSYMPCA trial with radium-223. *Ann. Oncol.* **2017**, *28*, 1090–1097. [CrossRef] [PubMed]
33. Gillessen, S.; Omlin, A.; Attard, G.; de Bono, J.S.; Efstathiou, E.; Fizazi, K.; Halabi, S.; Nelson, P.S.; Sartor, O.; Smith, M.R.; et al. Management of patients with advanced prostate cancer: Recommendations of the St Gallen Advanced Prostate Cancer Consensus Conference (APCCC) 2015. *Ann. Oncol.* **2015**, *26*, 1589–1604. [CrossRef] [PubMed]
34. Scher, H.I.; Morris, M.J.; Stadler, W.M.; Higano, C.; Basch, E.; Fizazi, K.; Antonarakis, E.S.; Beer, T.M.; Carducci, M.A.; Chi, K.N.; et al. Trial design and objectives for castration-resistant prostate cancer: Updated recommendations from the prostate cancer clinical trials working group 3. *J. Clin. Oncol.* **2016**, *34*, 1402–1418. [CrossRef] [PubMed]
35. Poeppel, T.D.; Handkiewicz-Junak, D.; Andreeff, M.; Becherer, A.; Bockisch, A.; Fricke, E.; Geworski, L.; Heinzel, A.; Krause, B.J.; Krause, T.; et al. EANM guideline for radionuclide therapy with radium-223 of metastatic castration-resistant prostate cancer. *Eur. J. Nucl. Med. Mol. Imaging* **2018**, *45*, 824–845. [CrossRef] [PubMed]
36. Heinrich, D.; Gillessen, S.; Heidenreich, A.; Keizman, D.; O'Sullivan, J.M.; Carles, J.; Wirth, M.; Miller, K.; Procopio, G.; Gratt, J.; et al. Changes in alkaline phosphatase (ALP) dynamics and overall survival (OS) in metastatic castration-resistant prostate cancer (mCRPC) patients treated with radium-223 in an international early access program (EAP). *Ann. Oncol.* **2016**, *27*, 751P. [CrossRef]
37. Keizman, D.; Fosboel, M.O.; Reichegger, H.; Peer, A.; Rosenbaum, E.; Desax, M.C.; Neiman, V.; Petersen, P.M.; Mueller, J.; Cathomas, R.; et al. Imaging response during therapy with radium-223 for castration-resistant prostate cancer with bone metastases-analysis of an international multicenter database. *Prostate Cancer Prostatic Dis.* **2017**, *20*, 289–293. [CrossRef]
38. McNamara, M.A.; George, D.J. Pain, PSA flare, and bone scan response in a patient with metastatic castration-resistant prostate cancer treated with radium-223, a case report. *BMC Cancer* **2015**, *15*, 371. [CrossRef]
39. Yoneyama, S.; Miyoshi, Y.; Tsutsumi, S.; Kawahara, T.; Hattori, Y.; Yokomizo, Y.; Hayashi, N.; Yao, M.; Uemura, H. Value of bone scan index for predicting overall survival among patients treated with radium-223 for bone metastatic castration-resistant prostate cancer. *J. Clin. Oncol.* **2018**, *36*, 216. [CrossRef]
40. O'Sullivan, G.J.; Carty, F.L.; Cronin, C.G. Imaging of bone metastasis: An update. *World J. Radiol.* **2015**, *7*, 202–211. [CrossRef]
41. Perez-Lopez, R.; Mateo, J.; Mossop, H.; Blackledge, M.D.; Collins, D.J.; Rata, M.; Morgan, V.A.; Macdonald, A.; Sandhu, S.; Lorente, D.; et al. Diffusion-weighted imaging as a treatment response biomarker for evaluating bone metastases in prostate cancer: A pilot study. *Radiology* **2017**, *283*, 168–177. [CrossRef]
42. Etchebehere, E.; Brito, A.E.; Rezaee, A.; Langsteger, W.; Beheshti, M. Therapy assessment of bone metastatic disease in the era of 223radium. *Eur. J. Nucl. Med. Mol. Imaging* **2017**, *44*, 84–96. [CrossRef] [PubMed]
43. Evangelista, L.; Zorz, A. Re: Response Assessment of 223Ra Treatment: Should a Fluorocholine PET/CT Be Performed? *Clin. Nucl. Med.* **2018**, *43*, 867–868. [PubMed]
44. Thomas, L.; Balmus, C.; Ahmadzadehfar, H.; Essler, M.; Strunk, H.; Bundschuh, R.A. Assessment of Bone Metastases in Patients with Prostate Cancer-A Comparison between 99mTc-Bone-Scintigraphy and [68Ga]Ga-PSMA PET/CT. *Pharmaceuticals* **2017**, *10*, 68. [CrossRef] [PubMed]
45. Uprimny, C.; Kroiss, A.; Nilica, B.; Buxbaum, S.; Decristoforo, C.; Horninger, W.; Virgolini, I.J. (68)Ga-PSMA ligand PET versus (18)F-NaF PET: Evaluation of response to (223)Ra therapy in a prostate cancer patient. *Eur. J. Nucl. Med. Mol. Imaging* **2015**, *42*, 362–363. [CrossRef]
46. Maruyama, K.; Utsunomia, K.; Nakamoto, T.; Kawakita, S.; Murota, T.; Tanigawa, N. Utility of F-18 FDG PET/CT for Detection of Bone Marrow Metastases in Prostate Cancer Patients Treated with Radium-223. *Asia Ocean. J. Nucl. Med. Biol.* **2018**, *6*, 61–67.
47. Iizuka, J. Evaluating radium-223 response in metastatic castration-resistant prostate cancer with imaging. *Asia Pac. J. Clin. Oncol.* **2018**, *14*, 16–23. [CrossRef]

48. Coleman, R.; Aksnes, A.K.; Naume, B.; Garcia, C.; Jerusalem, G.; Piccart, M.; Vobecky, N.; Thuresson, M.; Flamen, P. A phase IIa, nonrandomized study of radium-223 dichloride in advanced breast cancer patients with bone-dominant disease. *Breast Cancer Res. Treat.* **2014**, *145*, 411–418. [CrossRef]
49. Suominen, M.I.; Fagerlund, K.M.; Rissanen, J.P.; Konkol, Y.M.; Morko, J.P.; Peng, Z.; Alhoniemi, E.J.; Laine, S.K.; Corey, E.; Mumberg, D.; et al. Radium-223 inhibits osseous prostate cancer growth by dual targeting of cancer cells and bone microenvironment in mouse models. *Clin. Cancer Res.* **2017**, *23*, 4335–4346. [CrossRef]
50. Suominen, M.I.; Rissanen, J.P.; Käkönen, R.; Fagerlund, K.M.; Alhoniemi, E.; Mumberg, D.; Ziegelbauer, K.; Halleen, J.M.; Käkönen, S.M.; Scholz, A. Survival benefit with radium-223 dichloride in a mouse model of breast cancer bone metastasis. *J. Natl. Cancer Inst.* **2013**, *105*, 908–916. [CrossRef]
51. Lange, P.H.; Vessella, R.L. Mechanisms, hypotheses and questions regarding prostate cancer micrometastases to bone. *Cancer Metastasis Rev.* **1998**, *17*, 331–336. [CrossRef]
52. Fiz, F.; Dittman, H.; Campi, C.; Morbelli, S.; Marini, C.; Brignone, M.; Bauckneht, M.; Piva, R.; Massone, A.M.; Piana, M.; et al. Assessment of Skeletal Tumor Load in Metastasized Castration-Resistant Prostate Cancer Patients: A Review of Available Methods and an Overview on Future Perspectives. *Bioengineering (Basel)* **2018**, *5*, 58. [CrossRef] [PubMed]

11

A Resident's Perspective of Ovarian Cancer

Christopher G. Smith

Department of Obstetrics & Gynecology, University of Kentucky Medical Center, 800 Rose Street, Lexington, KY 40536-0293, USA; christophergsmith@uky.edu

Academic Editor: Andreas Kjaer

Abstract: Identifying, understanding, and curing disease is a lifelong endeavor for any medical practitioner. Equally as important is to be cognizant of the impact a disease has on the individual suffering from it, as well as on their family. Ovarian cancer is the leading cause of death from gynecologic malignancies. Symptoms are vague, and the disease is generally at an advanced stage at diagnosis. Efforts have been made to develop methods to identify ovarian cancer at earlier stages, thus improving overall mortality. Transvaginal ultrasound (TVUS), with and without laboratory tests, can be used to screen for ovarian cancer. For over thirty years, the University of Kentucky Markey Cancer Center Ovarian Cancer Screening Program has been studying the efficacy of TVUS for detecting early stage ovarian cancer. After 285,000+ TVUS examinations provided to over 45,000 women, the program has demonstrated that regular TVUS examinations can detect ovarian cancer at early stages, and that survival is increased in those women whose ovarian cancer was detected with screening and who undergo standard treatment. These results demonstrate the utility of TVUS as an efficacious method of ovarian cancer screening.

Keywords: ovarian cancer; screening; transvaginal ultrasound; quality of life

---

1. Introduction

As a first-year resident in Obstetrics and Gynecology, I am relating my perspective on ovarian cancer at this stage of my career. This disease has received modest attention during medical school and during residency. Having been to weekly didactics dedicated to this disease, as well as opportunities to scrub in on complex pelvic surgeries, I am beginning to understand more about the nuances of this disease process, its diagnosis, and management. Much of what I am relating here I have learned in my own efforts to eventually prepare me for a career in Gynecologic Oncology.

Cancer is the second most common cause of death among women in the United States of America and is the leading cause of death among women 40 to 79 years of age. Among the types of cancers affecting women, ovarian cancer is considered uncommon, yet it causes severe morbidity and mortality [1]. Abdominal ascites, bowel obstructions, venous thromboses, and adverse effects from chemotherapy are the realities faced by women diagnosed with ovarian cancer. Ovarian cancer is most often diagnosed at an advanced stage, which has led to investigations of screening tests to detect the disease at early stages. Transvaginal ultrasonography (TVUS) has been studied as a means to characterize and categorize adnexal masses. Since 1987, the University of Kentucky Markey Cancer Center Ovarian Cancer Screening Program has been studying the efficacy of TVUS for detecting early stage ovarian cancer. After over 285,000+ TVUS examinations provided to over 45,000 women, the program has demonstrated that regular TVUS examinations can detect ovarian cancer at early stages, and that survival increased in those women whose ovarian cancer was detected with screening and underwent standard treatment [2,3].

Histologically, ovarian cancer is any neoplasm arising from ovarian cells. Historically, these cells can either be those that line the surface of the ovary (epithelial) or those that originate from the ovary as non-epithelial cancers (embryonic or extra-embryonic (germ), hormone-producing, or structural cells [sex-cord stromal]) [4–8]. In recent years, numerous reports have proposed a unified hypothesis about the origin of high-grade serous ovarian cancer, implicating the Fallopian tubes fimbria as the point of origin [9–18]. In this hypothesis, invasive or serous tubal intraepithelial carcinoma (STIC) originating in the Fallopian fimbria is responsible for seeding the ovaries and peritoneal cavity with malignant cells [19]. However, STIC is not present in many high-grade serous carcinomas [20].

Ovarian cancer generally affects older women, the average age being 63 [21]. Ovarian cancer is the eleventh most common cause of cancer among women, with a lifetime risk of one in 70 to develop disease [22]. It is also the leading cause of death from gynecological malignancy. Nearly two thirds of ovarian carcinomas are diagnosed with disease located outside of the pelvis and thereby impose the consequences of advanced stage disease. Overall, the five-year survival rate for women diagnosed with ovarian cancer is 46%. When ovarian cancer spreads to distant sites, five-year survival decreases to 28%, and decreases to nearly 16% with Stage 4 disease [1].

2. Ovarian Cancer Risk Factors

2.1. Inherent Risk Factors

Over her lifetime, a woman has a nearly one in 70 chance of developing ovarian cancer [17]. However, certain risk factors confer an increased chance of developing ovarian cancer. Nulligravidity, or never becoming pregnant, can increase the risk for ovarian cancer. The basis for the increased risk is that repetitive ovulation can cause cellular damage, inflammation, and cellular repair, all processes that increase the likelihood of introducing DNA mutations. Multiple pregnancies, using contraception methods that interrupt ovulation, and ovulation suppression due to extended lactation can reduce the risk of developing ovarian cancer [23].

2.2. Genetic Risk Factors

The most significant risk factor for ovarian cancer is a strong family history of gynecological, breast, or colon cancers. These women generally have an underlying genetic predisposition to developing ovarian cancer and have mutations in tumor suppressor genes that prevent cancer [24]. Mutations that lead to the loss of function of tumor suppressor genes are recessive; therefore, they must be passed on by both parents to their daughter, resulting in an increased risk of cancer. However, in the case of ovarian cancer, there are mutations that are dominant, so that only one copy of the mutated gene needs to be inherited from either parent. BRCA-1 and -2 are tumor suppressor genes, specifically caretaker genes, that encode proteins involved in DNA repair that prevent the accumulation of mistakes encoded in DNA [25,26]. Ovarian cancer associated with BRCA-1/2 mutations is more indolent and affects younger women. Among women with mutations in BRCA-1, the risk of ovarian cancer can range from 39% to 44%, while the risk with BRCA-2 mutations 12% to 20% [27–29].

Lynch Syndrome is a disorder that predisposes women to right sided non-polyposis colon cancer and ovarian and endometrial cancers. There are five tumor suppressor genes mutations associated with Lynch Syndrome: MSH2, MLH1, MLH6, PMS1, and PMS2. Mutations in these genes are inherited in a dominant fashion, and result in increased microsatellite instability, or regions of DNA with incorrectly transcribed DNA. Ovarian cancer risk in women with Lynch Syndrome is six to 8% [30]. It is quite clear that women with inherited genetic mutations are at a greater risk of developing ovarian cancer, with a nearly three to fifteen-fold increase in risk for different gene mutations [31].

3. Clinical Presentation

3.1. Symptoms

Ovarian cancer is considered a "silent killer", meaning most women have no symptoms from the disease. Symptoms reported to be associated with ovarian cancer [32,33] are more often non-specific and associated with other conditions [26]. Sometimes, patients may present to their clinician with pelvic pain secondary to ovarian torsion. It is rare that any symptoms are associated with early stage ovarian cancer [34,35], and even when they do occur it is possible that they are coincidental. Women with advanced disease, however, are likely to have complaints of pelvic pain, abdominal fullness, early satiety, and bloating when tumor burden inflames abdominal structures.

3.2. Physical Examination Findings

A clinician may have an increased index of suspicion for ovarian cancer following their physical examination of the patient. A palpable pelvic mass, ascites with a fluid wave, or diminished breath sounds from pleural effusions can be identified on a physical examination. Rarely, a Sister-Mary Joseph nodule, resulting from ovarian cancer metastasized to the umbilicus, or the Sign of Leser-Trelat, which is an abrupt increase in seborrheic keratoses, can be indicative of occult cancer.

3.3. Ovarian Cancer Paraneoplastic Syndromes

Various paraneoplastic syndromes are infrequently associated with ovarian cancer. Hypercalcemia, usually due to increased levels of circulating parathyroid hormone releasing protein, can occur and cause altered mental status, increased thirst, urination, fatigue, constipation, and abdominal pain. Subacute cerebellar degeneration presenting as ataxia, dysarthria, vertigo, nystagmus, and double vision is due to cross-reactivity of antibodies to tumor antigens to cerebellar tissue. This condition usually precedes tumor occurrence by months to years, and can be associated with severe morbidity and mortality. Finally, Trousseau's syndrome, or unexplained thromboses, has been associated with ovarian cancer [36].

4. Diagnosis of Ovarian Cancer

4.1. Diagnostic Schema

If there is a high clinical index of suspicion, diagnostic evaluation can be undertaken. This begins with a transvaginal ultrasound (TVUS). TVUS is highly sensitive and provides morphological information about the ovary. Abnormal cystic findings on TVUS are broadly defined as simple or complex, with echogenic components in complex cysts more indicative of malignancy. Ultrasound findings can then be paired with blood tests that measure levels of tumor markers.

4.2. Tumor Markers

Discovered over 30 years ago, CA-125 is one of the most utilized biomarkers for ovarian cancer [37,38]. When circulating levels of the CA-125 glycoprotein are elevated, it is often indicative of ovarian cancer, although benign conditions like pregnancy, menstruation, endometriosis, and pelvic inflammation can also be responsible for elevated CA-125 levels [39]. CA-125 can be used to calculate the risk of malignancy index (RMI) for an individual patient. The RMI consists of a score assigned to TVUS findings, menopausal status, and CA-125 level. RMI values greater than 200 indicate high risk of malignancy [40].

A biomarker reported to be more sensitive for identifying ovarian cancer is HE-4, which is expressed on multiple organs but, surprisingly, not on the ovary. Elevations in HE-4 are found in nearly 100% of serous and endometrioid ovarian cancers and are sensitive in diagnosing early ovarian cancer. Compared to CA-125, HE-4 is not elevated in benign processes, allowing the biomarker to be specific for ovarian malignancy. The caveat for utilizing HE-4 is that normal values are not established. With the high specificity of HE-4, and the high sensitivity of CA-125, the utility of combining the two for diagnosing ovarian cancer has been implemented as the Risk of Malignancy algorithm (ROMA). The ROMA uses a mathematical formula utilizing HE-4 and CA-125 concentrations adjusted for pre- and post-menopausal status. Elevated ROMA values place women in a high risk of malignancy category. The ROMA serves as a good screening test that also has specificity for epithelial ovarian cancer. It not only detects more patients with ovarian cancer than the RMI, but also those with early stages of ovarian cancer [41].

In 2009, the Food and Drug Administration approved the clinical use of OVA-1, a serum test analyzing five biomarkers: CA-125, II-microglobulin (both elevated in ovarian cancer), apolipoprotein A1, prealbumin (transthyretin), and transferrin (which are decreased in ovarian cancer). Biomarker levels are used in a computer algorithm to provide a result between zero and ten and are stratified based on menopausal status. Patients with higher scores should be evaluated by a gynecologic oncologist because the complexity of their disease is expected to be greater than those with lower scores. To date, there are no studies directly comparing the performance of OVA-1 and ROMA [42].

5. Ovarian Cancer Staging

Once a woman is considered to be at high risk for ovarian malignancy, a referral to a gynecologic oncologist is made. Surgery is generally undertaken to properly assess the extent of the disease. An exploratory laparotomy through a midline incision allows for gross evaluation of the abdominal and pelvic cavities for disease. If staging of ovarian cancer is found to be necessary, saline is initially used to irrigate the pelvis and collected as "pelvic washings". This is followed by the surgical removal of the uterus, cervix, both Fallopian tubes, ovaries, lymph nodes that drain the ovaries (para-aortic lymph nodes), and the fat pad that insulates the intestines (omentum). Tissue is sent to the pathologist for final diagnosis of histological type, grade, and staging [31].

6. Treatment of Ovarian Cancer and Side Effects

6.1. Side Effects of Surgery

There are multiple side effects in the treatment of ovarian cancer. With surgery, potential risks generally include infection, hemorrhage, blood transfusion, pain, prolonged hospitalization, readmission, anesthesia complications, and death. Ovarian cancer surgical staging is often considered to be an "intermediate-complex surgery" and is associated with a 20% risk of morbidity and mortality occurring within the first 30 days following the operation [43]. Additionally, there is a ten to 15% risk of surgical site infections [44].

6.2. Chemotherapy and Associated Side Effects

Following surgery, most women receive some sort of chemotherapy treatment to eradicate any residual microscopic disease. More advanced stage ovarian cancer will have a greater likelihood of being associated with residual disease. Various platinum-based chemotherapy regimens have been used and are dependent on the stage of the cancer. These agents are not without side effects that can include nausea, renal and ototoxicity, myalgia, alopecia, bone marrow toxicity with resulting pancytopenia, mouth sores, swelling, redness, and chronic pain in the hands and feet (hand-foot syndrome) [45,46].

7. Psychosocial Effects of Ovarian Cancer

There can be considerable emotional and physical burdens associated with ovarian cancer. Anxiety and depression can develop from the distress over the pending removal of organs that represent a woman's femininity, motherhood, and sexuality [47]. Recurrence of disease is common, nearly 80% with advanced stage, serving as another nidus for stress. In a study from the Dana-Farber Cancer Institute, 56% of ovarian cancer survivors surveyed were concerned about recurrence [48]. Anxiety and depression is nearly two times more likely in women with ovarian cancer, and higher if there are other underlying health issues. Additionally, nearly 33% of ovarian cancer patients experience high levels of psychological distress [49]. The burden of ovarian cancer can be extended to caregivers. The Australian Ovarian Cancer Study Group investigated the effects of ovarian cancer on the quality of life of ovarian cancer caregivers. This study found that in the last year of life, caregivers had lower quality of life measures as well as higher distress than those who were not taking care of ovarian cancer partners. Additionally, mental and physical well-being worsened the closer their partner came to the end-of-life. The most reported unmet needs of caregivers in the last six months were found to be concerned with managing emotions surrounding prognosis, fear of worsening disease, balancing of both the needs of themselves and their partners, the impact of caring for their partner had on their career, and making decisions in an environment of uncertainty [50].

8. Ovarian Cancer Screening

8.1. Overview of Early Detection of Ovarian Cancer

Advanced ovarian cancer is associated with decreased survival, and increased morbidity with not only the disease itself, but also surgery and the effects of chemotherapy. A recent study found that if 75% of ovarian cases can be detected as Stage I or II disease, there would be a 50% reduction in ovarian cancer related deaths [3]. Therefore, there have been multiple investigations to improve detection of ovarian at earlier stages.

8.2. Disease Screening Principles

One method is to screen women for ovarian cancer. Disease that benefits from screening is one that is (1) highly prevalent in the population, (2) a major health problem, (3) has a significant preclinical stage during which detection by screening is possible, and (4) is significantly more curable at earlier stages. Ovarian cancer satisfies these conditions, but does challenge the condition of prevalence.

Screening for a disease is the process by which an asymptomatic population is evaluated for the likelihood of having the disease before there are symptoms or any indication of disease. Screening has two outcomes: positive (likely has the disease) or negative (does not have the disease). The ideal screening test will have:

A. High sensitivity: the ability to identify everyone with disease who tests positive (true positive) from everyone with disease (true positives + false negatives). Ideally, a highly sensitive test will have a low rate of false negative results so the test rarely misses subjects with the disease;

B. High specificity: the ability to correctly identify subjects *without* the disease (true negatives) from everyone without disease (true negatives + false positives). A highly specific screening test will have a low false positive rate;

C. High positive predictive value: the portion of subjects with disease that tested positive (true positives) relative to all who tested positive (true positives + false positives), a value dependent on the prevalence of the disease;

D. High negative predictive value: the portion without disease that tested negative (true negatives) relative to everyone testing negative (true negatives + false negatives), which is *inversely* dependent on disease prevalence;

E. Low cost: to allow maximum test affordability.

Table 1 summarizes these terms and relates them to ovarian cancer screening.

Table 1. Statistical terms and definitions used in ovarian cancer screening [51].

Term	Screening Result	Findings
True Positive (TP)	Positive	Histologically-proven ovarian cancer
False Positive (FP)	Positive	Benign ovarian histology
True Negative (TN)	Negative	No evidence of ovarian cancer 12 months after a negative screen
False Negative (FN)	Negative	Ovarian cancer diagnosed within 12 months of a negative screen

Sensitivity = TP/(TP + FN); Specificity = TN/(TN + FP); Positive Predictive Value = TP/(TP + FP); Negative Predictive Value = TN/(TN + FN). Reproduced from [51] with permission from publisher.

Screening tests are compared to an acceptable "gold standard" test, which is usually a definitive diagnostic test. It is typically invasive, unpleasant, expensive, or impractical for wide use. Considered the best test under "reasonable conditions", the "gold standard" test provides 100% sensitivity and specificity [52]. Regarding ovarian cancer, there is no current "gold standard" screening test. However, TVUS performs with the highest sensitivity and specificity. A TVUS is performed with a 5–7.5 mHz vaginal probe that generates accurate images of the ovary used to detect changes in ovarian morphology and volume that are subtle and usually inappreciable on physical examination.

8.3. Ovarian Cancer Screening Trials

8.3.1. University of Kentucky Ovarian Cancer Screening Program

There have been four large ovarian cancer screening trials with TVUS as the primary screening modality, one of which is the University of Kentucky Markey Cancer Center Ovarian Cancer Screening Program. Originally initiated in 1987 by Dr. John R. van Nagall, this project has enrolled over 45,000 women, and investigators have performed over 280,000 scans. The project includes two groups: asymptomatic women ≥50 years old, and asymptomatic women ≥25–49 years old with a documented history of ovarian cancer in at least one primary or secondary family member. Both groups of women are compared to an unscreened control group of women from the same geographic area who received the same treatment protocols over the same period. The groups undergoing screening undergo evaluation based on an established algorithm (Figure 1).

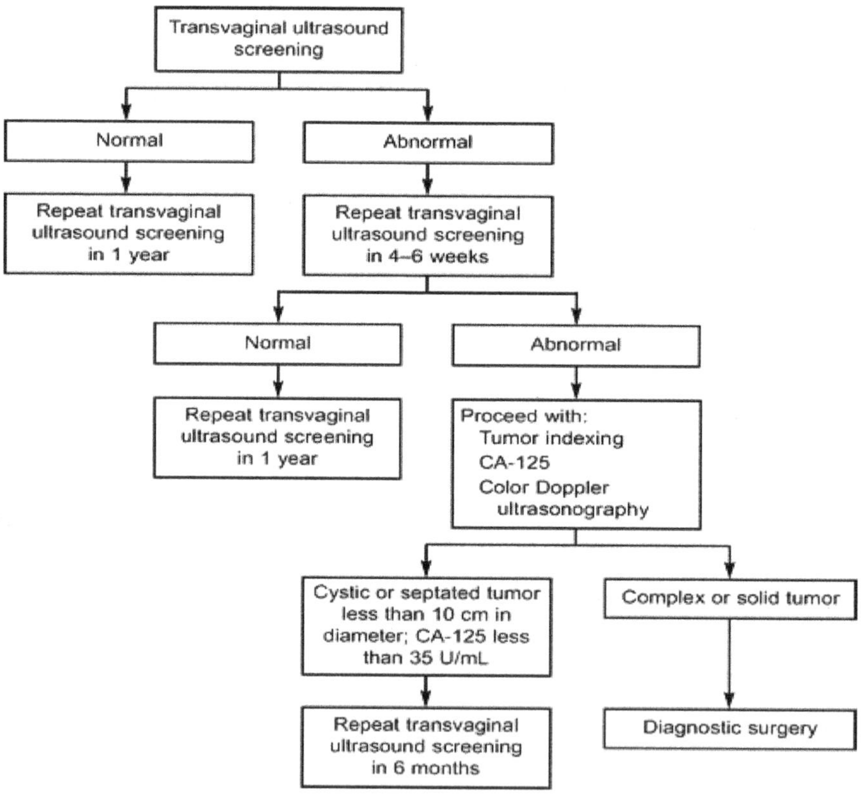

Figure 1. University of Kentucky Ovarian Cancer Screening Trial screening, evaluation, and treatment algorithm [53]. Reproduced with permission from publisher.

Using the algorithm, the detection of 53 primary epithelial ovarian malignancies has been reported [2]. Women who had ovarian cancer diagnosed by screening had earlier-stage disease (Stage 1 or 2) than those who did not receive screening (68% vs. 27%). The five-year survival rate of all women whose ovarian cancer was detected by screening compared to those not undergoing screening was

74.8% ± 6.6% and 53.7% ± 2.3%, a statistically significant difference. To date, the overall sensitivity, specificity positive and negative predictive values, and false positive rate are 86.4%, 98.8%, 14.53% to 20.17%, 99.97%, and 1.2%, respectively [54–57].

8.3.2. Prostate, Lung, Colon, and Ovarian Cancer Screening Trial

The Prostate, Lung, Colon, and Ovarian Cancer Screening Trial (PLCO) is a large, population-based randomized trial designed and sponsored by the National Cancer Institute starting in 1993 to determine the effects of screening on cancer-related mortality and secondary outcomes in men and women aged 55 to 74. Regarding ovarian cancer screening, women were assigned to undergo either annual screening with CA-125 and TVUS or usual care. There was no statistically significant reduction in ovarian cancer–related deaths between those screened and those who underwent usual care. There was a minimal increase in the detection of early stage ovarian cancer with screening than with usual care (22% vs. 21%). The five-year survival rate was 47.4% in the screening group compared to 36.0% in the group receiving usual care. The sensitivity, specificity, positive and negative predictive values, and false positive rate were 85.14%, 90.34%, 6.06%, 99.88%, and 9.6%, respectively [58,59].

8.3.3. United Kingdom Collaborative Trial of Ovarian Cancer Screening Trial

The United Kingdom Collaborative Trial of Ovarian Cancer Screening (UKCTOCS) trial recruited 200,000 women beginning in 2001 and randomized them into a usual care group, annual screening with TVUS group, or annual multimodal screening with CA-125 and risk for ovarian cancer algorithm (ROCA) group. The ROC utilizes an individual's CA-125 level profile (initial values and trends over time) and compares it to populations of women with and without cancer. The more a woman's ROC looks like profiles of women who have ovarian cancer, the greater her risk of having ovarian cancer [60]. Women found to have a high ROC scores were subsequently screened with TVUS per their algorithm. Results demonstrated an increased detection of low-volume disease (Stage 1, 2, and 3a) in the multimodal screening group than by TVUS alone (40% vs. 24%). There was no reduction in mortality regardless of the type of screening. Regarding the detection of any primary ovarian, tubal, or peritoneal cancers, the sensitivity, specificity, and positive predictive value for the TVUS group were found to be 84.9%, 98.2%, and 5.3%, respectively. The multimodal screening had a sensitivity of 89.4%, specificity of 99.8%, and a positive predictive value of 43.3%, respectively. When detecting primary invasive ovarian, tubal, and peritoneal malignancies, the sensitivity and positive predictive value of TVUS decreased to 75% and 2.8%. The multimodal screening was essentially unchanged, yet the positive predictive value decreased to 35% [61,62].

8.3.4. Multi-Center Japan University Trial

The final, large-scale ovarian cancer screening trial is the Multi-center Japan University trial. Over 80,000 asymptomatic women were divided into either a control group consisting of usual care following a physical examination or a screening group. Screening involved an annual pelvic examination, TVUS and/or transabdominal ultrasound, and measurement of CA-125 levels. The study showed that screening could detect Stage I and II disease at a higher rate compared to usual care (67% and 44%, respectively). Using the published data, the sensitivity, specificity, and positive and negative predictive values were 68.6%, 99.8%, 23.3% and 99.9%, respectively. The analysis of this screening protocol for the long-term effect on ovarian cancer mortality is presently in progress [63].

9. Life Is More Than Death: An Interview with the Husband of a Recently Deceased Woman Suffering from Advanced Stage Ovarian Cancer

In my short time in medical school and residency, I have made myself familiar with the pathophysiology of ovarian cancer, its treatments, the status of screening for the disease, and the survival curves that serve as the ultimate sterile summary of this disease. In all actuality, survival curves are the measure of time from diagnosis to death, conveying nothing more than the math of mortality. I have looked into the faces of women at various stages of this disease and have seen the suffering in their eyes as their mortality approaches them.

I felt compelled to convey only one story, a story that is much larger than the deaths due to ovarian cancer, because it is the journey on the terrifying road that women travel from their diagnosis to their death. I received permission to discuss the final stages of ovarian cancer with the husband and subsequent caregiver of a patient who died from ovarian cancer. To preserve patient confidentiality, identities are de-identified with pseudonyms.

9.1. Pre-Diagnosis Life

Mr. and Mrs. Johnson (pseudonyms) were college sweethearts who met through a mutual friend. Their first date consisted of a lovely bike ride across their college campus. Eventually, they wed and had three children. Mrs. Johnson primarily took care of their children and homeschooled them much of the time. Eventually, the children grew up and left home. She enjoyed working with her hands and loved embroidery, designing children's clothing, and creating smocking designs.

Mrs. Johnson took very good care of herself and never missed her annual gynecologic examinations. However, one day she noticed changes in her body. She mentioned this to her husband and said she "felt like she was filling up with water". Initially, they dismissed the complaint as something that would resolve itself. However, two days later, she again commented on how bloated she felt, and lifted her shirt, showing her husband how distended her abdomen was. She began to shake her hips, and they both could hear "water sloshing around her abdomen". Mrs. Johnson called a physician friend, who urged her to set up an appointment with her gynecologist.

At the discretion of her gynecologist, she underwent a CT scan and had a CA-125 level drawn. When her doctor entered the room with the results, he "had a complete change in his demeanor". Her CA-125 was over 15,000, and imaging showed some sort of gynecologic malignancy. Her gynecologist counseled her that she needed to be evaluated by a gynecologic oncologist and suggested she be evaluated at the Markey Cancer Center, located on the University of Kentucky Medical Center campus.

The gynecologic oncologist was certain she was suffering from at least Stage IIIC ovarian cancer and that a staging surgery was necessary. Surgery revealed extensive disease throughout the abdomen including involvement of the liver and diaphragm. A ureter obstruction required a ureter re-anastomosis by a urology consultation team. Post-operatively, she spent 11 days in the hospital, which was complicated by a right pleural effusion. The final pathology was consistent with high-grade Stage IVA papillary serous adenocarcinoma of the ovary arising from both ovaries. According to her husband, revelation of her diagnosis was "like being hit between the eyes".

9.2. Life after Diagnosis for Both Individuals

Though the chances of a five-year survival had been quoted as 15%, Mrs. Johnson had always been a strongminded individual, and she was determined to beat her disease. Chemotherapy options were discussed, and she elected to proceed with dose-dense carboplatin and taxol.

9.3. Life during Treatment for Both Individuals

Life during chemotherapy was a struggle, though she did not let those struggles dampen her faith and determination. Fatigue was the worst side effect from her chemotherapy to the point that she was unable to enjoy her usual embroidery activities. Faith played a large role in keeping her will to beat cancer alive. Her family and church members prayed constantly that she would not suffer from neuropathy in her hands so she could continue knitting, and thankfully, their prayers were answered. She had mild neuropathy in her feet with sparing of her hands.

Mrs. Johnson experienced recurrent pleural effusions, eventually showing evidence of malignancy and recurrence. She had the the lining of her right hemi-thorax removed, which did not show evidence of disease. Additionally, a new area of suspected malignancy on her spleen was evident on a repeat CT scan, along with a rise in her CA-125 to a maximum level of 4000. She received various chemotherapy regimens including, gemcitabine, Avastin with vinorelbine, taxotere, cyclophosphamide, and etoposide. External beam radiation therapy was utilized to address the malignant area of her spleen. She had 13 radiation treatments, but decided to decline any more radiation treatments because they caused more fatigue than her chemotherapy. Her cancer responded to the cyclophosphamide, but eventually her CA-125 began to rise. She declined further chemotherapy, and the topic of hospice was approached. She decided that she did not want hospice at that point.

9.4. Life during the Final Months for Both Individuals

The final months of Mrs. Johnson's life were filled with overwhelming difficulties resulting from her recurrent ovarian cancer. She suffered greatly from recurrent pleural effusions and abdominal ascites. She had nearly eight liters of ascites removed as an outpatient. She would continue to have paracenteses whenever she became symptomatic. She decided to resume chemotherapy treatment with etoposide. Two days later, she was admitted to the hospital with chemotherapy induced nausea and vomiting. She was discharged after five days, but was readmitted for intractable symptoms. She wanted to have a Denver drain placed to allow personal drainage of her ascites whenever she was symptomatic. This improved her quality of life considerably.

However, she suffered another setback when she was diagnosed with a small bowel obstruction. She elected to forego aggressive surgical treatment to address the obstruction and decided instead to go home to be treated with intravenous fluids. The topic of hospice was brought up multiple times, but she did not want to give in to her cancer. She was unable to tolerate any food, but she was determined to eat. The thought of food became an obsession, as she would "watch cooking shows and read every page of every cookbook in her kitchen". She developed a routine of self-induced emesis in the morning and evenings so that she could at least eat something. She continued to be symptomatic from her small bowel obstruction, utilizing outpatient intravenous fluid hydration and electrolyte replacements. Through all of this, she still declined hospice, with hope still alive of overcoming her disease.

Mrs. Johnson died in November 2016. From the time of diagnosis, she lived 33 months, underwent 66 chemotherapy treatments with 10 different chemotherapy agents, 13 external radiation treatments, five thoracenteses to relieve recurrent pleural effusions, and four paracentesis procedures that removed nearly eight liters of ascites. Mrs. Johnson did not live without pain, nor die without immense suffering.

9.5. Feelings of the Family (Husband) after the Woman's Death

Mrs. Johnson's family had a very peaceful Thanksgiving with her son and his wife assuming the cooking responsibilities that Mrs. Johnson had traditionally performed. Christmas was "a 'new' Christmas, but not a sad one". Mr. Johnson said that he did not regret anything about his wife's fight with cancer, and though it was the most terrible time for them, they would do nothing different if they had to go through it again.

10. Conclusions

It is estimated that a woman's lifetime risk of developing ovarian cancer is one in 70. Many ovarian cancers are diagnosed at an advanced stage, with only 15% of cases diagnosed in early stages. Ovarian cancer screening trials have attempted to diagnose women with early stage disease because survival is significantly greater in those patients. With screening programs like the University of Kentucky Markey Cancer Center Ovarian Cancer Screening Program, transvaginal ultrasound is effective for discovering early stage ovarian cancer. With continued efforts and determination, more ovarian cancers can be diagnosed at earlier, more curable stages, avoiding the pain and suffering associated with advanced stage disease like that endured by Mrs. Johnson.

References

1. Siegel, R.L.; Miller, K.D.; Jemal, A. Cancer statistics, 2016. *Cancer J. Clin.* **2016**, *66*, 7–30. [CrossRef] [PubMed]
2. Van Nagell, J.R.; Miller, R.W.; DeSimone, C.P.; Ueland, F.R.; Podzielinski, I.; Goodrich, S.T.; Elder, J.W.; Huang, B.; Kryscio, R.J.; Pavlik, E.J. Long-term survival of women with epithelial ovarian cancer detected by ultrasonographic screening. *Obstet. Gynecol.* **2011**, *118*, 1212–1221. [CrossRef] [PubMed]
3. Van Nagell, J.R.; Pavlik, E.J. Ovarian cancer screening. *Clin. Obstet. Gynecol.* **2012**, *55*, 43–51. [CrossRef] [PubMed]
4. Bridgewater, J.A.; Rustin, G.J.S. Management of Non-Epithelial Ovarian Tumours. *Oncology* **1999**, *57*, 89–98. [CrossRef] [PubMed]
5. Sundar, S.; Neal, R.D.; Kehoe, S. Diagnosis of ovarian cancer. *BMJ* **2015**, *351*, h4443. [CrossRef] [PubMed]
6. Boussios, S.; Zarkavelis, G.; Seraj, E.; Zerdes, I.; Tatsi, K.; Pentheroudakis, G. Non-epithelial Ovarian Cancer: Elucidating Uncommon Gynaecological Malignancies. *Anticancer Res.* **2016**, *36*, 5031–5042. [CrossRef] [PubMed]
7. Karnezis, A.N.; Cho, K.R.; Gilks, B.; Pearce, C.L.; Huntsman, D.G. The disparate origins of ovarian cancers: Pathogenesis and prevention strategies. *Nat. Rev. Cancer* **2017**, *17*, 65–74. [CrossRef] [PubMed]
8. National Comprehensive Cancer Network. Ovarian Cancer Including Fallopian Tube Cancer and Primary Peritoneal Cancer (Version 1.2016). OV-D. Available online: https://www.nccn.org/professionals/physician_gls/pdf/ovarian.pdf (accessed on 4 November 2017).
9. Alvarado-Cabrero, I.; Navani, S.S.; Young, R.H.; Scully, R.E. Tumors of the Fimbriated End of the Fallopian Tube: A Clinicopathologic Analysis of 20 Cases, Including Nine Carcinomas. *Int. J. Gynecol. Pathol.* **1997**, *16*, 189–196. [CrossRef] [PubMed]
10. Colgan, T.J.; Murphy, J.; Cole, D.E.; Narod, S.; Rosen, B. Occult Carcinoma in Prophylactic Oophorectomy Specimens: Prevalence and Association with BRCA Germline Mutation Status. *Am. J. Surg. Pathol.* **2001**, *25*, 1283–1289. [CrossRef] [PubMed]
11. Cass, I.; Holschneider, C.; Datta, N.; Barbuto, D.; Walts, A.E.; Karlan, B.Y. BRCA-Mutation-Associated Fallopian Tube Carcinoma: A Distinct Clinical Phenotype? *Obstet. Gynecol.* **2005**, *106*, 1327–1334. [CrossRef] [PubMed]
12. Medeiros, F.; Muto, M.G.; Lee, Y.; Elvin, J.A.; Callahan, M.J.; Feltmate, C.; Garber, J.E.; Cramer, D.W.; Crum, C.P. The Tubal Fimbria Is a Preferred Site for Early Adenocarcinoma in Women With Familial Ovarian Cancer Syndrome. *Am. J. Surg. Pathol.* **2006**, *30*, 230–236. [CrossRef] [PubMed]
13. Kindelberger, D.W.; Lee, Y.; Miron, A.; Hirsch, M.S.; Feltmate, C.; Medeiros, F.; Callahan, M.J.; Garner, E.O.; Gordon, R.W.; Birch, C.; et al. Intraepithelial Carcinoma of the Fimbriae and Pelvic Serous Carcinoma: Evidence for a Causal Relationship. *Am. J. Surg. Pathol.* **2007**, *31*, 161–169. [CrossRef] [PubMed]
14. Crum, C.R.; Drapkin, R.; Miron, A.; Ince, T.A.; Muto, M.; Kindelberger, D.W.; Lee, Y. The distal fallopian tube: A new model for pelvic serous carcinogenesis. *Curr. Opin. Obstet. Gynecol.* **2007**, *19*, 3–9. [CrossRef] [PubMed]
15. Landen, C.N.; Birrer, M.J.; Sood, A.K. Early Events in the Pathogenesis of Epithelial Ovarian Cancer. *J. Clin. Oncol.* **2008**, *26*, 995–1005. [CrossRef] [PubMed]
16. Lengyel, E. Ovarian Cancer Development and Metastasis. *Am. J. Pathol.* **2010**, *177*, 1053–1064. [CrossRef] [PubMed]
17. Kurman, R.J.; Shih, L.M. The Origin and Pathogenesis of Epithelial Ovarian Cancer: A Proposed Unifying Theory. *Am. J. Surg. Pathol.* **2010**, *34*, 433–443. [CrossRef] [PubMed]
18. Crum, C.P.; Mckeon, F.D.; Xian, X. The Oviduct and Ovarian Cancer: Causality, Clinical Implications, and "Targeted Prevention". *Clin. Obstet. Gynecol.* **2012**, *55*, 24–35. [CrossRef] [PubMed]
19. Nezhat, F.R.; Aposto, R.l.; Nezha, C.T.; Pejovic, T. New insights in the pathophysiology of ovarian cancer and implications for screening and prevention. *Am. J. Obstet. Gynecol.* **2015**, *213*, 262–267. [CrossRef] [PubMed]
20. Schneider, S.; Heikaus, S.; Harter, P.; Heitz, F.; Grimm, C.; Ataseven, B.; Prader, S.; Kurzeder, C.; Ebel, T.; Traut, A.; et al. Serous Tubal Intraepithelial Carcinoma Associated With Extraovarian Metastases. *Int. J. Gynecol. Cancer* **2017**, *27*, 444–451. [CrossRef] [PubMed]
21. Surveillance, Epidemiology, and End Results (SEER) Program. Cancer of the Ovary—SEER Stat Facts Sheet. National Cancer Institute, DCCPS, Surveillance Research Program, Surveillance Systems Branch. Available online: https://seer.cancer.gov/statfacts/html/ovary.html (accessed on 9 November 2016).
22. Cancer of the Ovary: SEER Stat Fact Sheets. Available online: http://seer.cancer.gov/statfacts/html/ovary.html (accessed on 27 December 2016).
23. Webb, P.M.; Jordan, S.J. Epidemiology of epithelial ovarian cancer. *Best Pract. Res. Clin. Obstet. Gynaecol.* **2016**. [CrossRef] [PubMed]
24. Weinberg, R.A. *The Biology of Cancer*; Garland Science: New York, NJ, USA, 2014; Volume 231.

25. Duncan, J.A.; Reeves, J.R.; Cooke, T.G. BRCA1 and BRCA2 proteins: Roles in health and disease. *Mol. Pathol.* **1998**, *51*, 237–247. [CrossRef] [PubMed]
26. Yoshida, K.; Miki, Y. Role of BRCA1 and BRCA2 as regulators of DNA repair, transcription, and cell cycle in response to DNA damage. *Cancer Sci.* **2004**, *95*, 866–871. [CrossRef] [PubMed]
27. American College of Obstetricians and Gynecologists. *Hereditary Breast and Ovarian Cancer Syndrome*; ACOG Practice Bulletin No. 103; American College of Obstetricians and Gynecologists: Washington, DC, USA, 2009; Volume 113, pp. 957–966.
28. Antoniou, A.; Pharoah, P.D.P.; Narod, S.; Risch, H.A.; Eyfjord, J.E.; Hopper, J.L.; Loman, N.; Olsson, H.; Johannsson, O.; Borg, A.; et al. Average Risks of Breast and Ovarian Cancer Associated with BRCA1 or BRCA2 Mutations Detected in Case Series Unselected for Family History: A Combined Analysis of 22 Studies. *Am. J. Hum. Genet.* **2003**, *72*, 1117–1130. [CrossRef] [PubMed]
29. Brose, M.S.; Rebbeck, T.R.; Calzone, K.A.; Stopfer, J.E.; Nathanson, K.L.; Weber, B.L. Cancer Risk Estimates for BRCA1 Mutation Carriers Identified in a Risk Evaluation Program. *J. Natl. Cancer Inst.* **2002**, *94*, 1365–1372. [CrossRef] [PubMed]
30. American College of Obstetricians and Gynecologists. *Lynch Syndrome*; Practice Bulletin No. 147; American College of Obstetricians and Gynecologists: Washington, DC, USA, 2014; Volume 124, pp. 1042–1054.
31. National Academies of Sciences, Engineering, and Medicine. *Ovarian Cancers: Evolving Paradigms in Research and Care*; The National Academies Press: Washington, DC, USA, 2016.
32. Goff, B.A.; Mandel, L.S.; Drescher, C.W.; Urban, N.; Gough, S.; Schurman, K.M.; Patras, J.; Mahony, B.S.; Andersen, M.R. Development of an ovarian cancer symptom index: Possibilities for earlier detection. *Cancer* **2007**, *109*, 221–227. [CrossRef] [PubMed]
33. Goff, B. Symptoms associated with ovarian cancer. *Clin. Obstet. Gynecol.* **2012**, *55*, 36–42. [CrossRef] [PubMed]
34. Pavlik, E.J.; Saunders, B.A.; Doran, S.; McHugh, K.W.; Ueland, F.R.; Desemone, C.P.; Depriest, P.D.; Ware, R.A.; Kryscio, R.J.; van Nagell, J.R., Jr. The search for meaning—Symptoms and transvaginal sonography screening for ovarian cancer. *Cancer* **2009**, *115*, 3689–3698. [CrossRef] [PubMed]
35. Rossing, M.A.; Wicklund, K.G.; Cushing-Haugen, K.L.; Weiss, N.S. Predictive value of symptoms for early detection of ovarian cancer. *J. Natl. Cancer Inst.* **2010**, *102*, 222–229. [CrossRef] [PubMed]
36. Cannistra, S.A. Cancer of the Ovary. *N. Engl. J. Med.* **2004**, *351*, 2519–2529. [CrossRef] [PubMed]
37. Bast, R.C.; Feeney, M.; Lazarus, H.; Nadler, L.M.; Colvin, R.B.; Knapp, R.C. Reactivity of a monoclonal antibody with human ovarian carcinoma. *J. Clin. Investig.* **1981**, *68*, 1331–1337. [CrossRef] [PubMed]
38. Gupta, D.; Lis, C.G. Role of CA125 in predicting ovarian cancer survival—A review of the epidemiological literature. *J. Ovarian Res.* **2009**, *2*, 13. [CrossRef] [PubMed]
39. Fritsche, H.A.; Bast, R.C. CA 125 in ovarian cancer: Advances and controversy. *Clin. Chem.* **1998**, *44*, 1379–1380. [PubMed]
40. Jayson, G.C.; Kohn, E.C.; Kitchener, H.C.; Ledermann, J.A. Ovarian Cancer. *Lancet* **2014**, *384*, 1376–1388. [CrossRef]
41. Moore, R.G.; Jabre-Raughley, M.; Brown, A.K.; Robison, K.M.; Miller, M.C.; Allard, W.J.; Kurman, R.J.; Bast, R.C.; Skates, S.J. Comparison of a novel multiple marker assay vs. the Risk of Malignancy Index for the prediction of epithelial ovarian cancer in patients with a pelvic mass. *Am. J. Obstet. Gynecol.* **2010**, *203*, 1–6. [CrossRef] [PubMed]
42. Novak, M.; Lukasz, J.; Stachowiak, G.; Stetkiewicz, T.; Wilczynski, J.R. Current clinical application of serum biomarkers to detect ovarian cancer. *Prz. Menopauzalny* **2015**, *14*, 254–259.
43. Thrall, M.M.; Goff, B.A.; Symons, R.G.; Flum, D.R.; Gray, H.J. Thirty-day mortality after primary cytoreductive surgery for advanced ovarian cancer in the elderly. *Obstet. Gynecol.* **2011**, *118*, 537–547. [CrossRef] [PubMed]
44. Gerestein, C.G.; Nieuwenhuyzen-de Boer, G.M.; Eijekmans, M.J.; Kooi, G.S.; Burger, C.W. Prediction of 30-day morbidity after primary cytoreductive surgery for advanced stage ovarian cancer. *Eur. J. Cancer* **2010**, *46*, 102–109. [CrossRef] [PubMed]
45. Sun, C.C.; Bodurka, D.C.; Weaver, C.B.; Rasu, R.; Wolf, J.K.; Bevers, M.W.; Smith, J.A.; Wharton, J.T.; Rubenstein, E.B. Rankings and symptom assessments of side effects from chemotherapy: Insights from experienced patients with ovarian cancer. *Support. Care Cancer* **2005**, *13*, 219–227. [CrossRef] [PubMed]
46. American Cancer Society. Chemotherapy for Ovarian Cancer. Available online: https://www.cancer.org/cancer/ovarian-cancer/treating/chemotherapy.html (accessed on 9 November 2016).

47. Guidozzi, F. Living with Ovarian Cancer. *Gynecol. Oncol.* **1992**, *50*, 202–207. [CrossRef] [PubMed]
48. Matulonis, U.A.; Kornblith, A.; Lee, H.; Bryan, J.; Gibson, C.; Wells, C.; Lee, J.; Sullivan, L.; Penson, R. Long-term adjustment of early-stage ovarian cancer survivors. *Int. J. Gynecol. Cancer* **2008**, *18*, 1183–1193. [CrossRef] [PubMed]
49. Bodurka-Bevers, D.; Basen-Engquist, K.; Carmack, C.L.; Fitzgerald, M.A.; Wolf, J.K.; de Moor, C.; Gershenson, D.M. Depression, anxiety, and quality of life in patients with epithelial ovarian cancer. *Gynecol. Oncol.* **2000**, *78*, 302–308. [CrossRef] [PubMed]
50. Butow, P.N.; Price, M.A.; Bell, M.L.; Webb, P.M.; DeFazio, A.; Australian Ovarian Cancer Study Group; Australian Ovarian Cancer Study Quality of Life Study Investigators; Friedlander, M. Caring for women with ovarian cancer in the last year of life: A longitudinal study of caregiver quality of life, distress and unmet needs. *Gynecol. Oncol.* **2014**, *132*, 690–697. [PubMed]
51. Van Nagell, J.R.; Depriest, P.D.; Gallion, H.H.; Pavlik, E.J. Ovarian cancer screening. *Cancer* **1993**, *71*, 1523–1528. [CrossRef] [PubMed]
52. Maxim, L.D.; Niebo, R.; Utell, M.J. Screening tests: A review with examples. *Inhal. Toxicol.* **2014**, *26*, 811–828. [CrossRef] [PubMed]
53. Van Nagell, J.R., Jr.; DePriest, P.D.; Ueland, F.R.; DeSimone, C.P.; Cooper, A.L.; McDonald, J.M.; Pavlik, E.J.; Kryscio, R.J. Ovarian cancer screening with annual transvaginal sonography: Findings of 25,000 women screened. *Cancer* **2007**, *109*, 1887–1896. [CrossRef] [PubMed]
54. Van Nagell, J.R.; Gallion, H.H.; Pavlik, E.J.; DePriest, P.D. Ovarian cancer screening. *Cancer* **1995**, *76*, 2086–2091. [CrossRef]
55. Pavlik, E.J.; Ueland, F.R.; Miller, R.W.; Ubellacker, J.M.; DeSimone, C.P.; Elder, J.; Hoff, J.; Baldwin, L.; Kryscio, R.J.; van Nagell, J.R., Jr. Frequency and disposition of ovarian abnormalities followed with serial transvaginal ultrasonography. *Obstet. Gynecol.* **2013**, *122*, 210–217. [CrossRef] [PubMed]
56. Van Nagell, J.R.; Hoff, J.T. Transvaginal ultrasonography in ovarian cancer screening: Current perspectives. *Int. J. Women Health* **2014**, *6*, 25–33. [CrossRef] [PubMed]
57. Elder, J.W.; Pavlik, E.J.; Long, A.; Miller, R.W.; DeSimone, C.P.; Hoff, J.T.; Ueland, W.R.; Kryscio, R.J.; van Nagell, J.R., Jr. Serial ultrasonographic evaluation of ovarian abnormalities with morphology index. *Gynecol. Oncol.* **2014**, *135*, 8–12. [CrossRef] [PubMed]
58. Buys, S.S.; Partridge, E.; Black, A.; Johnson, C.C.; Lamerato, L.; Isaacs, C.; Reding, D.J.; Greenlee, R.T.; Yokochi, L.A.; Kessel, B.; et al. Effect of screening on ovarian cancer mortality: The prostate, lung, colorectal and ovarian (PLCO) cancer screening randomized controlled trial. *JAMA* **2011**, *305*, 2295–2303. [CrossRef] [PubMed]
59. Pinsky, P.F.; Yu, K.; Kramer, B.S.; Black, A.; Buys, S.S.; Partridge, E.; Gohagan, J.; Berg, C.D. Extended mortality results for ovarian cancer screening in the PLCO trial with median 15 years follow-up. *Gynecol. Oncol.* **2016**, *135*, 270–275. [CrossRef] [PubMed]
60. Skates, S.S. OCS: Development of the Risk of Ovarian Cancer Algorithm (ROCA) and ROCA screening trials. *Int. J. Gynecol. Cancer* **2012**, *22*, S24–S26. [CrossRef] [PubMed]
61. Jacobs, I.J.; Menon, U.; Ryan, A.; Gentry-Maharaj, A.; Burnell, A.; Kalsi, J.K.; Amso, N.N.; Apostolidou, S.; Benjamin, E.; Cruickshank, D.; et al. Ovarian cancer screening and mortality in the UK collaborative trial of ovarian cancer screening (UKCTOCS): A randomized controlled trial. *Lancet* **2016**, *387*, 945–956. [CrossRef]
62. Wentzensen, N. Large ovarian cancer screening trial shows modest mortality reduction, but does not justify population-based ovarian cancer screening. *Evid. Based Med.* **2016**, *21*, 159. [CrossRef] [PubMed]
63. Kobayashi, H.; Yamada, Y.; Sado, T.; Sakata, M.; Yoshida, S.; Kawaguchi, R.; Kanayama, S.; Shigetomi, J.; Haruta, S.; Tsuji, Y.; et al. A randomized study of screening for ovarian cancer: A multicenter study in Japan. *Int. J. Gynecol. Cancer* **2008**, *18*, 414–420. [CrossRef] [PubMed]

12

Consensus Procedures in Oncological Imaging: The Case of Prostate Cancer

Stefano Fanti [1], Wim Oyen [2,3] and Elisabetta Lalumera [4,*]

1 Department of Experimental, Diagnostic and Specialty Medicine—DIMES, University of Bologna, and Nuclear Medicine Division, Policlinico S.Orsola, 40138 Bologna, Italy; stefano.fanti@aosp.bo.it
2 Department of Radiology and Nuclear Medicine, Rijnstate Hospital, 6815 Arnhem, The Netherlands; wjg.oyen@gmail.com
3 Department of Biomedical Sciences, Humanitas University and Department of Nuclear Medicine, Humanitas Clinical and Research Center, 20126 Milan, Italy
4 Psychology Department, Milano-Bicocca University, 20126 Milan, Italy
* Correspondence: elisabetta.lalumera@unimib.it

Abstract: Recently, there has been increasing interest in methodological aspects of advanced imaging, including the role of guidelines, recommendations, and experts' consensus, the practice of self-referral, and the risk of diagnostic procedure overuse. In a recent Delphi study of the European Association for Nuclear Medicine (EANM), panelists were asked to give their opinion on 47 scientific questions about imaging in prostate cancer. Nine additional questions exploring the experts' attitudes and opinions relating to the procedure of consensus building itself were also included. The purpose was to provide insights into the mechanism of recommendation choice and consensus building as seen from the experts' point of view. Results: Regarding the factors likely to influence the willingness to refer a patient for imaging, the most voted were incorporation into guidelines and data from scientific literature, while personal experience and personal relationship were chosen by a small minority. Regarding the recommendations more relevant to prescribe an imaging procedure, it resulted the incorporation into guidelines promoted by scientific societies (59% of votes); these guidelines also resulted the more trusted. With respect to patients' preferences considered when prescribing an imaging procedure, the most voted was accuracy, resulted more important than easy access and time to access to the procedure. The majority of the experts expressed the opinion that there is a scarce use of imaging procedures in prostate cancer. With respect to the most relevant factor to build consensus, it resulted the transparency of the process (52% of votes), followed by multidisciplinarity of contributors. The main obstacle to incorporation of modern imaging procedures into guidelines resulted the lack of primary literature on clinical impact. Conclusions: Firstly, the panelists portray themselves as having Evidence-Based Medicine oriented and scientifically inclined attitudes and preferences. Secondly, guidelines and recommendations from scientific societies, especially clinical ones, are positively taken into account as factors influencing decisions, but panelists tend to consider their own appraisal of the scientific literature as more relevant. Thirdly, in respect of overuse, panelists do not think that advanced diagnostic procedures are overutilized in the specific case of Prostate Cancer, but rather they are underutilized.

Keywords: nuclear medicine; guidelines; prostate cancer; overutilization; epistemology; consensus

---

1. Introduction

Production of clinical practice guidelines (hereinafter "guidelines") and consensus statements is of paramount importance for the medical community. This is because the availability of an increasing number of therapeutic and diagnostic options for many diseases requires careful choices, and evidence-based data such as meta-analyses are not always sufficient to drive appropriate use of medical options [1,2]. This is arguably more relevant in the field of advanced medical imaging, where the evaluation of a new diagnostic technique is often not obtainable from evidence cased on randomized controlled trials (RCT), for both conceptual and practical reasons [3].

Even though conspicuous efforts have been made recently to improve and standardize guidelines [4,5], they are still far from being a perfect tool, as philosophers of medicine and methodologists have outlined. They are inevitably outdated in respect of the development of new technologies, they are seldom followed in clinical practice, and they intrinsically need further clinical judgment in order to be appropriately applied to the individual patient's case [6–9]. Moreover, it has recently been pointed out that scarce adherence to guidelines and recommendations favors self-referral and excessive compliance with patients' requests, factors that may cause overuse of diagnostic procedures [10,11]. In addition to these problematic aspects, guidelines are likely to be affected by bias as they are promoted by professional organizations which may tend to select experts from among their members [12,13].

Literature on the functioning of guideline development groups and their attitudes (the view from inside) is relatively scarce [14–16]. Here we take Prostate Cancer (PC) as a case study and illustrate and discuss how experts themselves involved in a consensus conference judge the procedures of consensus building, referral, and compliance with guidelines.

Available diagnostic options at various stages of the disease require careful consideration. A number of imaging methods to study PC have been suggested. These include methods which have been available for decades, for example, computed tomography (CT), bone scintigraphy (BS), and trans rectal ultrasound (TRU), as well as methods which have been introduced more recently, such as whole-body magnetic resonance imaging (MRI), multiparametric MRI, and positron emission tomography (PET). However, there is significant disagreement about the usefulness of such approaches [17–19].

In light of this, the European Association for Nuclear Medicine (EANM), representing nuclear medicine specialists who have been at the forefront of advances in molecular imaging techniques for PC, launched EANM Focus 1 to develop consensus statements in PC. EANM Focus 1 was held in February 2018 and resulted in a consensus on molecular imaging for diagnosis and treatment of prostate cancer. The findings were published in Lancet Oncology in December 2018 [20].

The organizers of EANM focus 1 were also interested in knowing the experts' attitudes and opinions relating to the procedure of consensus building itself as well as guidelines and their problematic aspects. For this reason, the final questionnaire included nine questions specifically focusing on these issues. This article reports and discusses the results of the aforementioned survey. Our goal is to provide insights into the mechanism of recommendation choice and consensus building as seen from the experts' point of view. We are aware that experts' declared attitudes and opinions may not be identical to the actual reasons motivating their decisions in practice. Nevertheless, we believe that their perception of their own role may be of interest in understanding the epistemology of consensus procedures, especially in the relatively new field of imaging epistemology. Moreover, we submit that experts' reflection and self-appraisal on methodological and ethical issues may enhance their commitment to their scientific role.

2. Materials and Methods

EANM Focus 1 was based on a clinical questionnaire proposed and then agreed among the panelists. A modified Delphi process was used to generate consensus on the topics identified. Overall, the questionnaire contained 47 questions, and a 70% cut-off was adopted to determine consensus [21–25]. Three Delphi rounds were conducted, and consensus was achieved in 36 out of 47 clinical questions (77%), as detailed in [20].

In order to address the specific problem of bias from affiliation to a scientific society, a multidisciplinary expert panel was established (hereinafter "the panelists"). The panel consisted of

24 people with representation from all fields involved to ensure a similar number of oncologists (5), urologists (5), radiation oncologists (2), radiologists (4), and nuclear medicine specialists (7). All the panelists were selected on the basis of their international reputation. Furthermore, one pathologist, one molecular biologist, and one radio pharmacist were involved, as well as two patient advocates. The full list of panelists is enclosed in Appendix A.

During the first Delphi round, in addition to the 47 clinical questions, panelists were given nine additional questions specifically designed to evaluate the role of guidelines in respect of clinical practice and the overall approach to consensus building. Questions 48 to 55 are grouped by topic, and their results are shown below. An informal discussion of the findings, without statistical analysis, then follows.

3. Results and Discussion

3.1. Factors to Refer PC Patients for Imaging

Question number 48 was, "Which factors are likely to influence your willingness to refer a patient for an imaging procedure, assuming that availability is not limited?", and panelists were asked to choose all that apply. Results are reported in Table 1.

Table 1. Consensus outcomes for question number 48.

Which Factors are Likely to Influence your Willingness to Refer a Patient for an Imaging Procedure, Assuming that Availability is not Limited?	
Incorporation into guidelines	76.2%
Data from scientific literature	90.5%
Study on cost-effectiveness	52.4%
Patients preferences	42.8%
Personal relationship with imaging professionals	19.0%
Personal experience	23.8%
Out of pocket cost to patient	19.0%
Abstain	4.3%
Unqualified to answer	4.3%

Before moving to further consideration, it is necessary to clarify some possible implications deriving from this question (number 48), as well as from the next (number 49). Some of the answers, and in particular "personal relationship" and "personal experience", may raise an ethical issue. If a "personal relationship" between a medical professional and the imaging professional has the ability to influence the outcome of the patient care, then we could have a major ethical violation. However, this was not the meaning of the answers and rather referred to professional trust that is developed when you personally know the imaging specialist and you are used to personally contacting him in case of any doubtful findings. Wording may seem somewhat vague, and therefore it is important to emphasize that all questions were reviewed and approved by all panelists, before being submitted, and no ethical concern was raised. The main reason to offer those possible answers was related to awareness that doctors may prescribe imaging exams not recommended by guidelines, for nonscientific reasons [26], and we were aimed at evaluating such possibility.

The panelists considered all the possible factors as potential influencers, but some of them were chosen by a small minority. In particular, the personal relationship with imaging professionals was regarded as a possible influencer by less than 20% of the panel. This indicates strong independence from a factor that may have either positive or negative implications.

Indeed, the personal relationship does not have much scientific value. It may be speculated that long-lasting collaboration may result in a fruitful professional relationship. Nonetheless, this factor seems less reliable than others. Surprisingly, the out of pocket cost of the examination for the patient gained the same low percentage of votes, while being a more relevant factor for appropriateness. It could be speculated that the experts regarded as minor the expense of an imaging procedure as compared with the overall costs of treatment. Further considerations regarding patient preference are detailed in question number 51 (see below).

A relatively low number of votes was also scored by the influence of the prescriber's personal experience, confirming that all the factors relating to nonscientific data were regarded as less relevant. Indeed, the first three answers are clearly related to objective scientific facts and gained a clear preference among the experts, while the two answers relating to individual personal perception did not obtain many votes. Factors relating to patient perspective scored somewhere in between. These results are in line with a scientifically oriented approach of the panelists, who clearly preferred rational, evidence-based factors to less measurable issues.

Question number 49 was as question 48, but in this case, panelists were asked to choose one answer only: results are reported in Table 2.

Table 2. Consensus outcomes for question number 49.

Which is the most Relevant Factor Influencing Referral to Imaging? Choose One	
Incorporation into guidelines	23.8%
Data from scientific literature	81.9%
Study on cost-effectiveness	9.5%
Patients preferences	4.7%
Personal relationship with imaging professionals	4.7%
Personal experience	0.0%
Out of pocket cost to patient	0.0%
Abstain	4.3%
Unqualified to answer	4.3%

When it comes to identifying the most relevant factor among the many proposed, there was a clear winner in data from scientific literature. Please note the sum of percentages is greater than 100% because several panelists, despite the question explicitly asking them not to, chose more than one answer. A formal consensus was reached regarding the most relevant factor (data from scientific literature), with almost 82% of the panelists voting for it. This consensus is in line with the principles of EBM (Evidence-based medicine) which consider scientific articles published in peer-reviewed journals as the most valuable source of evidence to decide whether to use a certain imaging procedure or not.

The panelists also considered incorporation into guidelines as a relevant factor, but to a minor extent. It should be mentioned that data from the literature is the prerequisite for proper incorporation into guidelines. Therefore, this factor implies the existence of the previous and most selected factor. The impression is that experts tend to prefer their own evaluation of original articles over guidelines, given that guidelines are only updated several months later.

There is much debate about the problems of timing required to have a new imaging method incorporated into PC guidelines. Previously, before the development of an EBM culture, conventional imaging methods such as CT and BS were incorporated without any formal evaluation of the positive effects on patient outcome. In the 1970's, these methods were simply introduced and rapidly considered mandatory without a specifically designed clinical trial being undertaken. Thirty years later, rapid developments in the field of imaging still pose issues for guideline development. Indeed, new methods such as MRI and PET are available and have been adopted in clinical practice before evidence-generating clinical trials have been performed, resulting in a significant increase in their use. With the growth of medical imaging, the concern that not all examinations are necessary has increased, and it is argued that up to 40% of diagnostic imaging studies may be inappropriate[17-18]. Furthermore, as mentioned, there are intrinsic problems in building EBM literature for diagnostic imaging[11] and this fact has led to significant disagreement in the field of PC imaging. At the Advanced Prostate Cancer Consensus Conference held in St. Gallen there was no consensus on most questions relating to advanced PC imaging [27]. The problem of reliability in the sources of recommendations was further investigated in the next question.

3.2. Source of Recommendations

Question number 50 was, "Which recommendations are more relevant for you when prescribing an imaging procedure?": results are reported in Table 3.

Table 3. EANM (European Association for Nuclear Medicine) consensus outcomes for question number 50.

Which Recommendations are more Relevant for you when Prescribing an Imaging Procedure?	
Guidelines published by Evidence-Based Medicine/Health Technology Assessment authorities	13.6%
Guidelines promoted by scientific societies (imaging)	19.2%
Guidelines promoted by scientific societies (clinical)	59.0%
Local healthcare recommendation	0.0%
Proceeding of consensus multidisciplinary congresses	13.6%
None of the above	9.9%
Abstain	0.0%
Unqualified to answer	4.3%

There could be several reasons why a minority of the panelists chose the option of EBM/Health Technology Assessment-promoted guidelines. Firstly, in the area of prostate cancer, there is a complete lack of such guidelines, and the panel was surely aware of that even if the question did not focus on PC. A more general reason might be the resistance of clinicians to guidelines developed outside their professional control. See also question no. 54.

It is interesting to note that experts regard published studies as the most reliable evidence to influence their willingness to refer a patient for imaging (see question no. 49). On the other hand, EBM guidelines resulting directly from scientific data review are perceived as less reliable than scientific society guidelines.

It is noteworthy that not a single panelist considers local healthcare recommendations as relevant. Once again, this result could relate to the composition of the panel, which is made up of clinicians selected on the basis of their international reputation. This means they may not be keen to adhere to local rules that often tend to limit access to expensive and innovative imaging methods.

3.3. Patients' Preferences

Question number 51 was "Which part of patients' preference are you considering when prescribing an imaging procedure?", and panelists were asked to choose all that apply: results are reported in Table 4.

The suggested answers to this question were slightly tricky because only the first four are genuinely related to patient preference and the fifth (accuracy of the procedure) relates to a scientific point of view. Indeed, it was this answer that received the largest majority of preferences (almost 82%), with the others being selected, but not to such a great extent. It is clear that this finding is related to the paternalistic approach of doctors to patients. When a final decision has to be taken, all patient preferences are duly taken into account, but the most relevant factor remains purely scientific evidence. In other words, the doctor is deciding in favor of the best diagnostic option, the value of which is more important than other factors.

Table 4. EANM consensus outcomes for question number 51.

Which Part of Patients' Preference are you Considering when Prescribing an Imaging Procedure?	
Easy access to the procedure (distance and availability)	54.5%
Time to access to the procedure (waiting list)	45.4%
Cost of the procedure (irrespective whether or not it is covered by healthcare system or insurance)	22.7%
Out of pocket cost to patient	22.7%
Accuracy of the procedure (best available option)	81.8%
None of the above	9.9%
Abstain	0.0%
Unqualified to answer	4.3%

3.4. Degree of Use of Imaging Procedures (See Below)

Question number 52 was, "Which is your overall opinion about the use of imaging procedures in PC?": results are reported in Table 5.

Table 5. EANM consensus outcomes for question number 52.

Which is your Overall Opinion about the Use of Imaging Procedures in PC?	
Overall there is excessive use of imaging procedures in PC	25.0%
There is excessive use of modern imaging procedures in PC	20.0%
Overall there is scarce use of imaging procedures in PC	10.0%
There is scarce use of modern imaging procedures in PC	60.0%
Use of imaging procedures in PC is optimal	10.0%
Abstain	8.7%
Unqualified to answer	4.3%

Question 53 was, "Which is your overall opinion about the use of imaging procedures in PC for BCR/APC (Biochemical Recurrence/Advanced Prostate Cancer)?": results are reported in Table 6.

Table 6. EANM consensus outcomes for question number 53.

Which is your Overall Opinion about the Use of Imaging Procedures in PC for Biochemical Recurrence (BCR)/Advanced Prostate Cancer(APC)?	
Overall there is excessive use of imaging procedures in PC for BCR/APC	10.5%
There is excessive use of modern imaging procedures in PC for BCR/APC	15.8%
Overall there is scarce use of imaging procedures in PC for BCR/APC	5.2%
There is scarce use of modern imaging procedures in PC for BCR/APC	52.6%
Use of imaging procedures in PC is quite optimal for BCR/APC	15.8%
Abstain	9.0%
Unqualified to answer	4.5%

3.5. *Trustworthiness of Recommendations*

Question 54 was, "Which recommendations do you consider more trustworthy regarding imaging usage?". Results are reported in Table 7.

Table 7. EANM consensus outcomes for question number 54.

Which Recommendations do you Consider more Trustworthy Regarding Imaging Usage?	
Guidelines promoted by clinical scientific societies (European Association of Urology, or similar)	52.4%
Guidelines promoted by imaging scientific societies (European Association for Nuclear Medicine or similar)	19.2%
Guidelines promoted by EBM/HTA authorities	4.7%
Proceeding of consensus multidisciplinary congresses	14.3%
Equally all of the above	14.3%
Abstain	4.5%

This question is closely linked to question number 50, but with the emphasis placed on trustworthiness of recommendations. Once again there is a clear preference for guidelines promoted by clinical scientific societies. This point deserves further consideration. It seems that overall results are mainly influenced by the actual scenario of existing recommendations in the field. As already mentioned, guidelines promoted by clinical scientific societies are more common and more usual.

3.6. *Building Consensus*

Question number 55 was, "Which factor do you consider most relevant to build consensus on imaging procedures?". Results are reported in Table 8.

The issue of consensus building is complex and controversial, with a number of factors involved and significant consequences for any healthcare system. Despite the fact that only one question in this questionnaire specifically covered the issue, some comments are necessary. The panelists clearly considered transparency of the process as the most relevant factor, thus favoring an EBM-oriented procedure. This is undoubtedly in line with current scientific opinion but contradicts the answers to question nos. 50 and 54, where EBM guidelines gained limited preferences. In other words, EBM methodology is widely recognized as the best option when making a recommendation, but there is resistance to guidelines promoted by EBM/HTA authorities. This fact is easily recognizable in the current practice of preparation of EAU guidelines, which are the most widely used in the treatment of PC.

Table 8. EANM consensus outcomes for question number 55.

Which Factor do you Consider most Relevant to Build Consensus on Imaging Procedures?	
Transparency of the process (evidence based medicine oriented)	52.4%
Participation of expert panelists (imaging specialist)	9.5%
Participation of multidisciplinary expert panelists (clinical specialist)	19.0%
Contribution of all stakeholders (specialists, patients, healthcare)	28.6%
Cost-effectiveness analysis	4.7%
Translational and primary literature data	9.5%
Abstain	0.0%
Unqualified to answer	4.5%

3.7. *Incorporation of Imaging into Guidelines*

Question 56 was, "Which factor do you consider the most relevant obstacle for the lack of incorporation of modern imaging procedures into guidelines and clinical practice?". Results are reported in Table 9.

Table 9. EANM consensus outcomes for question number 56.

Which Factor do you Consider the most Relevant Obstacle for the Lack of Incorporation of Modern Imaging Procedures into Guidelines and Clinical Practice?	
Lack of primary literature on accuracy (Multicentric Prospective Trials)	9.5%
Lack of primary literature on clinical impact (Multicentric Prospective Trials)	66.6%
Lack of secondary literature (systematic reviews and meta-analyses)	4.7%
Lack of cost-effectiveness analyses	0.0%
Difficulties of access to modern imaging methods	19.0%
Difficulties in communications with imaging specialists	0.0%
Abstain	0.0%
Unqualified to answer	4.5%

This question is based on recognition that modern imaging procedures, such as MRI and PET, have gained widespread use in some countries despite a lack of incorporation into guidelines. Lack of primary literature on the clinical impact of modern imaging procedures is identified as the most relevant factor.

4. Conclusions

We cautiously assume that the panelists' answers to the meta-questions show what they consider to be the right attitudes and preferences to have rather than the attitudes and preferences they actually have. The general picture that emerges is that experts, in their role as panelists, are adequately conscious of their role, that is, of which factors should be taken into account in deciding on imaging procedures within an EBM framework.

The results reported so far can be summarized as follows.

Firstly, the panelists show themselves to have EBM-oriented and scientifically inclined attitudes and preferences (questions 49, 55, and 56).

Secondly, guidelines and recommendations from scientific societies, especially clinical ones, are positively taken into account as factors influencing decisions, but panelists tend to consider their own appraisal of the scientific literature as more relevant and reliable. This is in line with a widespread need to rethink guidelines.

Thirdly, in relation to overutilization, panelists do not think that advanced diagnostic procedures are overutilized in the specific case of PC, but rather they are underutilized. Moreover, in line with the EBM-inclined attitude, they do not consider patient preferences as factors that should influence their decision whether to prescribe a test or not. This result suggests that the issue of overutilization of diagnostic procedures should be considered on a case-by-case basis. Furthermore, additional research should be done to compare the inclinations of medical specialists with those of general practitioners and patients with regard to this topic.

Fourthly, various problems specific to the field have also emerged. These include the relative scarcity of primary literature on the clinical effectiveness of some imaging tests and the predominance of the clinical importance of the procedure over its intrinsic diagnostic accuracy in evaluation and recommendation.

As a final and general suggestion, we submit that questions such as the ones we have posed and analyzed may, in general, enhance the experts' self-appraisal of their role when actively participating in Delphi and consensus procedures, may act as a reminder of good scientific practices, and, therefore, may contribute to better performance on their part.

Author Contributions: Conceptualization, S.F. and W.O.; methodology, S.F.; writing—original draft preparation, S.F. and E.L.; writing—review and editing, S.F. and E.L.

Acknowledgments: The authors wish to thank Silvia Minozzi for Delphi supervision and data analysis; Susanne Koebe, Andreas Felser, and Henrik Silber (EANM) for project management. We would also like to thank all the panelists for their contribution.

Appendix A. —Expert Panel

Name of Expert	Institute	Field of Expertise
Gerald Antoch	University Hospital Düsseldorf, Germany	Radiology
Ian Banks	ECCO & European Men's Health Forum	Patient Advocate
Alberto Briganti	San Raffaele University Hospital, Milan, Italy	Urology
Ignasi Carriò	Hospital de la Santa Creu i Sant Pau, Barcelona, Spain	Nuclear Medicine
Arturo Chiti	Instituto Clinico Humanitas, Milan, Italy	Nuclear Medicine
Noel Clarke	The Christie Hospital	Urological Oncology
Johann De Bono	The Institute of Cancer Research, London, United Kingdom	Medical Oncology
Matthias Eiber	Klinikum rechts der Isar, TUM, München, Germany	Nuclear Medicine
Karim Fizazi	Institut Gustave Roussy, Paris, France	Medical Oncology
Silke Gillessen	Kantonsspital St. Gallen, Switzerland	Medical Oncology
Sam Gledhill	Movember Foundation	Patient Advocate
Uwe Haberkorn	University Hospital Heidelberg, Germany	Nuclear Medicine
Ken Herrmann	Universitätsklinikum Essen, Germany	Nuclear Medicine
Rodney Hicks	Peter Mac Callum Cancer Institute, Melbourne, Australia	Nuclear Medicine
Frédéric Lecouvet	Clinique Universitaires Saint-Luc UCL, Brussels, Belgium	Radiology
Rodolfo Montironi	Ospedali Riuniti Ancona, Italy	Pathology
Joe O'Sullivan	Queen's University Belfast, United Kingdom	Radiation Oncology
Piet Ost	Ghent University Hospital, Belgium	Radiation Oncology
Anwar Padhani	Mount Vernon Cancer Centre, London, United Kingdom	Radiology
Jack Schalken	Radboud UMC, Netherland	Molecular Biology
Howard Scher	Memorial Sloan Kettering Cancer Center, New York, USA	Medical Oncology
Bertrand Tombal	Cliniques Universitaires Saint-Luc; Belgium	Urology
Jeroen van Moorselaar	VU Medisch Centrum, Netherland	Urology
Hendrik Van Poppel	KU Leuven	Urology
Herbert Alberto Vargas	Memorial Sloan Kettering Cancer Center, New York, USA	Radiology
Jochen Walz	Institute Paoli-Calmettes, Marseille, France	Urology
Wolfgang Weber	Memorial Sloan Kettering Cancer Center, New York, USA	Nuclear Medicine
Hans-Jürgen Wester	Technische Universität München, Germany	Radiochemistry

References

1. Woolf, S.H.; Grol, R.; Hutchinson, A.; Eccles, M.; Grimshaw, J. Potential benefits, limitations, and harms of clinical guidelines. *BMJ* **1999**, *318*, 527–530. [CrossRef] [PubMed]
2. Qaseem, A.; Forland, F.; Macbeth, F.; Ollenschläger, G.; Phillips, S.; van der Wees, P. Guidelines International Network: Toward international standards for clinical practice guidelines. *Ann. Intern. Med.* **2012**, *156*, 525–531. [CrossRef] [PubMed]

3. Lalumera, E.; Fanti, S. Randomized Controlled Trials for Diagnostic Imaging: Conceptual and Pratical Problems. *Topoi* **2017**, 1–6. [CrossRef]
4. Brouwers, M.C.; Kho, M.E.; Browman, G.P.; Burgers, J.S.; Cluzeau, F.; Feder, G.; Littlejohns, P. AGREE II: Advancing guideline development, reporting and evaluation in health care. *Cmaj* **2010**, *182*, E839–E842. [CrossRef]
5. Eccles, M.P.; Grimshaw, J.M.; Shekelle, P.; Schünemann, H.J.; Woolf, S. Developing clinical practice guidelines: Target audiences, identifying topics for guidelines, guideline group composition and functioning and conflicts of interest. *Implement. Sci.* **2012**, *7*, 60. [CrossRef]
6. Upshur, R.E. Do clinical guidelines still make sense? No. *Ann. Fam. Med.* **2014**, *12*, 202–203. [CrossRef]
7. Cartwright, N. A philosopher's view of the long road from RCTs to effectiveness. *Lancet* **2011**, *377*, 1400–1401. [CrossRef]
8. Cartwright, N. What evidence should guidelines take note of? *J. Evaluat. Clin. Pract.* **2018**, *24*, 1139–1144. [CrossRef]
9. Cabana, M.D.; Rand, C.S.; Powe, N.R.; Wu, A.W.; Wilson, M.H.; Abboud, P.A.C.; Rubin, H.R. Why don't physicians follow clinical practice guidelines? A framework for improvement. *Jama* **1999**, *282*, 1458–1465. [CrossRef]
10. Hendee, W.R.; Becker, G.J.; Borgstede, J.P.; Bosma, J.; Casarella, W.J.; Erickson, B.A.; Wallner, P.E. Addressing overutilization in medical imaging. *Radiology* **2010**, *257*, 240–245. [CrossRef]
11. Hofmann, B. Too much of a good thing is wonderful? A conceptual analysis of excessive examinations and diagnostic futility in diagnostic radiology. *Med. Health Care Philos.* **2010**, *13*, 139–148. [CrossRef] [PubMed]
12. Grilli, R.; Magrini, N.; Penna, A.; Mura, G.; Liberati, A. Practice guidelines developed by specialty societies: The need for a critical appraisal. *Lancet* **2000**, *355*, 103–106. [CrossRef]
13. Shekelle, P.G. Clinical practice guidelines: what's next? *Jama* **2018**, *320*, 757–758. [CrossRef] [PubMed]
14. Atkins, L.; Smith, J.A.; Kelly, M.P.; Michie, S. The process of developing evidence-based guidance in medicine and public health: A qualitative study of views from the inside. *Implement. Sci.* **2013**, *8*, 101. [CrossRef] [PubMed]
15. Sundberg, L.R.; Garvare, R.; Nyström, M.E. Reaching beyond the review of research evidence: A qualitative study of decision making during the development of clinical practice guidelines for disease prevention in healthcare. *BMC Health Serv. Res.* **2017**, *17*, 344.
16. Raine, R.; Sanderson, C.; Hutchings, A.; Carter, S.; Larkin, K.; Black, N. An experimental study of determinants of group judgments in clinical guideline development. *Lancet* **2004**, *364*, 429–437. [CrossRef]
17. American Urological Association—Clinically Localized Prostate Cancer: AUA/ASTRO/SUO Guideline. Available online: http://www.auanet.org/guidelines/clinically-localized-prostate-cancer-new-(aua/astro/suo-guideline-2017) (accessed on 5 September 2019).
18. Cornford, P.; Bellmunt, J.; Bolla, M.; Briers, E.; De Santis, M.; Gross, T.; Henry, A.M.; Joniau, S.; Lam, T.B.; Mason, M.D.; et al. EAU-ESTRO-SIOG Guidelines on Prostate Cancer. Part II: Treatment of Relapsing, Metastatic, and Castration-Resistant Prostate Cancer. *Eur. Urol.* **2017**, *71*, 630–642. [CrossRef]
19. Mottet, N.; Bellmunt, J.; Bolla, M.; Briers, E.; Cumberbatch, M.G.; De Santis, M.; Fossati, N.; Gross, T.; Henry, A.M.; Joniau, S.; et al. EAU-ESTRO-SIOG Guidelines on Prostate Cancer. Part I: Screening, Diagnosis, and Local Treatment with Curative Intent. *Eur. Urol.* **2017**, *71*, 618–629. [CrossRef]
20. Fanti, S.; Minozzi, S.; Antoch, G.; Banks, I.; Briganti, A.; Carrio, I.; Fizazi, K. Consensus on molecular imaging and theranostics in prostate cancer. *Lancet Oncol.* **2018**, *19*, e696–e708. [CrossRef]
21. Delphi Method/RAND. Available online: https://www.rand.org/topics/delphi-method.html (accessed on 22 September 2019).
22. Landis, J.R.; Koch, G.G. The measurement of observer agreement for categorical data. *Biometrics* **1977**, *33*, 159–174. [CrossRef]
23. Bruinsma, S.M.; Roobol, M.J.; Carroll, P.R.; Klotz, L.; Pickles, T.; Moore, C.M.; Gnanapragasam, V.J.; Villers, A.; Rannikko, A.; Valdagni, R.; et al. Expert consensus document: Semantics in active surveillance for men with localized prostate cancer—Results of a modified Delphi consensus procedure. *Nat. Rev. Urol.* **2017**, *14*, 312–322. [CrossRef] [PubMed]
24. Zafar, S.Y.; Currow, D.C.; Cherny, N.; Strasser, F.; Fowler, R.; Abernethy, A.P. Consensus-based standards for best supportive care in clinical trials in advanced cancer. *Lancet Oncol.* **2012**, *13*, e77–e82. [CrossRef]

25. Hasson, F.; Keeney, S.; McKenna, H. Research guidelines for the Delphi survey technique. *J. Adv. Nurs.* **2000**, *32*, 1008–1015. [PubMed]
26. Simos, D.; Hutton, B.; Graham, I.D.; Arnaout, A.; Caudrelier, J.M.; Clemons, M. Imaging for metastatic disease in patients with newly diagnosed breast cancer: Are doctor's perceptions in keeping with the guidelines? *J. Eval. Clin. Pract.* **2015**, *21*, 67–73. [CrossRef] [PubMed]
27. Gillessen, S.; Attard, G.; Beer, T.M.; Beltran, H.; Bossi, A.; Bristow, R.; Carver, B.; Castellano, D.; Chung, B.H.; Clarke, N.; et al. Management of Patients with Advanced Prostate Cancer: The Report of the Advanced Prostate Cancer Consensus Conference APCCC 2017. *Eur. Urol.* **2018**, *73*, 178–211. [CrossRef] [PubMed]

13

Validation of the Performance of International Ovarian Tumor Analysis (IOTA) Methods in the Diagnosis of Early Stage Ovarian Cancer in a Non-Screening Population

Wouter Froyman [1,2], Laure Wynants [1], Chiara Landolfo [1,2], Tom Bourne [1,2,3], Lil Valentin [4], Antonia Testa [5], Povilas Sladkevicius [4], Dorella Franchi [6], Daniela Fischerova [7], Luca Savelli [8], Ben Van Calster [1] and Dirk Timmerman [1,2,*]

1. Department of Development and Regeneration, KU Leuven, Leuven post code3000, Belgium; wouter.froyman@uzleuven.be (W.F.); laure.wynants@kuleuven.be (L.W.); chiara.landolfo@kuleuven.be (C.L.); t.bourne@imperial.ac.uk (T.B.); ben.vancalster@kuleuven.be (B.V.C.)
2. Department of Obstetrics and Gynecology, University Hospitals Leuven, Leuven 3000, Belgium
3. Queen Charlotte's and Chelsea Hospital, Imperial College, London W12 0HS, UK
4. Department of Obstetrics and Gynecology, Skåne University Hospital Malmö, Lund University, Malmö 20502, Sweden; lil.valentin@med.lu.se (L.V.); povilas.sladkevicius@med.lu.se (P.S.)
5. Department of Oncology, Catholic University of the Sacred Heart, Rome 00168, Italy; atesta@rm.unicatt.it
6. Preventive Gynecology Unit, Division of Gynecology, European Institute of Oncology, Milan 20141, Italy; dorella.franchi@ieo.it
7. Gynecological Oncology Center, Department of Obstetrics and Gynecology, Charles University, Prague 12108, Czech Republic; Daniela.Fischerova@seznam.cz
8. Department of Obstetrics and Gynecology, S. Orsola-Malpighi Hospital, University of Bologna, Bologna 40138, Italy; luca.savelli@aosp.bo.it

* Correspondence: dirk.timmerman@uzleuven.be

Academic Editor: Edward J. Pavlik

Abstract: Background: The aim of this study was to assess and compare the performance of different ultrasound-based International Ovarian Tumor Analysis (IOTA) strategies and subjective assessment for the diagnosis of early stage ovarian malignancy. Methods: This is a secondary analysis of a prospective multicenter cross-sectional diagnostic accuracy study that included 1653 patients recruited at 18 centers from 2009 to 2012. All patients underwent standardized transvaginal ultrasonography by experienced ultrasound investigators. We assessed test performance of the IOTA Simple Rules (SRs), Simple Rules Risk (SRR), the Assessment of Different NEoplasias in the adneXa (ADNEX) model and subjective assessment to discriminate between stage I-II ovarian cancer and benign disease. Reference standard was histology after surgery. Results: 230 (13.9%) patients proved to have stage I–II primary invasive ovarian malignancy, and 1423 (86.1%) had benign disease. Sensitivity and specificity with respect to malignancy (95% confidence intervals) of the original SRs (classifying all inconclusive cases as malignant) were 94.3% (90.6% to 96.7%) and 73.4% (71.0% to 75.6%). Subjective assessment had a sensitivity and specificity of 90.0% (85.4% to 93.2%) and 86.7% (84.9% to 88.4%), respectively. The areas under the receiver operator characteristic curves of SRR and ADNEX were 0.917 (0.902 to 0.933) and 0.905 (0.920 to 0.934), respectively. At a 1% risk cut-off, sensitivity and specificity for SRR were 100% (98.4% to 100%) and 38.0% (35.5% to 40.6%), and for ADNEX were 100% (98.4% to 100%) and 19.4% (17.4% to 21.5%). At a 30% risk cut-off, sensitivity and specificity for SRR were 88.3% (83.5% to 91.8%) and 81.1% (79% to 83%), and for ADNEX were 84.5% (80.5% to 89.6%) and 84.5% (82.6% to 86.3%). Conclusion: This study shows that all three IOTA strategies have good ability to discriminate between stage I-II ovarian malignancy and benign disease.

Keywords: ovary; ovarian neoplasms; early detection of cancer; diagnostic imaging; ultrasonography; risk assessment; logistic models

1. Introduction

Ovarian tumors are common in women of all ages [1–3]. It has been estimated that in the female population, the lifetime risk of undergoing surgery for a suspected ovarian neoplasm is 5–10% [4]. However, the incidence of ovarian cancer is low. In Europe, there were 65,538 new cases during 2012, with an age-adjusted incidence rate of 13.1 per 100,000 women. Still, ovarian cancer is an important health problem in gynecology, as it is the most lethal gynecological malignancy, with 42,700 deaths occurring in 2012 in Europe (mortality rate 7.6 per 100,000) [5]. This accounts for 5% of all cancer deaths in women, which makes ovarian cancer the sixth most lethal cancer in females in Europe [6].

In recent decades, despite advances in cytoreductive radical surgery and cytotoxic chemotherapy, we have seen only a marginal improvement in the overall survival of patients with ovarian cancer [7].

Almost 60% of patients are diagnosed with advanced disease with regional or distant spread and an unfavorable long-term prognosis. Five-year relative survival is 46% for all International Federation of Gynecology and Obstetrics (FIGO) stages [8], but ranges from 90% at Stage I to 4% for Stage IV disease [6,8]. Therefore, attention for the development of strategies to detect ovarian malignancy at an early stage using imaging and/or biomarkers is increasing, in order to improve patient survival. This idea is reflected in the conduction of several large ovarian cancer screening trials [9–11], but also plays an important role in clinical management of the non-screening population.

Early detection of cancer means that treatment is not delayed and that appropriate staging can be carried out in specialized surgical centers, which is known to improve survival [12–15].

The best ultrasound method for discrimination between benign and malignant adnexal masses is the subjective assessment of ultrasound findings by an experienced ultrasound examiner [16–18]. However, as such expert knowledge is not available in each center, the International Ovarian Tumor Analysis (IOTA) study aims to develop diagnostic algorithms to assist clinicians in characterizing adnexal pathology, irrespective of their level of expertise. The IOTA group initially published a consensus paper in order to standardize terms, definitions, and measurements used to assess ovarian pathology [19]. By prospectively investigating patients presenting with an adnexal mass (i.e., non-screening population), this formed the basis for the development of different IOTA methods such as the Simple Rules (SRs), which are based on five ultrasound features suggestive for a benign lesion (B-features) and five features suggestive for a malignant lesion (M-features) [20]. The IOTA SRs have become very popular because they are easy to use, without the need for any calculation. They have been extensively validated and are incorporated in international guidelines [21,22]. Two systematic reviews and meta-analyses have concluded that the IOTA SRs are one of the best performing available diagnostic methods for differentiating between benign and malignant adnexal masses [18,23]. Shortcomings of the SRs are that there are inconclusive results in a proportion of cases (when B and M features apply or when no features apply) and the absence of an estimated risk of malignancy. Therefore, the ultrasound features used in the SRs have recently been used to calculate a risk of malignancy, leading to the Simple Rules Risk (SRR) model [24]. Another logistic regression model developed by the IOTA group is the Assessment of Different NEoplasias in the adneXa (ADNEX) model. As a multiclass prediction model, ADNEX not only calculates the likelihood of malignancy in adnexal masses, but also divides this into the likelihood that the mass is borderline malignant, stage I primary invasive ovarian cancer, stage II–IV primary invasive ovarian cancer, or a metastasis in the ovary from another primary tumor [25]. The performance of ADNEX is at least as good as the performance of previous IOTA methods, as confirmed by external validation studies [26–30]. The ADNEX model is available online and in mobile applications (www.iotagroup.org/adnexmodel/).

Given the good performance of IOTA strategies in discriminating between benign and malignant disease in patients presenting with an adnexal mass prior to surgery, we are often confronted with the question on how IOTA methods could potentially improve detection in ovarian cancer screening. For the purpose of this special issue of Diagnostics, we assessed and compared the test performance of various diagnostic IOTA methods and subjective assessment to identify early stage, i.e., FIGO stage I and II [8], primary invasive ovarian malignancy in a non-screening population.

2. Materials and Methods

2.1. Patients

This study was performed on data of IOTA phase 3 [31], a multicenter cross-sectional diagnostic accuracy study with prospective data collection. Patients were recruited in 18 centers in six countries (Sweden, Belgium, Italy, Poland, Spain, and Czech Republic) between October 2009 and May 2012. The participating centers were either oncology referral centers (i.e., tertiary centers with a specific gynecological oncology unit) or general hospitals and units with a special interest in gynecological ultrasound. Ethics approval for IOTA 3 was obtained by the ethics committee of the University Hospitals Leuven (B32220095331/S51375 approved 21 January 2009) as the main investigating center as well of the local ethics committees of all contributing centers.

Patients were eligible for IOTA 3 if they presented with at least one adnexal mass (ovarian, para-ovarian, or tubal), underwent standardized transvaginal ultrasonography by a principal investigator at one of the participating centers, and were then selected for surgical intervention by the managing clinician. All examiners were experienced in gynecologic ultrasound. Details on the ultrasound examination technique and the IOTA terms and definitions used to describe adnexal pathology have been published elsewhere [19]. More information on data collection can be found in the original IOTA 3 publication [31]. The pathologist was blinded to the predicted outcomes of the index tests being compared.

For the purpose this study, only patients having a histopathology diagnosis of a benign mass or FIGO stage I and II [8] invasive (epithelial or non-epithelial) ovarian malignancy were considered for analysis.

2.2. Diagnostic Models

Three diagnostic IOTA methods for the assessment of adnexal masses (the original SRs, SRR and ADNEX) were evaluated in terms of their ability to discriminate between benign disease and stage I–II primary ovarian malignancy. These methods were developed on data of earlier IOTA phases. Hence, this is a temporal validation study, including new centers. The original IOTA SRs result in a classification of ovarian masses as benign, malignant, or inconclusive. In this work, we classified inconclusive cases as malignant. The SRR yields a predicted probability of ovarian malignancy. The ADNEX model provides the predicted risks of four different subclasses of malignant adnexal tumors (borderline, stage I invasive, stage II-IV invasive or metastatic cancer). When using the ADNEX model, the probability of malignancy is computed as the sum of the predicted probabilities for all malignant subtypes (including borderline tumors). We validated the version of ADNEX that does not use serum cancer antigen 125 (CA125) measurements as a predictor, because CA125 results are not always available in women with benign or stage I–II tumors (results for serum CA125 measurements were missing for 45% of women in our database). ADNEX with and without CA125 has similar ability to predict malignancy [25]. Both SRR and ADNEX were initially developed on data from IOTA phases 1 and 2, validated on data from IOTA 3, and then refitted on all data [24,25]. In this study, we used the initial versions of SRR and ADNEX that were not refitted using IOTA 3 data. We also evaluated the performance of subjective assessment.

2.3. Statistical Methods

All strategies were evaluated in terms of their ability to discriminate between benign and malignant masses. The area under the receiver-operator characteristic curve (AUC) was computed for ADNEX and the SRR. We also calculated the sensitivity and specificity for ADNEX and the SRR at risk thresholds of 1%, 10%, 20%, and 30%, as well the sensitivity and specificity of the original SRs (classifying inconclusive results as malignant) and subjective assessment. Subgroup analyses were performed for pre- and postmenopausal women. R software (version 3.3.1.) was used for all calculations (R: A language and environment for statistical computing. R Foundation for Statistical Computing, Vienna, Austria, Available online: http/www.r-project.org/). The pROC package and binom packages were used to calculate Delong [32] and Wilson [33] confidence intervals for AUCs and sensitivity/specificity, respectively. The Transparent Reporting of a multivariable prediction model for Individual Prognosis or Diagnosis (TRIPOD) guidelines [34] were used for reporting in this study.

3. Results

In total, 2541 women with adnexal masses were enrolled in IOTA phase 3. We excluded 138 women from the final data set after the application of exclusion criteria [31].

Of the remaining 2403 patients, 1423 had a benign mass. Patients with borderline tumors, stage III–IV primary invasive malignancies, and metastatic cancer were excluded from the analysis. The resulting database for analysis consisted of 1653 women from 18 centers, 230 of which had stage I–II invasive ovarian malignancy. Patient and tumor characteristics are represented in Table 1. Of the women included, 34.6% were postmenopausal. Histology findings are listed in Table 2.

Table 1. Descriptive statistics of the sample.

Variable	Result	
	Benign Tumor	**Early Stage Malignancy (I and II)**
N	1423 (86.1%)	230 (13.9%)
Age (years)	44 (33 to 56)	55 (42 to 66)
Postmenopausal	447 (31.4%)	125 (54.3%)
CA125 (IU/L), if available [a]	21 (12 to 46)	55 (20 to 207)
Maximum tumor diameter (mm)	64 (47 to 90)	103 (68 to 143)
Presence of solid components	474 (33.3%)	214 (93.0%)
Maximum diameter of the solid component (if any, mm)	28 (13 to 54)	62 (37 to 93)
Locularity		
Unilocular	595 (41.8%)	2 (0.9%)
Unilocular-solid	141 (9.9%)	34 (14.8%)
Multilocular	354 (24.9%)	14 (6.1%)
Multilocular-solid	179 (12.6%)	93 (40.4%)
Solid	154 (10.8%)	87 (37.8%)
Number of locules (if any)	1 (1 to 3)	5 (1.5 to 6)
Acoustic shadows	265 (18.6%)	17 (7.4%)
Intratumoral blood flow		
No blood flow	574 (40.3%)	5 (2.2%)
Minimal blood flow	563 (39.6%)	54 (23.5%)
Moderate blood flow	239 (16.8%)	95 (41.3%)
Very strong blood flow	47 (3.3%)	76 (33.0%)
Irregular internal cyst wall	385 (27.1%)	151 (65.7%)
Presence of ascites	18 (1.3%)	33 (14.3%)
Presence of papillary structures	180 (12.6%)	54 (23.5%)
Number of papillary structures (if present)	1 (1 to 3)	3 (2 to 4)

[a] CA125: cancer antigen 125. There were 683 (48%) missing values for CA125 for benign tumors and 64 (28%) for early stage tumors.

Results are shown as medians (interquartile range) for continuous and ordinal variables, and as *N* (%) for categorical variables. Possible values for "Number of locules" are 1 = presence of one locule,

2 = presence of two locules, 3 = presence of three locules, 4 = presence of four locules, 5 = presence of five to ten locules, 6 = presence of more than ten locules. Possible values for "Number of papillary structures" are 1 = presence of one papillary structure, 2 = presence of two papillary structures, 3 = presence of three papillary structures, 4 = presence of more than three papillary structures.

Table 2. Overview of histologic outcomes (*N*, %).

Histology	*N* (%)
Endometrioma	344 (20.8%)
Teratoma	231 (14.0%)
Simple cyst + parasalpingeal cyst	106 (6.4%)
Functional cyst	40 (2.4%)
Hydrosalpinx + salpingitis	47 (2.8%)
Peritoneal pseudocyst	18 (1.1%)
Abscess	17 (1.0%)
Fibroma	130 (7.9%)
Serous cystadenoma	259 (15.7%)
Mucinous cystadenoma	183 (11.1%)
Rare benign	48 (2.9%)
Primary invasive (epithelial) cancer stage I	128 (7.7%)
Primary invasive (epithelial) cancer stage II	47 (2.8%)
Rare primary invasive malignancy stage I or II *	55 (3.3%)

* Includes germ cell tumors and sex cord-stromal tumors.

Regarding the identification of stage I–II primary ovarian malignancy as malignant disease, the original SRs (classifying inconclusive cases as malignant) had a sensitivity and specificity (95% confidence intervals) of 94.3% (90.6% to 96.7%) and 73.4% (71.0% to 75.6%). Subjective assessment had a sensitivity and specificity of 90.0% (85.4% to 93.2%) and 86.7% (84.9% to 88.4%), respectively. Considering the discrimination of benign and malignant disease in the study population of patients with benign masses and stage I–II primary ovarian malignancy the AUCs of the SRR and ADNEX model were 0.917 (0.902 to 0.933) and 0.920 (0.905 to 0.934), respectively. The sensitivity and specificity for these risk prediction models differ depending on the selected risk threshold to predict malignancy. Table 3 summarizes the sensitivity and specificity for the two models at different risk thresholds.

Table 3. Sensitivity and specificity for Assessment of Different NEoplasias in the adneXa (ADNEX) model and Simple Rules Risk (SRR) model at various risk thresholds (percent (95% confidence interval)).

Risk Threshold	Statistic	ADNEX	SRR
1%	Sensitivity	100.0% (98.4% to 100.0%)	100.0% (98.4% to 100.0%)
	Specificity	19.4% (17.4% to 21.5%)	38.0% (35.5% to 40.6%)
10%	Sensitivity	97.4% (94.4% to 98.8%)	97.0% (93.9% to 98.5%)
	Specificity	69.5% (67.1% to 71.8%)	65.1% (62.6% to 67.6%)
20%	Sensitivity	91.3% (87.0% to 94.3%)	94.3% (90.6% to 96.7%)
	Specificity	79.7% (77.5% to 81.7%)	74.3% (71.9% to 76.5%)
30%	Sensitivity	84.5% (80.5% to 89.6%)	88.3% (83.5% to 91.8%)
	Specificity	84.5% (82.6% to 86.3%)	81.1% (79.0% to 83.0%)

When stratifying for menopausal status, the original SRs (classifying inconclusive cases as malignant) had a sensitivity and specificity of 94.3% (88.1% to 97.4%) and 77.3% (74.5% to 79.8%) in premenopausal patients, and 94.4% (88.9% to 97.3%) and 64.9% (60.3% to 69.2%) in postmenopausal patients. Subjective assessment had a sensitivity and specificity of 87.6% (80.0% to 92.6%) and 89.0% (86.9% to 90.8%) in premenopausal patients, and 92.0% (85.9% to 95.6%) and 81.7% (77.8% to 85.0%) in postmenopausal patients.

In premenopausal women, the AUCs of the SRR and ADNEX model were 0.932 (0.913 to 0.950) and 0.932 (0.913 to 0.950), respectively. In postmenopausal women, the AUCs of the SRR and ADNEX model were 0.882 (0.853 to 0.912) and 0.885 (0.858 to 0.912), respectively.

Table 4 summarizes the sensitivity and specificity for the two models at different risk thresholds for pre- and postmenopausal women.

Table 4. Sensitivity and specificity by menopausal status for Assessment of Different NEoplasias in the adneXa (ADNEX) model and Simple Rules Risk (SRR) model at various risk thresholds (percent (95% confidence interval)).

Risk Threshold	Statistic	ADNEX		SRR	
		Premenopausal	Postmenopausal	Premenopausal	Postmenopausal
1%	Sens	100.0% (96.5% to 100.0%)	100.0% (97.0% to 100%)	100.0% (96.5% to 100.0%)	100% (97.0% to 100.0%)
	Spec	25.8% (23.2% to 28.7%)	5.4% (3.6% to 7.9%)	41.4% (38.3% to 44.5%)	30.6% (26.6% to 35.1%)
10%	Sens	94.3% (88.1% to 97.4%)	100% (97.0% to 100%)	98.1% (93.3% to 99.5%)	96.0% (91.0% to 98.3%)
	Spec	77.8% (75.1% to 80.3%)	51.5% (46.8% to 56.1%)	70.6% (67.7% to 73.4%)	53.2% (48.6% to 57.8%)
20%	Sens	86.7% (78.9% to 91.9%)	95.2% (89.9% to 97.8%)	94.3% (88.1% to 97.4%)	94.4% (88.9% to 97.3%)
	Spec	85.6% (83.2% to 87.6%)	66.9% (62.4% to 71.1%)	78.5% (75.8% to 80.9%)	65.1% (60.6% to 69.4%)
30%	Sens	78.1% (69.3% to 84.9%)	92.0% (85.9% to 95.6%)	84.8% (76.7% to 90.4%)	91.2% (84.9% to 95.0%)
	Spec	89.5% (87.5% to 81.3%)	73.6% (96.3% to 77.5%)	84.1% (81.7% to 86.3%)	74.5% (70.3% to 78.3%)

4. Discussion

This validation of IOTA ultrasound-based rules and risk prediction models showed good test performance to discriminate between benign disease and stage I–II ovarian malignancy before surgery.

The strength of this study is the use of a large international database in which information was prospectively collected using well-defined terms, definitions, and measurement methods [19]. The large sample size and the participation of different types of centers are likely to yield generalizable results.

A limitation of our study is that the diagnostic methods were validated exclusively on patients who underwent surgery. This does not reflect clinical practice, where some masses are managed expectantly, but it allowed us to use histological diagnosis as the gold standard. We are awaiting the results of IOTA phase 5, in which IOTA methods are validated on consecutively collected adnexal masses of all kinds, including those managed conservatively. A second limitation is that all ultrasound examiners in the study were very experienced. Our results might not necessarily be applicable to less experienced operators. However, published studies have shown that the IOTA SRs and ADNEX retain their performance in the hands of less experienced examiners [27,28,35–41]. This is likely to be true also for the SRR model, because the same ultrasound variables are used in the original SRs are used to calculate the risks of the SRR model. A third limitation of our study is that not all histopathology information necessary to classify the tumors into type I and type II epithelial malignancies had been collected. This is explained by the fact that patient recruitment for IOTA 3 started in 2009, before the dualistic model of ovarian carcinogenesis [42] was widely accepted.

The findings of our study show that the performance of IOTA methods for differentiating benign disease from stage I–II primary ovarian malignancy is not much lower than the performance for the discrimination of benign from all malignant disease (all malignant subtypes grouped together) [24,25,31]. In the original publications including all IOTA 3 patients, validation AUCs (95% confidence intervals) regarding discrimination between benign and malignant disease for SRR and ADNEX (without CA125) were 0.917 (0.902–0.930) [24] and 0.932 (0.922–0.941) [25], respectively. Sensitivity and specificity for the original SRs on validation in the same population were 95.3% (93.1% to 96.9%) and 74.1% (67.7% to 79.7%), respectively [24,25,31].

Borderline malignant tumors were excluded from our analysis. These tumors are known to be more difficult to classify as benign or malignant [25,43,44]. On the other hand, borderline (i.e., non-invasive malignant) ovarian tumors rarely precede invasive epithelial ovarian carcinoma [45,46]. More clinically relevant is the correct identification of early stage primary invasive tumors, where prompt and adequate surgical staging is important for improving survival [47]. Detection of stage I-II ovarian cancer is particularly important for screening for ovarian cancer to be successful. The aim of screening for ovarian cancer is to decrease ovarian cancer mortality. For this to be possible, screening should result in a shift towards earlier stages at detection, i.e., the detection rate of stage I–II ovarian cancer should be high. However, a shift towards earlier detection of ovarian cancer has been shown in only two [9,11] of three randomized controlled trials [9–11] on ovarian cancer screening, and none of the two completed screening trials has shown conclusive evidence of decreased ovarian cancer mortality in the screened group [10,11]. In the two completed randomized trials on ovarian cancer screening [10,11], the ultrasound criteria to define an abnormal screening result were subjective or arbitrary. As a result, many patients with benign disease were scheduled for surgery, i.e., a large number of operations were performed to detect one cancer case. We speculate that the positive predictive value of an abnormal screen result could be improved if the IOTA methods were used to define an abnormal scan result. To the best of our knowledge, the discriminative or predictive performance of the IOTA methods has never been assessed in a screening population.

About 90% of invasive malignant ovarian tumors are epithelial [48]. The dualistic model proposed by Shih and Kurman highlights the heterogeneity of ovarian carcinoma and implies that ultrasound-based screening will not be effective in detecting all types of ovarian carcinoma. Type I tumors (low-grade serous, low-grade endometrioid, clear cell, and mucinous) are slow growing, attain a large size while still confined to the ovary, and are thus likely to be detected early by transvaginal ultrasound. Unfortunately, these lesions constitute only 25% of ovarian cancers and account for only approximately 10% of ovarian cancer deaths. On the other hand, type II tumors (high-grade serous and undifferentiated carcinomas, and malignant mixed mesodermal tumors (carcinosarcomas)) represent 75% of all ovarian carcinomas, are responsible for 90% of ovarian cancer deaths, and may originate outside the ovary. These tumors are almost never confined to the ovary at diagnosis, making their diagnosis at an early point in the disease course challenging [42,49]. To allow detection of this aggressive type of ovarian cancer, there is ongoing search for sensitive biomarkers expressed early in ovarian carcinogenesis. More recently, there is increasing interest in the use of genomic profiling as a potential candidate for the detection of ovarian malignancies [50,51]. Further research should explore whether IOTA methods may serve as a second stage test in a program of ovarian cancer screening to avoid unnecessary surgery without delaying a diagnosis of ovarian cancer.

5. Conclusions

This analysis shows that the IOTA methods have good ability to discriminate between stage I–II ovarian malignancy and benign adnexal lesions prior to surgery. The potential use of IOTA methods as a second stage test in ovarian cancer screening should be the subject of further investigation.

Acknowledgments: This study was supported by the Flemish government (Research Foundation–Flanders (FWO) project G049312N and G0B4716N, Flanders' Agency for Innovation by Science and Technology (IWT) project IWT-TBM 070706-IOTA3, and iMinds 2015) and Internal Funds KU Leuven (University of Leuven) (project C24/15/037). Dirk Timmerman is a senior clinical investigator of Fonds Wetenschappelijk Onderzoek (FWO). Tom Bourne is supported by the National Institute for Health Research (NIHR) Biomedical Research Centre based at Imperial College Healthcare National Health Service (NHS) Trust and Imperial College London.

The views expressed are those of the authors and not necessarily those of the NHS, NIHR or Department of Health, Lil Valentin is supported by the Swedish Medical Research Council (grants K2001-72X-11605-06A, K2002-72X-11605-07B, K2004-73X-11605-09A, and K2006-73X-11605-11-3), funds administered by Malmö University Hospital and Skåne University Hospital, Allmänna Sjukhusets i Malmö Stiftelse för bekämpande av cancer (the Malmö General Hospital Foundation for fighting against cancer), and two Swedish governmental grants (Avtal om läkarutbildning och forskning (ALF)-medel and Landstingsfinansierad Regional Forskning). Laure Wynants holds a postdoctoral mandate from Internal Funds KU Leuven. The sponsors had no role in study design; in the collection, analysis, and interpretation of data; in the writing of the report; and in the decision to submit the work for publication. The researchers performed this work independently of the funding sources.

Author Contributions: Wouter Froyman, Laure Wynants, Chiara Landolfo, Ben Van Calster and Dirk Timmerman conceived and designed the study, with additional support from Tom Bourne, Lil Valentin and Antonia Testa; Lil Valentin, Antonia Testa, Povilas Sladkevicius, Dorella Franchi, Daniela Fischerova, Luca Savelli and Dirk Timmerman enrolled patients and acquired data; Ben Van Calster and Dirk Timmerman were involved in data cleaning; Laure Wynants analyzed the data, with support from Ben Van Calster; Wouter Froyman, Laure Wynants, Chiara Landolfo, Tom Bourne, Lil Valentin, Antonia Testa, Ben Van Calster and Dirk Timmerman were involved in data interpretation; Wouter Froyman, Laure Wynants, Chiara Landolfo, Ben Van Calster and Dirk Timmerman wrote the first draft of the manuscript, which was then critically reviewed and revised by the other coauthors. All authors approved the final version of the manuscript for submission; Laure Wynants, Ben Van Calster and Dirk Timmerman had full access to all the data in the study and take responsibility for the integrity of the data and the accuracy of the data analysis.

References

1. Pavlik, E.J.; Ueland, F.R.; Miller, R.W.; Ubellacker, J.M.; DeSimone, C.P.; Elder, J.; Hoff, J.; Baldwin, L.; Kryscio, R.J.; van Nagell, J.R., Jr. Frequency and disposition of ovarian abnormalities followed with serial transvaginal ultrasonography. *Obstet. Gynecol.* **2013**, *122*, 210–217. [CrossRef] [PubMed]
2. Castillo, G.; Alcazar, J.L.; Jurado, M. Natural history of sonographically detected simple unilocular adnexal cysts in asymptomatic postmenopausal women. *Gynecol. Oncol.* **2004**, *92*, 965–969. [CrossRef] [PubMed]
3. Borgfeldt, C.; Andolf, E. Transvaginal sonographic ovarian findings in a random sample of women 25–40 years old. *Ultrasound Obstet. Gynecol.* **1999**, *13*, 345–350. [CrossRef] [PubMed]
4. Curtin, J.P. Management of the Adnexal Mass. *Gynecol. Oncol.* **1994**, *55*, S42–S46. [CrossRef] [PubMed]
5. Ferlay, J.; Steliarova-Foucher, E.; Lortet-Tieulent, J.; Rosso, S.; Coebergh, J.W.; Comber, H.; Forman, D.; Bray, F. Cancer incidence and mortality patterns in Europe: Estimates for 40 countries in 2012. *Eur. J. Cancer* **2013**, *49*, 1374–1403. [CrossRef] [PubMed]
6. Cancer Research UK. Available online: www.cancerresearchuk.org (accessed on 20 November 2016).
7. Vaughan, S.; Coward, J.I.; Bast, R.C., Jr.; Berchuck, A.; Berek, J.S.; Brenton, J.D.; Coukos, G.; Crum, C.C.; Drapkin, R.; Etemadmoghadam, D.; et al. Rethinking ovarian cancer: Recommendations for improving outcomes. *Nat. Rev. Cancer* **2011**, *11*, 719–725. [CrossRef] [PubMed]
8. Heintz, A.P.M.; Odicino, F.; Maisonneuve, P.; Quinn, M.A.; Benedet, J.L.; Creasman, W.T.; Ngan, H.Y.S.; Pecorelli, S.; Beller, U. Carcinoma of the Ovary. *Int. J. Gynecol. Obstet.* **2006**, *95*, S161–S192. [CrossRef]
9. Kobayashi, H.; Yamada, Y.; Sado, T.; Sakata, M.; Yoshida, S.; Kawaguchi, R.; Kanayama, S.; Shigetomi, H.; Haruta, S.; Tsuji, Y.; et al. A randomized study of screening for ovarian cancer: A multicenter study in Japan. *Int. J. Gynecol. Cancer* **2008**, *18*, 414–420. [CrossRef] [PubMed]
10. Buys, S.S. Effect of Screening on Ovarian Cancer Mortality. *JAMA* **2011**, *305*, 2295. [CrossRef] [PubMed]
11. Jacobs, I.J.; Menon, U.; Ryan, A.; Gentry-Maharaj, A.; Burnell, M.; Kalsi, J.K.; Amso, N.N.; Apostolidou, S.; Benjamin, E.; Cruickshank, D.; et al. Ovarian cancer screening and mortality in the UK Collaborative Trial of Ovarian Cancer Screening (UKCTOCS): A randomised controlled trial. *Lancet* **2016**, *387*, 945–956. [CrossRef]
12. Paulsen, T.; Kjaerheim, K.; Kaern, J.; Tretli, S.; Tropé, C. Improved short-term survival for advanced ovarian, tubal, and peritoneal cancer patients operated at teaching hospitals. *Int. J. Gynecol. Cancer* **2006**, *16*, 11–17. [CrossRef] [PubMed]
13. Engelen, M.J.; Kos, H.E.; Willemse, P.H.; Aalders, J.G.; de Vries, E.G.; Schaapveld, M.; Otter, R.; van der Zee, A.G. Surgery by consultant gynecologic oncologists improves survival in patients with ovarian carcinoma. *Cancer* **2006**, *106*, 589–598. [CrossRef] [PubMed]
14. Earle, C.C.; Schrag, D.; Neville, B.A.; Yabroff, K.R.; Topor, M.; Fahey, A.; Trimble, E.L.; Bodurka, D.C.; Bristow, R.E.; Carney, M.; et al. Effect of surgeon specialty on processes of care and outcomes for ovarian cancer patients. *J. Natl. Cancer Inst.* **2006**, *98*, 172–180. [CrossRef] [PubMed]

15. Woo, Y.L.; Kyrgiou, M.; Bryant, A.; Everett, T.; Dickinson, H.O. Centralisation of services for gynaecological cancer—A Cochrane Systematic Review. *Gynecol. Oncol.* **2012**, *126*, 286–290. [CrossRef] [PubMed]
16. Valentin, L.; Hagen, B.; Tingulstad, S.; Eik-Nes, S. Comparison of "pattern recognition" and logistic regression models for discrimination between benign and malignant pelvic masses: A prospective cross validation. *Ultrasound Obstet. Gynecol.* **2001**, *18*, 357–365. [CrossRef] [PubMed]
17. Timmerman, D. The use of mathematical models to evaluate pelvic masses; can they beat an expert operator? *Best Pract. Res. Clin. Obstet. Gynaecol.* **2004**, *18*, 91–104. [CrossRef] [PubMed]
18. Meys, E.M.; Kaijser, J.; Kruitwagen, R.F.; Slangen, B.F.; van Calster, B.; Aertgeerts, B.; Verbakel, J.Y.; Timmerman, D.; van Gorp, T. Subjective assessment versus ultrasound models to diagnose ovarian cancer: A systematic review and meta-analysis. *Eur. J. Cancer* **2016**, *58*, 17–29. [CrossRef] [PubMed]
19. Timmerman, D.; Valentin, L.; Bourne, T.; Collins, W.P.; Verrelst, H.; Vergote, I. Terms, definitions and measurements to describe the sonographic features of adnexal tumors: A consensus opinion from the International Ovarian Tumor Analysis (IOTA) group. *Ultrasound Obstet. Gynecol.* **2000**, *16*, 500–505. [CrossRef] [PubMed]
20. Timmerman, D.; Testa, A.C.; Bourne, T.; Ameye, L.; Jurkovic, D.; van Holsbeke, C.; Paladini, D.; van Calster, B.; Vergote, I.; van Huffel, S.; et al. Simple ultrasound-based rules for the diagnosis of ovarian cancer. *Ultrasound Obstet. Gynecol.* **2008**, *31*, 681–690. [CrossRef] [PubMed]
21. Royal College of Obstetricians and Gynaecologists. *Management of Suspected Ovarian Masses in Premenopausal Women*; Green-top Guideline No. 62; Royal College of Obstetricians and Gynaecologists: London, UK, 2011.
22. The American College of Obstetricians and Gynecologists. Practice bulletin—Evaluation and Management of Adnexal Masses. *Obstet. Gynecol.* **2016**, *128*, e210–e226.
23. Kaijser, J.; Sayasneh, A.; van Hoorde, K.; Ghaem-Maghami, S.; Bourne, T.; Timmerman, D.; van Calster, B. Presurgical diagnosis of adnexal tumours using mathematical models and scoring systems: A systematic review and meta-analysis. *Hum. Reprod. Update* **2014**, *20*, 449–462. [CrossRef] [PubMed]
24. Timmerman, D.; van Calster, B.; Testa, A.; Savelli, L.; Fischerova, D.; Froyman, W.; Wynants, L.; van Holsbeke, C.; Epstein, E.; Franchi, D.; et al. Predicting the risk of malignancy in adnexal masses based on the Simple Rules from the International Ovarian Tumor Analysis group. *Am. J. Obstet. Gynecol.* **2016**, *214*, 424–437. [CrossRef] [PubMed]
25. Van Calster, B.; van Hoorde, K.; Valentin, L.; Testa, A.C.; Fischerova, D.; van Holsbeke, C.; Savelli, L.; Franchi, D.; Epstein, E.; Kaijser, J.; et al. International Ovarian Tumour Analysis, G. Evaluating the risk of ovarian cancer before surgery using the ADNEX model to differentiate between benign, borderline, early and advanced stage invasive, and secondary metastatic tumours: Prospective multicentre diagnostic study. *BMJ* **2014**, *349*, g5920. [CrossRef] [PubMed]
26. Meys, E.M.; Jeelof, L.S.; Achten, N.M.; Slangen, B.F.; Lambrechts, S.; Kruitwagen, R.F.; van Gorp, T. Estimating the risk of malignancy in adnexal masses: An external validation of the ADNEX model and comparison with other frequently used ultrasound methods. *Ultrasound Obstet. Gynecol.* **2016**. [CrossRef] [PubMed]
27. Sayasneh, A.; Ferrara, L.; de Cock, B.; Saso, S.; Al-Memar, M.; Johnson, S.; Kaijser, J.; Carvalho, J.; Husicka, R.; Smith, A.; et al. Evaluating the risk of ovarian cancer before surgery using the ADNEX model: A multicentre external validation study. *Br. J. Cancer* **2016**, *115*, 542–548. [CrossRef] [PubMed]
28. Szubert, S.; Wojtowicz, A.; Moszynski, R.; Zywica, P.; Dyczkowski, K.; Stachowiak, A.; Sajdak, S.; Szpurek, D.; Alcazar, J.L. External validation of the IOTA ADNEX model performed by two independent gynecologic centers. *Gynecol. Oncol.* **2016**, *142*, 490–495. [CrossRef] [PubMed]
29. Araujo, K.G.; Jales, R.M.; Pereira, P.N.; Yoshida, A.; de Angelo Andrade, L.; Sarian, L.O.; Derchain, S. Performance of the IOTA ADNEX model in the preoperative discrimination of adnexal masses in a gynecologic oncology center. *Ultrasound Obstet. Gynecol.* **2016**. [CrossRef]
30. Joyeux, E.; Miras, T.; Masquin, I.; Duglet, P.E.; Astruc, K.; Douvier, S. Before surgery predictability of malignant ovarian tumors based on ADNEX model and its use in clinical practice. *Gynecol. Obstet. Fertil.* **2016**, *44*, 557–564. [CrossRef] [PubMed]
31. Testa, A.; Kaijser, J.; Wynants, L.; Fischerova, D.; van Holsbeke, C.; Franchi, D.; Savelli, L.; Epstein, E.; Czekierdowski, A.; Guerriero, S.; et al. Strategies to diagnose ovarian cancer: New evidence from phase 3 of the multicentre international IOTA study. *Br. J. Cancer* **2014**, *111*, 680–688. [CrossRef] [PubMed]

32. DeLong, E.R.; DeLong, D.M.; Clarke-Pearson, D.L. Comparing the areas under two or more correlated receiver operating characteristic curves: A nonparametric approach. *Biometrics* **1988**, *44*, 837–845. [CrossRef] [PubMed]
33. Wilson, E.B. Probable inference, the law of succession, and statistical inference. *J. Am. Stat. Assoc.* **1927**, *22*, 209–212. [CrossRef]
34. Collins, G.S.; Reitsma, J.B.; Altman, D.G.; Moons, K.G. Transparent reporting of a multivariable prediction model for individual prognosis or diagnosis (TRIPOD): The TRIPOD statement. *BMJ* **2015**, *350*, g7594. [CrossRef] [PubMed]
35. Hartman, C.A.; Juliato, C.R.; Sarian, L.O.; Toledo, M.C.; Jales, R.M.; Morais, S.S.; Pitta, D.D.; Marussi, E.F.; Derchain, S. Ultrasound criteria and CA 125 as predictive variables of ovarian cancer in women with adnexal tumors. *Ultrasound Obstet. Gynecol.* **2012**, *40*, 360–366. [CrossRef] [PubMed]
36. Alcazar, J.L.; Pascual, M.A.; Olartecoechea, B.; Graupera, B.; Auba, M.; Ajossa, S.; Hereter, L.; Julve, R.; Gaston, B.; Peddes, C.; et al. IOTA simple rules for discriminating between benign and malignant adnexal masses: Prospective external validation. *Ultrasound Obstet. Gynecol.* **2013**, *42*, 467–471. [CrossRef] [PubMed]
37. Sayasneh, A.; Wynants, L.; Preisler, J.; Kaijser, J.; Johnson, S.; Stalder, C.; Husicka, R.; Abdallah, Y.; Raslan, F.; Drought, A.; et al. Multicentre external validation of IOTA prediction models and RMI by operators with varied training. *Br. J. Cancer* **2013**, *108*, 2448–2454. [CrossRef] [PubMed]
38. Nunes, N.; Ambler, G.; Foo, X.; Naftalin, J.; Widschwendter, M.; Jurkovic, D. Use of IOTA simple rules for diagnosis of ovarian cancer: Meta-analysis. *Ultrasound Obstet. Gynecol.* **2014**, *44*, 503–514. [CrossRef] [PubMed]
39. Tinnangwattana, D.; Vichak-ururote, L.; Tontivuthikul, P.; Charoenratana, C.; Lerthiranwong, T.; Tongsong, T. IOTA Simple Rules in Differentiating between Benign and Malignant Adnexal Masses by Non-expert Examiners. *Asian Pac. J. Cancer Prev.* **2015**, *16*, 3835–3838. [CrossRef] [PubMed]
40. Ruiz de Gauna, B.; Rodriguez, D.; Olartecoechea, B.; Auba, M.; Jurado, M.; Gomez Roig, M.D.; Alcazar, J.L. Diagnostic performance of IOTA simple rules for adnexal masses classification: A comparison between two centers with different ovarian cancer prevalence. *Eur. J. Obstet. Gynecol. Reprod. Biol.* **2015**, *191*, 10–14. [CrossRef] [PubMed]
41. Knafel, A.; Banas, T.; Nocun, A.; Wiechec, M.; Jach, R.; Ludwin, A.; Kabzinska-Turek, M.; Pietrus, M.; Pitynski, K. The Prospective External Validation of International Ovarian Tumor Analysis (IOTA) Simple Rules in the Hands of Level I and II Examiners. *Ultraschall Med.* **2015**, *37*, 516–523. [CrossRef] [PubMed]
42. Shih, I.-M.; Kurman, R. Ovarian Tumorigenesis—A Proposed Model Based on Morphological and Molecular Genetic Analysis. *Am. J. Pathol.* **2004**, *164*, 1511–1518. [CrossRef]
43. Valentin, L.; Ameye, L.; Jurkovic, D.; Metzger, U.; Lecuru, F.; van Huffel, S.; Timmerman, D. Which extrauterine pelvic masses are difficult to correctly classify as benign or malignant on the basis of ultrasound findings and is there a way of making a correct diagnosis? *Ultrasound Obstet. Gynecol.* **2006**, *27*, 438–444. [CrossRef] [PubMed]
44. Valentin, L.; Ameye, L.; Savelli, L.; Fruscio, R.; Leone, F.P.; Czekierdowski, A.; Lissoni, A.A.; Fischerova, D.; Guerriero, S.; van Holsbeke, C.; et al. Adnexal masses difficult to classify as benign or malignant using subjective assessment of gray-scale and Doppler ultrasound findings: Logistic regression models do not help. *Ultrasound Obstet. Gynecol.* **2011**, *38*, 456–465. [CrossRef] [PubMed]
45. Vergote, I.; Amant, F.; Ameye, L.; Timmerman, D. Screening for ovarian carcinoma: Not quite there yet. *Lancet Oncol.* **2009**, *10*, 308–309. [CrossRef]
46. Fischerova, D.; Zikan, M.; Dundr, P.; Cibula, D. Diagnosis, treatment, and follow-up of borderline ovarian tumors. *Oncologist* **2012**, *17*, 1515–1533. [CrossRef] [PubMed]
47. Vergote, I.; de Brabander, J.; Fyles, A.; Bertelsen, K.; Einhorn, N.; Sevelda, P.; Gore, M.; Kaern, J.; Verrelst, H.; Sjövall, K.; et al. Prognostic importance of degree of differentiation and cyst rupture in stage I invasive epithelial ovarian carcinoma. *Lancet* **2001**, *357*, 176–182. [CrossRef]
48. Ledermann, J.A.; Raja, F.A.; Fotopoulou, C.; Gonzalez-Martin, A.; Colombo, N.; Sessa, C.; Group, E.G.W. Newly diagnosed and relapsed epithelial ovarian carcinoma: ESMO Clinical Practice Guidelines for diagnosis, treatment and follow-up. *Ann. Oncol.* **2013**, *24* (Suppl. S6), vi24–vi32. [CrossRef] [PubMed]
49. Kurman, R.J.; Shih, I.-M. Molecular pathogenesis and extraovarian origin of epithelial ovarian cancer—Shifting the paradigm. *Hum. Pathol.* **2011**, *42*, 918–931. [CrossRef] [PubMed]
50. Amant, F.; Verheecke, M.; Wlodarska, I.; Dehaspe, L.; Brady, P.; Brison, N.; van Den Bogaert, K.; Dierickx, D.;

Vandecaveye, V.; Tousseyn, T.; et al. Presymptomatic Identification of Cancers in Pregnant Women During Noninvasive Prenatal Testing. *JAMA Oncol.* **2015**, *1*, 814–819. [CrossRef] [PubMed]

51. Vanderstichele, A.; Busschaert, P.; Smeets, D.; Landolfo, C.; van Nieuwenhuysen, E.; Leunen, K.; Neven, P.; Amant, F.; Mahner, S.; Braicu, E.I.; et al. Chromosomal Instability in Cell-Free DNA as a Highly Specific Biomarker for Detection of Ovarian Cancer in Women with Adnexal Masses. *Clin. Cancer Res.* **2016**. [CrossRef] [PubMed]

14

Prognostic Significance of CT-Attenuation of Tumor-Adjacent Breast Adipose Tissue in Breast Cancer Patients with Surgical Resection

Jeong Won Lee [1], Sung Yong Kim [2], Hyun Ju Lee [3], Sun Wook Han [2], Jong Eun Lee [2] and Sang Mi Lee [4,*]

1 Department of Nuclear Medicine, International St. Mary's Hospital, Catholic Kwandong University College of Medicine, 25 Simgok-ro 100 beon-gil, Seo-gu, Incheon 22711, Korea
2 Department of Surgery, Soonchunhyang University Cheonan Hospital, 31 Suncheonhyang 6-gil, Dongnam-gu, Cheonan, Chungcheongnam-do 31151, Korea
3 Department of Pathology, Soonchunhyang University Cheonan Hospital, 31 Suncheonhyang 6-gil, Dongnam-gu, Cheonan, Chungcheongnam-do 31151, Korea
4 Department of Nuclear Medicine, Soonchunhyang University Cheonan Hospital, 31 Suncheonhyang 6-gil, Dongnam-gu, Cheonan, Chungcheongnam-do 31151, Korea
* Correspondence: c91300@schmc.ac.kr

Abstract: The purpose of this study was to evaluate the prognostic significance of computed tomography (CT)-attenuation of tumor-adjacent breast adipose tissue for predicting recurrence-free survival (RFS) in patients with breast cancer. We retrospectively enrolled 287 breast cancer patients who underwent pretreatment ^{18}F-fluorodeoxyglucose (FDG) positron emission tomography (PET)/CT. From non-contrast-enhanced CT images of PET/CT, CT-attenuation values of tumor-adjacent breast adipose tissue (TAT HU) and contralateral breast adipose tissue (CAT HU) were measured. Difference (HU difference) and percent difference (HU difference %) in CT-attenuation values between TAT HU and CAT HU were calculated. The relationships of these breast adipose tissue parameters with tumor factors and RFS were assessed. TAT HU was significantly higher than CAT HU ($p < 0.001$). TAT HU, HU difference, and HU difference % showed significant correlations with T stage and estrogen receptor and progesterone receptor status ($p < 0.05$), whereas CAT HU had no significant relationships with tumor factors ($p > 0.05$). Patients with high TAT HU, HU difference, and HU difference % had significantly worse RFS than those with low values ($p < 0.001$). In multivariate analysis, TAT HU and HU difference % were significantly associated with RFS after adjusting for clinico-pathologic factors ($p < 0.05$). CT-attenuation of tumor-adjacent breast adipose tissue was significantly associated with RFS in patients with breast cancer. The findings seem to support the close contact between breast cancer cells and tumor-adjacent adipocytes observed with imaging studies.

Keywords: breast cancer; Hounsfield unit; computed tomography; prognosis; adipose tissue

---

1. Introduction

Adipose tissue is one of the major components of the human body, found all around the body [1]. In non-lactating human breast tissue, up to 56% of the total breast volume consists of adipose tissue [2]. Although adipose tissue is mainly composed of adipocytes, it is also comprised of various other kinds of cell types including immune cells, endothelial cells, pre-adipocytes, and fibroblasts [1,3]. For a long time, adipose tissue was considered to function as a simple storage organ of excessive energy;

however, evidence showed that adipose tissue also function as an endocrine organ secreting hundreds of cell signaling proteins, called adipokines [4]. Previous studies published over the last decade have continuously demonstrated that adipose tissue could play a role in cancer growth, progression, and metastasis by secreting multiple kinds of adipokines, inducing inflammatory micro-environment, remodeling the extracellular matrix, and providing energy to tumor cells [1,3,5]. Furthermore, adipocytes in the close vicinity of cancer cells can have crosstalk with cancer cells, which increases the potential of tumor progression and metastasis [1,3,6]. Because of the close localization between mammary epithelium and breast adipose tissue, breast cancer is considered as one of the most representative malignancies that is in close contact with adipose tissue, along with gastric, colon, and ovary cancers [1,3]. In previous cell-culture and histopathological studies of breast cancer, it has already been proven that breast cancer cells have active interaction with peritumoral adipose tissue, which further enhances aggressiveness and invasiveness of breast cancer cells [1,3,7–9].

In recent clinical studies with imaging examinations, the clinical implication of adipose tissue features on diagnostic images has been investigated in various diseases [10–12]. In addition to the amount of adipose tissue, the qualitative characteristics of adipose tissue has also been studied using imaging modalities such as computed tomography (CT) and positron emission tomography (PET) [10,12–15]. One of the most commonly used imaging features representing qualitative changes in adipose tissue is CT-attenuation of adipose tissue measured on non-contrast-enhanced CT images [10,12–14]. In recent clinical studies with diverse kinds of malignancies, increased CT-attenuation on unenhanced CT images has shown a significant association with worse clinical outcomes, suggesting that increased CT-attenuation might reflect a microenvironment of adipose tissue which promotes cancer cell progression [12–14]. Considering the close localization between breast cancer and breast adipose tissue, the qualitative characteristics of peritumoral breast adipose tissue might have a significant association with the characteristics and clinical outcomes of breast cancer [1]. However, few studies have evaluated the clinical significance of the peritumoral adipose tissue environment using imaging studies [16].

In breast cancer, previous studies have shown the clinical significance of ^{18}F-fluorodeoxyglucose (FDG) PET/CT for staging, differentiating molecular subtypes, and predicting clinical outcomes; therefore, currently, FDG PET/CT is widely used in patients with breast cancer [17–20]. In the present study, we used unenhanced CT images of pretreatment ^{18}F-fluorodeoxyglucose (FDG) PET/CT for measuring CT-attenuation of tumor-adjacent breast adipose tissue and investigated whether it has a significant association with recurrence-free survival (RFS) in patients with breast cancer who underwent curative surgical resection.

2. Results

2.1. Patient Characteristics

Baseline characteristics of the 287 patients enrolled in the present study are shown in Table 1. Of the enrolled patients, 33 (11.5%) were histopathologically confirmed as having triple negative breast cancer. Neoadjuvant chemotherapy was performed in 32 patients (11.1%), and, after curative surgical resection, 282 patients (98.3%) received adjuvant treatments. The median interval between FDG PET/CT and initial treatment was 5.0 days (range, 2–14 days). On PET/CT image analysis of primary breast cancer, 89 patients (31.0%) had a metabolic tumor volume (MTV) of 0.0 cm^3, because maximum standardized uptake values (SUVs) of the primary breast cancer were less than 2.50. The median follow-up duration of the patients was 55.1 months with a range of 6.1–88.9 months, and during the follow-up period, cancer recurrence was found in 30 patients (10.5%).

Table 1. Baseline characteristics of patients ($n = 287$).

Characteristics		Number (%)	Median (Range)
Age (years)			52 (30–85)
Body mass index			23.8 (16.4–35.2)
Menopausal status	Premenopausal	108 (37.6%)	
	Postmenopausal	179 (62.4%)	
Histopathology	Intraductal carcinoma	252 (87.8%)	
	Intralobular carcinoma	35 (12.2%)	
T stage	T1	136 (47.4%)	
	T2	128 (44.6%)	
	T3	23 (8.0%)	
N stage	N0	190 (66.2%)	
	N1	58 (20.2%)	
	N2	21 (7.3%)	
	N3	18 (6.3%)	
Tumor size (cm)			2.0 (0.4–8.0)
Histologic grade	Grade 1	67 (23.4%)	
	Grade 2	143 (49.7%)	
	Grade 3	77 (26.9%)	
Estrogen receptor statue	Positive	213 (74.2%)	
	Negative	74 (25.8%)	
Progesterone receptor status	Positive	177 (61.7%)	
	Negative	110 (38.3%)	
HER2 status	Positive	142 (49.5%)	
	Negative	145 (50.5%)	
Ki67 expression status	Positive	177 (61.7%)	
	Negative	110 (38.3%)	
Maximum SUV of primary tumor			4.06 (1.10–35.59)
MTV of primary tumor (cm^3)			1.14 (0.0–235.30)
TAT HU			−87.69 (−104.88––63.36)
CAT HU			−97.54 (−116.85––70.74)
HU difference			8.66 (−2.67–35.84)
HU difference %			8.94 (−3.15–30.67)
Neoadjuvant chemotherapy	Yes	32 (11.1%)	
	No	255 (88.9%)	
Adjuvant treatment	CTx + RTx + HTx	139 (48.4%)	
	RTx + HTx	82 (28.6%)	
	CTx + HTx	17 (5.9%)	
	CTx + RTx	3 (1.0%)	
	HTx	24 (8.4%)	
	CTx	16 (5.6%)	
	RTx	1 (0.3%)	
	No	5 (1.7%)	

HER2, human epidermal growth factor receptor 2; SUV, standardized uptake value; MTV, metabolic tumor volume; TAT HU, CT-attenuation of tumor-adjacent breast adipose tissue; CAT HU, CT-attenuation of contralateral breast adipose tissue; HU difference, difference of CT-attenuation; HU difference %, percent difference of CT-attenuation; CTx, chemotherapy; RTx, radiotherapy; HTx, hormonal therapy.

2.2. *Breast Adipose Tissue Measurement*

On the assessment of reproducibility of breast adipose tissue measurement, substantial agreement was shown between the two reviewers for CT-attenuation values, expressed in Hounsfield unit (HU), of tumor-adjacent breast adipose tissue (TAT HU) (concordance correlation coefficient: 0.953; 95% confidence interval: 0.934–0.968) and CT-attenuation values of contralateral breast adipose tissue (CAT HU) (concordance correlation coefficient: 0.951; 95% confidence interval: 0.924–0.972).

Among the enrolled patients, TAT HU was higher than CAT HU in 269 patients (93.7%), showing significant difference between TAT HU and CAT HU ($p < 0.001$). Body mass index (BMI) showed significant negative correlation with both TAT HU ($r = -0.136$, $p = 0.001$) and CAT HU ($r = -0.274$, $p < 0.001$) but showed weaker correlation with TAT HU and no significant correlation with the difference in CT-attenuation values between tumor-adjacent and contralateral breast adipose tissues (HU difference) ($p = 0.231$) and percent difference of CT-attenuation values between tumor-adjacent and contralateral breast adipose tissues (HU difference %) ($p = 0.425$).

In correlation analysis between breast adipose tissue parameters and tumor stage, increased CT-attenuation of peritumoral breast adipose tissue was related with advanced stage (Table 2). For T stage, significant differences of TAT HU, HU difference, and HU difference % were shown on Kruskal—Wallis test ($p < 0.001$ for all; Figure 1). On post-hoc analysis, each T stage group showed significant difference of TAT HU from each other, and HU difference and HU difference % in T2 and T3 stage groups were significantly higher than those in the T1 stage group ($p < 0.05$). For N stage, patients with regional lymph node metastasis had significantly higher HU difference and HU difference % than those with no lymph node metastasis ($p < 0.001$ for all). In contrast, there were no significant differences of CAT HU according to T stage and N stage ($p > 0.05$).

Table 2. Relationship between breast cancer adipose tissue parameters and clinico-histological factors.

Clinico-Histological Factors		TAT HU	CAT HU	HU Difference	HU Difference %
T stage	T1	−88.95 ± 6.53	−96.95 ± 6.61	7.99 ± 6.06	8.08 ± 6.02
	T2	−86.33 ± 5.72	−97.15 ± 7.22	10.82 ± 6.69	10.87 ± 6.23
	T3	−82.67 ± 5.68	−95.43 ± 7.39	12.76 ± 6.18	13.14 ± 5.66
	p-value	<0.001 *	0.505 *	<0.001 *	<0.001 *
N stage	N0	−87.64 ± 6.26	−96.95 ± 6.82	8.63 ± 6.43	8.76 ± 6.27
	N1-3	−86.56 ± 6.56	−98.06 ± 7.97	11.61 ± 6.34	11.63 ± 5.92
	p-value	0.176	0.203	<0.001	<0.001
Histologic grade	Grade 1	−87.62 ± 7.21	−96.28 ± 7.61	8.65 ± 7.11	8.76 ± 6.75
	Grade 2	−87.65 ± 6.23	−96.87 ± 6.71	9.23 ± 6.42	9.32 ± 6.21
	Grade 3	−86.27 ± 5.85	−97.58 ± 6.84	11.21 ± 6.09	11.29 ± 5.83
	p-value	0.288 *	0.391 *	0.013 *	0.013 *
ER status	Positive	−88.03 ± 6.26	−96.76 ± 6.91	8.73 ± 6.34	8.81 ± 6.09
	Negative	−85.11 ± 6.25	−97.36 ± 7.07	12.25 ± 6.46	12.36 ± 6.15
	p-value	<0.001	0.528	<0.001	<0.001
PR status	Positive	−87.94 ± 6.47	−96.60 ± 6.76	8.16 ± 5.73	8.34 ± 5.69
	Negative	−86.22 ± 6.09	−97.23 ± 7.06	12.01 ± 7.08	11.97 ± 6.58
	p-value	0.026	0.318	<0.001	<0.001
HER2 status	Positive	−87.54 ± 5.71	−97.56 ± 6.34	10.02 ± 6.79	10.03 ± 6.49
	Negative	−87.02 ± 6.97	−96.29 ± 7.45	9.27 ± 6.29	9.43 ± 6.10
	p-value	0.488	0.122	0.336	0.426
Ki67 expression status	Positive	−86.72 ± 6.10	−96.88 ± 6.83	10.16 ± 6.76	10.25 ± 6.42
	Negative	−88.01 ± 7.01	−96.72 ± 7.37	8.72 ± 6.25	8.82 ± 6.17
	p-value	0.115	0.856	0.083	0.076
Recurrence	No recur	−87.74 ± 6.27	−96.90 ± 6.74	9.16 ± 6.37	9.25 ± 6.17
	Recur	−83.35 ± 6.00	−97.10 ± 8.62	13.75 ± 6.71	13.85 ± 5.91
	p-value	<0.001	0.882	<0.001	<0.001

* Performed using Kruskal—Wallis test.; ER, estrogen receptor; PR, progesterone receptor; HER2, human epidermal growth factor receptor 2; TAT HU, CT-attenuation of tumor-adjacent breast adipose tissue; CAT HU, CT-attenuation of contralateral breast adipose tissue; HU difference, difference of CT-attenuation; HU difference %, percent difference of CT-attenuation.

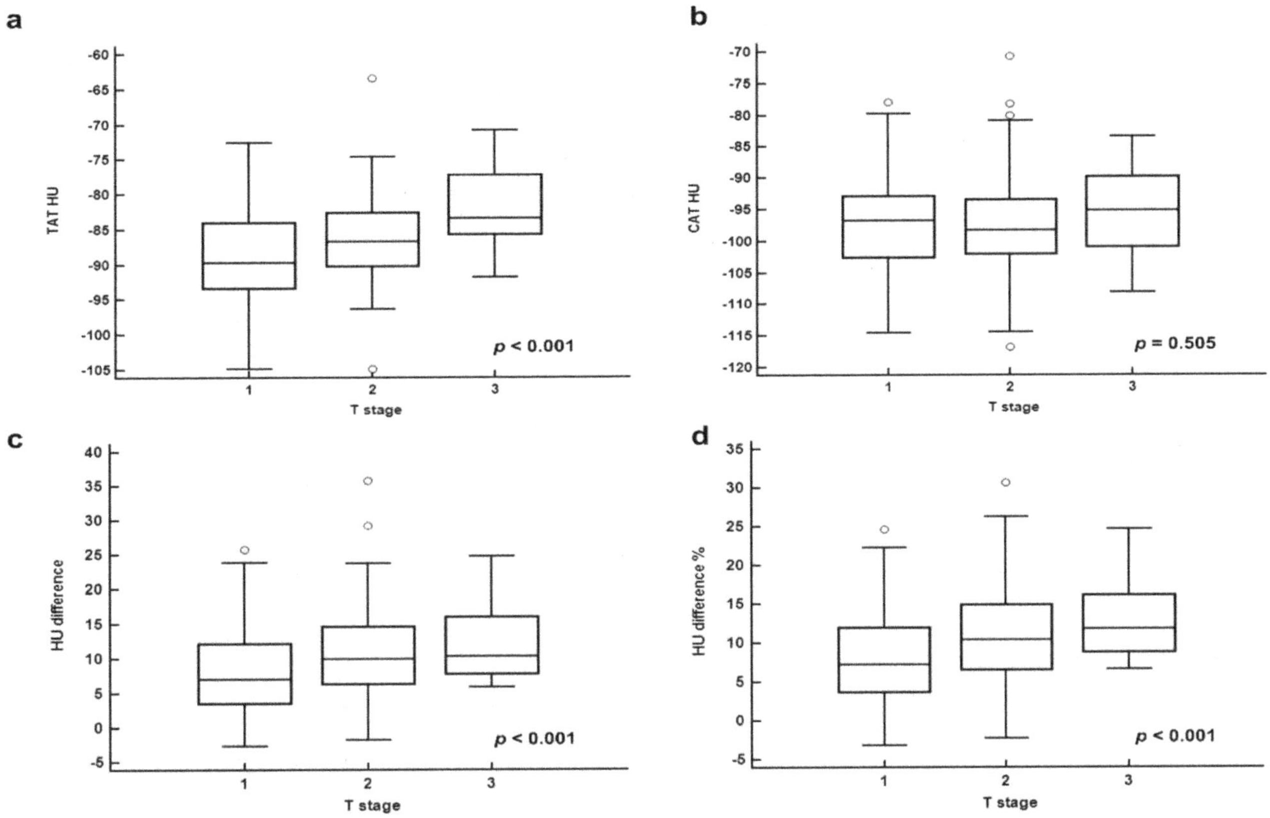

Figure 1. CT-attenuation of tumor-adjacent breast adipose tissue (TAT HU) (**a**), CT-attenuation of contralateral breast adipose tissue (CAT HU) (**b**), difference of CT-attenuation (HU difference) (**c**), and percent difference of CT-attenuation (HU difference %) (**d**), according to T stage.

In correlation analysis with histopathological results, increased CT-attenuation of peritumoral breast adipose tissue was related with aggressive features of breast cancer (Table 2). Patients with negative estrogen receptor (ER) and progesterone receptor (PR) showed higher values of TAT HU, HU difference, and HU difference % than those with positive ER and PR, respectively ($p < 0.05$). Moreover, significant differences of HU difference and HU difference % were observed according to the histologic grade of the primary tumor, showing significantly higher HU difference and HU difference % in patients with histologic grade 3 tumors than in those with grade 1 and grade 2 tumors on post-hoc analysis ($p < 0.05$). In contrast, human epidermal growth factor receptor 2 (HER2) status and Ki67 expression status had no significant correlation with any breast adipose tissue parameters ($p > 0.05$).

In correlation analysis with FDG PET/CT parameters of primary breast cancer lesions, TAT HU, HU difference, and HU difference % showed significant but weak positive correlations with maximum SUV ($r = 0.125$, $p = 0.034$ for TAT HU, $r = 0.266$, $p < 0.001$ for HU difference, and $r = 0.265$, $p < 0.001$ for HU difference %) and MTV of primary tumor ($r = 0.135$, $p = 0.023$ for TAT HU, $r = 0.248$, $p < 0.001$ for HU difference, and $r = 0.241$, $p < 0.001$ for HU difference %).

In comparison, the breast adipose tissue parameters of patients with recurrence showed significantly higher values of TAT HU, HU difference, and HU difference % than those with no recurrence ($p < 0.001$; Figure 2). In contrast, there is no significant difference in CAT HU between those two groups ($p = 0.882$; Figure 2)

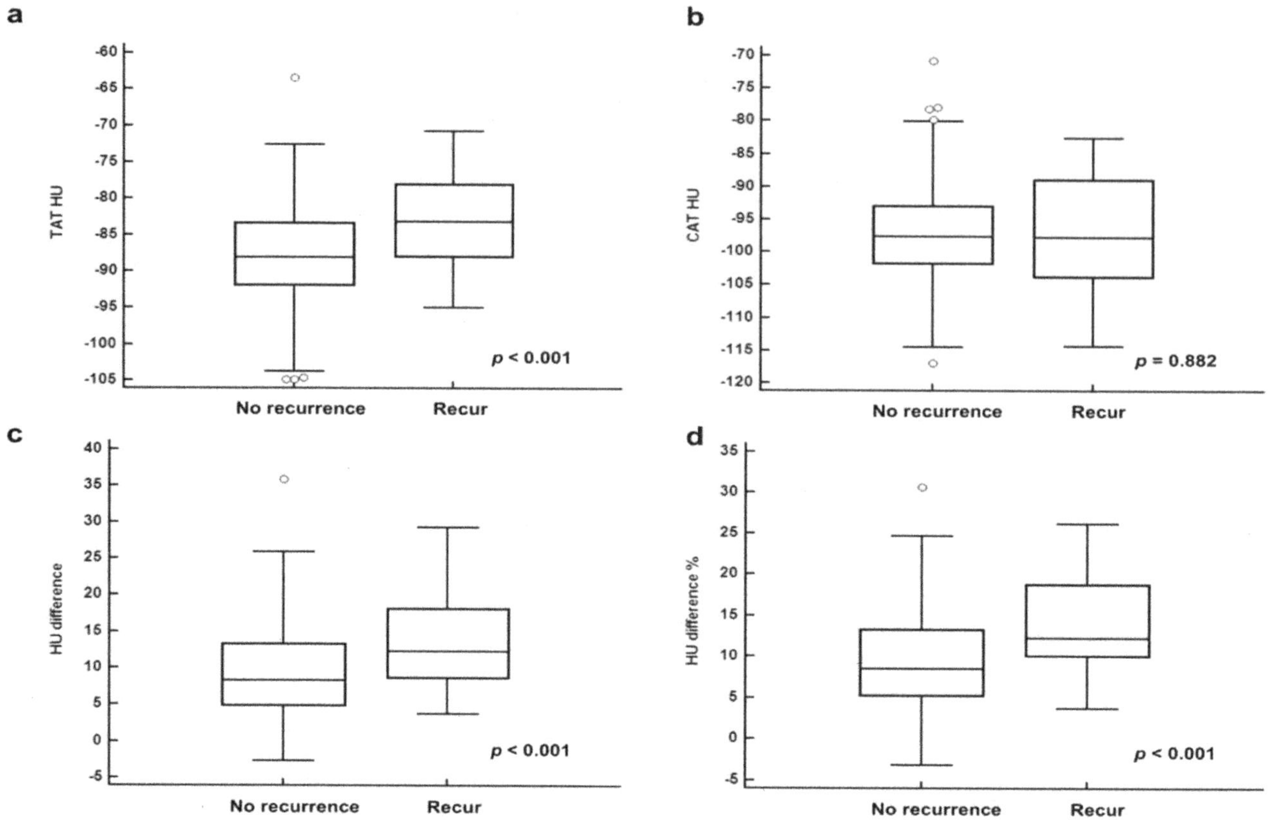

Figure 2. CT-attenuation of tumor-adjacent breast adipose tissue (TAT HU) (**a**), CT-attenuation of contralateral breast adipose tissue (CAT HU) (**b**), difference of CT-attenuation (HU difference) (**c**), and percent difference of CT-attenuation (HU difference %) (**d**) between patients with no recurrence and recurrence.

2.3. Survival Analysis

The prognostic values of breast adipose tissue parameters for predicting RFS were evaluated using univariate Cox regression analysis along with clinico-histological factors and PET/CT parameters of the primary breast cancer. In univariate analysis, TAT HU, HU difference, and HU difference % were significantly associated with RFS ($p < 0.001$ for all; Table 3), while CAT HU showed no statistical significance ($p = 0.786$). Among clinico-histological factors and PET/CT parameters, T stage, N stage, histologic grade, ER status, PR status, Ki67 index, triple negative tumor, and maximum SUV and MTV of primary tumor showed significance in predicting RFS ($p < 0.05$; Table 3).

TAT HU, HU difference, and HU difference % were included in the multivariate analysis for RFS with the addition of eight different covariates in three different models (Table 4). TAT HU and HU difference % remained as significant positive predictors for RFS in all three models after adjustment for age, T stage, N stage, ER status, PR status, Ki67 index, maximum SUV, and MTV ($p < 0.05$). On the other hand, HU difference showed significant association with RFS in models with adjustment for age, T stage, N stage, ER status, PR status, and Ki67 index ($p < 0.05$) but failed to show statistical significance after correcting for maximum SUV and MTV ($p = 0.054$).

Table 3. Univariate analysis for recurrence-free survival.

Variables		*p*-Value	Hazard Ratio (95% CI)
Age (1-year increase)		0.562	1.01 (0.98–1.04)
BMI (1 kg/m^2 increase)		0.283	0.93 (0.82–1.06)
Menopausal status (pre vs. post)		0.799	0.91 (0.44–1.89)
T stage	T1 stage	-	1.00
	T2 stage	0.001	11.24 (2.62–48.25)
	T3 stage	<0.001	37.90 (8.17–175.80)
N stage (N0 vs. N1-3)		0.004	2.92 (1.42–6.09)
Histologic grade	Grade 1	-	1.00
	Grade 2	0.873	1.10 (0.34–3.58)
	Grade 3	0.008	4.42 (1.48–13.16)
ER status (positive vs. negative)		<0.001	3.41 (1.66–7.00)
PR status (positive vs. negative)		<0.001	5.22 (2.32–11.74)
HER2 status (positive vs. negative)		0.254	0.65 (0.31–1.36)
Ki67 index (negative vs. positive)		0.005	7.79 (1.85–32.83)
Triple negative tumor (no vs. yes)		0.011	3.00 (1.28–7.03)
Maximum SUV (1.0 increase)		<0.001	1.08 (1.03–1.13)
MTV (1.0 cm^3 increase)		<0.001	1.03 (1.02–1.04)
TAT HU (1.0 HU increase)		<0.001	1.10 (1.05–1.16)
CAT HU (1.0 HU increase)		0.786	0.99 (0.94–1.05)
HU difference (1.0 HU increase)		<0.001	1.10 (1.05–1.16)
HU difference % (1.0% increase)		<0.001	1.12 (1.06–1.18)

BMI, body mass index; ER, estrogen receptor; PR, progesterone receptor; HER2, human epidermal growth factor receptor 2; SUV, standardized uptake value; MTV, metabolic tumor volume; TAT HU, CT-attenuation of tumor-adjacent breast adipose tissue; CAT HU, CT-attenuation of contralateral breast adipose tissue; HU difference, difference of CT-attenuation; HU difference %, percent difference of CT-attenuation; HU, Hounsfield units; CI, confidence interval.

Table 4. Multivariate models for recurrence-free survival.

Models		TAT HU (1.0 HU Increase)	HU Difference (1.0 HU Increase)	HU Difference % (1.0% Increase)
Model 1 *	*p*-value	0.012	0.001	0.001
	Hazard ratio (95% CI)	1.08 (1.02–1.15)	1.07 (1.02–1.19)	1.09 (1.02–1.15)
Model 2 †	*p*-value	0.018	0.044	0.033
	Hazard ratio (95% CI)	1.08 (1.01–1.16)	1.06 (1.00–1.12)	1.07 (1.01–1.14)
Model 3 ‡	*p*-value	0.014	0.054	0.038
	Hazard ratio (95% CI)	1.09 (1.02–1.16)	1.05 (1.00–1.11)	1.07 (1.00–1.13)

* Adjusted for age, T stage and N stage; † Adjusted for age, T stage, N stage, estrogen receptor status, progesterone receptor status, and Ki67 index; ‡ Adjusted for age, T stage, N stage, estrogen receptor status, progesterone receptor status, Ki67 index, maximum standardized uptake value, and metabolic tumor volume; CI, confidence interval; TAT HU, CT-attenuation of tumor-adjacent breast adipose tissue; HU difference, difference of CT-attenuation; HU difference %, percent difference of CT-attenuation; HU, Hounsfield units.

For Kaplan—Meier analysis, TAT HU, HU difference, and HU difference % were categorized into two groups according to the optimal cut-off values (−82.50 for TAT HU, 8.50 for HU difference, and 10.00 for HU difference %) determined by receiver operating characteristic (ROC) curve analysis. Kaplan—Meier analysis of enrolled patients stratified by TAT HU, HU difference, and HU difference % showed significantly worse RFS in patients with high values than in those with low values ($p < 0.001$ for all; Figure 3). Patients with high values of TAT HU (75.7% vs. 93.1%), HU difference (82.7% vs. 96.3%), and HU difference % (80.0% vs. 96.8%) showed lower 5-year RFS rates than those with low values.

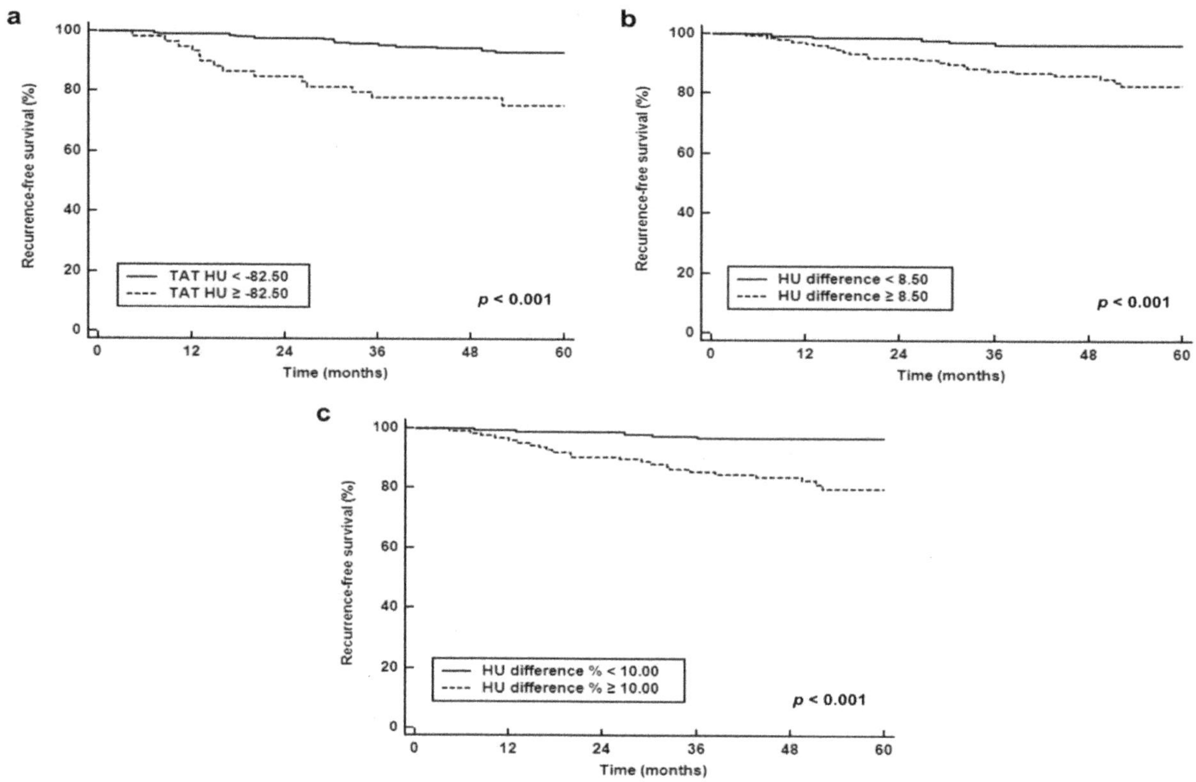

Figure 3. Survival curves. Recurrence-free survival stratified by CT-attenuation of tumor-adjacent breast adipose tissue (TAT HU) (**a**), difference of CT-attenuation (HU difference) (**b**), and percent difference of CT-attenuation (HU difference %) (**c**).

While comparing recurrence rates based on the combination of T stage and TAT HU (Table 5), patients with high TAT HU showed a higher recurrence rate than those with low TAT HU, irrespective of T stage (5.3% vs. 0.9% for T1 stage; 34.1% vs. 12.7% for T2–T3 stage).

Table 5. Recurrence rates according to the combination of T stage and TAT HU.

TAT HU		T Stage	
		T1 Stage	**T2–T3 Stage**
TAT HU	<−82.50 HU	1/117 (0.9%)	14/110 (12.7%)
	≥−82.50 HU	1/19 (5.3%)	14/41 (34.1%)
	p-value	0.260	0.003

TAT HU, CT-attenuation of tumor-adjacent breast adipose tissue; HU, Hounsfield units.

3. Discussion

In the present study, CT-attenuation of tumor-adjacent breast adipose tissue and difference of CT-attenuation between tumor-adjacent and contralateral breast adipose tissues showed significant association with T stage, tumor characteristics, and RFS in patients with breast cancer. In previous studies with histopathological analysis of resected breast cancer tissue, profound modifications of phenotype and biological features were found in the adipocytes that were present at the invasive front of the breast cancer cells [8,9]. The adipocytes in the vicinity of the breast cancer cells showed decreased cell size and less lipid content when compared to the adipocytes that are located far away from the breast cancer cells [8,9]. These alterations of adipocytes were reproduced in adipocytes which were co-cultivated with cancer cells, showing less differentiated features of adipocytes with decreased expression of adipocyte markers such as adiponectin and resistin and increased expression of matrix metalloproteinase 11, osteopontin, and pro-inflammatory cytokines including tumor necrosis factor-alpha and interleukin-6 [1,8,9,21]. These modified adipocytes are now called cancer-associated adipocytes [1,8,22]. The cancer-associated adipocytes are known to have an active bidirectional crosstalk with cancer cells, inducing fibrotic change in adipose tissue, stimulating tumor progression and metastasis by secreting multiple cytokines and adipokines, and releasing lipid content within the cell to provide source of energy to cancer cells [1,3,21–23]. Previous studies with breast cancer have also demonstrated that expressions of cancer-associated adipocytes-related protein are different according to the subtypes of breast cancer and the interactions between tumor cells and adipocytes can contribute to growth, proliferation, and epithelial-mesenchymal transition of breast cancer cells [23–26].

In a previous study that evaluated the correlation between CT-attenuation of adipose tissue and histopathological results of adipose tissue collected at necropsy in non-human primates, increased CT-attenuation of adipose tissue was significantly associated with smaller adipocytes and increased extracellular matrix fibrosis, which corresponded to the findings in the peritumoral adipose tissue affected by cancer cells [8,10,14]. Therefore, CT-attenuation of adipose tissue has been used as an imaging parameter for the qualitative alterations of adipose tissue in patients with malignant diseases [13,14]. In our study, we measured CT-attenuation in both tumor-adjacent and contralateral breast adipose tissue and tried to find out whether CT-attenuation of tumor-adjacent breast adipose tissue had different features compared to that of the contralateral side. The results of our study demonstrated that increased CT-attenuation was observed in tumor-adjacent breast adipose tissue compared to the contralateral side. Moreover, TAT HU, HU difference, and HU difference % had a significant correlation with the T stage, hormone receptor status, and FDG PET/CT parameters of the primary tumor, while CAT HU showed no significant association with them. These results suggested that qualitative changes had occurred in the peritumoral adipose tissue, which has a positive relationship with tumor aggressiveness.

Given that cancer-associated adipocytes conversely affect the growth and metastasis of cancer cells, it could be hypothesized that CT-attenuation of adipose tissue in patients with malignant diseases has significant prognostic significance for predicting clinical outcomes [5,7,13–15]. In previous studies, CT-attenuations of subcutaneous and visceral adipose tissue measured in the abdomen at the level of the lumbar spine were found to be significant predictors for disease progression-free survival and overall survival [12–15,27]. Previous studies consistently showed that increased CT-attenuation of adipose tissue was significantly associated with worse survival not only in malignant diseases that have close localization with adipose tissue such as pancreatic and prostate cancers, but also in malignant diseases that are remote from abdominal adipose tissue such as head and neck cancer and extremity sarcoma [12–14,27]. In a broad way, breast adipose tissue might be considered as a part of subcutaneous adipose tissue, but it permanently interacts with surrounding mammary epithelial cells consequently having distinctive characteristics from subcutaneous adipose tissue in other body compartments [7]. Considering that even the subcutaneous adipose tissue in remote location had association with cancer progression [13], it is no surprise that tumor-adjacent breast adipose tissue had significant association with cancer recurrence. The results of our study demonstrated that TAT HU and HU difference % were independently associated with RFS event after adjusting for age, tumor stage, ER and PR status, ki67 index, maximum SUV, and MTV, suggesting that perceiving the qualitative characteristics of peritumoral breast adipose tissue, as well as primary tumor features, might be of importance for predicting breast cancer recurrence after surgical resection. Furthermore, the combination of T stage and TAT HU can further improve the stratification of recurrence risk, suggesting that imaging features of tumor-adjacent breast adipose tissue might provide additional prognostic value to tumor stage. Recently, adipocytes have been considered as a new attractive treatment target for breast cancer [7,28,29]. The results of the present study might provide a clue for selecting candidates for future therapy that targets adipocytes in breast cancer patients.

Since the changes in the normal tissue surrounding breast cancer have drawn the attention of researchers, several recent studies have evaluated the clinical implication of imaging findings of tumor-adjacent breast parenchyma on magnetic resonance imaging (MRI) [30,31]. However, in the literature, only a single study has investigated the clinical significance of tumor-adjacent breast adipose tissue on imaging studies [16]. A previous study by Obeid et al. [16] retrospectively enrolled 63 patients with early breast cancer and investigated the association between imaging features of peritumoral breast adipose tissue on MRI images and axillary lymph nodal status. Similar to our study, they defined the peritumoral region as the area which is within a 1-cm spherical extension from the tumor contour. They generated peritumoral adipose volume using voxel intensity filtering and measured five imaging features of peritumoral tissue: mean voxel intensity, standard deviation of voxel intensity, total volume, fat-specific volume, and the fat ratio. Their study demonstrated that significant association was only shown between the fat ratio of peritumoral tissue and the ratio of positive-to-total axillary lymph nodes. On the other hand, the peritumoral fat ratio showed no significant correlation with other histopathologic features such as tumor grade, lymphovascular invasion, extracapsular extension, and tumor size, and the axillary lymph node status also showed no significant correlation with other imaging features of peritumoral tissue including mean voxel intensity. Because different imaging modalities were used in both studies, a direct comparison between our study and the previous studies would be limited. Although both CT and MRI are accurate and effective imaging modalities for adipose tissue measurement, each has different advantages and disadvantages [32,33]. CT is the most well-established method for adipose tissue measurement, and HU is consistent between images on difference scans, while CT scanning has the risk of exposure to high doses of ionizing radiation [32,33]. In contrast, adipose tissue measurements on MRI are expressed in arbitrary units that are difficult to compare between studies and are less reproducible than CT images [32,33]. Therefore, further studies using both CT and MRI in the same patients would be needed to compare the adipose tissue parameters of both modalities. Furthermore, CT-attenuation of only the breast adipose tissue was measured in our study, whereas voxel intensity of whole peritumoral breast tissue, including breast parenchyma and adipose tissue, was measured in the aforementioned study, which could cause differences in the results between the studies [16]. Nonetheless, our study also revealed no significant relationship between N stage and TAT HU, suggesting that the qualitative characteristics of tumor-adjacent breast tissue might have limited value for predicting axillary lymph node metastasis.

Recently, a dual-energy CT system has been introduced to improve tissue differentiation [34]. Using dual-energy CT, virtual non-contrast CT images can be synthesized, which could replace a precontrast CT scan, thereby reducing radiation exposure [34]. In previous studies, CT-attenuation values of various organs in virtual non-contrast CT images have shown close agreement with those in true unenhanced CT images [35,36]. Therefore, future studies are needed to clarify whether CT-attenuation of breast adipose tissue measured on virtual non-contrast CT images of dual-energy CT also has prognostic significance in breast cancer patients, which may form an imaging protocol for evaluating both tumor factors and tumor-adjacent breast tissue factors using a single CT scan.

There are several limitations to our study. Because the study was retrospectively performed in a single center and only the patients who had sufficient breast adipose tissue for the image analysis were included, selection bias is inevitable, which may limit the general application of the results of the present study. Furthermore, having a small number of patients who experienced recurrence could affect the results of survival analysis. Because of the retrospective nature of the study, we cannot compare the histopathological features of tumor-adjacent adipose tissue according to the CT-attenuation. Further studies with histopathological evaluation are needed to elucidate the mechanisms of our results. Lastly, as the present study is the first study to measure the tumor-adjacent breast adipose tissue, there is no established method of calculating CT-attenuation of breast adipose tissue [12,13]. A more sophisticated method, which could properly measure CT-attenuation of tumor-adjacent breast adipose tissue even in patients with a small amount of adipose tissue, would be helpful to confirm the association between breast adipose tissue parameters and clinical outcomes.

4. Materials and Methods

4.1. Study Population

This study was approved by the Institutional Review Board of Soonchunhyang University (Ethic code: SCHCA 2019-05-023, Date: 20 March 2019), and the requirement to obtain informed consent was waived by the board due to its retrospective nature. All procedures in this study were in accordance with the Declaration of Helsinki. Electronic medical records of 393 female patients who had biopsy proven invasive breast cancer and underwent pretreatment FDG PET/CT between February 2012 and December 2016 in our medical center were retrospectively reviewed. Among them, patients (1) who were diagnosed with distant metastasis on staging examinations, (2) who were diagnosed with ductal carcinoma in situ, (3) who had any kind of treatment before FDG PET/CT, (4) who had bilateral breast cancers, (5) who had a previous history of breast surgery, (6) who had a previous history of another malignancy, and (7) who were lost to follow-up within two years after the initial treatment without event were excluded from the study, and 355 patients met the initial eligibility criteria of the study. Of the 355 patients, 68 were excluded from the study during PET/CT image analysis due to insufficient breast adipose tissue for analysis ($n = 55$) and diffuse infiltration of breast cancer lesion ($n = 13$). Therefore, the remaining 287 female patients finally comprised the subjects of the study.

All enrolled patients underwent pretreatment staging examinations which consisted of blood tests, breast ultrasonography, breast MRI, bone scintigraphy, and FDG PET/CT. The BMI for each patient was calculated using the height and weight measured at the time of staging work-up. With the results of staging examinations, clinical TNM stage according to the 7th Edition of the American Joint Committee on Cancer staging system was determined for each patient. ER, PR, HER2, and Ki67 expression status were obtained from histopathological records. ER and PR positive tumors were defined as tumors with 10% or more positively stained cells using immunohistochemistry. A HER2 positive tumor was defined as a tumor with a 3+ score on immunohistochemistry or a tumor with gene amplification on fluorescence in situ hybridization. A tumor with 14% or more Ki67 expression using immunohistochemistry was defined as a Ki67 positive tumor. After staging examinations, all enrolled patients underwent curative surgical resection of breast cancer with or without neoadjuvant chemotherapy and/or adjuvant treatment. All patients were regularly followed up at intervals of 3–6 months with blood test and imaging studies. The duration of follow-up was calculated from the date of the initial treatment to the last date of clinical follow-up at our medical center or to the occurrence of cancer recurrence.

4.2. Image Analysis

All patients underwent FDG PET/CT scanning from the skull base to the proximal thigh in a supine position using a Biograph mCT 128 scanner (Siemens Healthcare, Knoxville, TN, USA) after at least six hours fasting. One hour after intravenous injection of approximately 4.07 MBq/kg of FDG, a non-contrast-enhanced attenuation correction CT scan was performed at 100 mA and 120 kV_p with a slice thickness of 5 mm followed by a PET scan at 1.5 min per bed position. PET images were reconstructed using point-spread-function modeling and time-of-flight reconstruction (2 iterations and 21 subsets) with attenuation correction.

Two expert readers independently reviewed FDG PET/CT images of all patients without knowing clinico-pathological and follow-up results. A United States Food and Drug Administration-approved medical image viewer (OsiriX MD 10.0.3, Pixmeo, Geneva, Switzerland) was used for image analyses. For breast adipose tissue measurement, non-contrast-enhanced CT images of FDG PET/CT were used. A total of four parameters (TAT HU, CAT HU, HU difference, and HU difference %) were measured from breast adipose tissue. We used a 1-cm distance from the tumor margin for defining tumor-adjacent breast adipose tissue. A spheroid-shaped volume-of-interest (VOI) that includes the entire breast cancer lesion and surrounding breast tissue within a 1-cm distance to the tumor margin was manually drawn (Figure 4). Afterwards, another spheroid-shaped VOI of the same size was drawn over the contralateral breast tissue in the same quadrant of the breast tissue (Figure 4). A CT-attenuation range of −200 and −50 HU was used to define breast adipose tissue within VOIs. The mean CT-attenuation value of the area within the CT-attenuation range of breast adipose tissue was measured for each VOI and defined as TAT HU and CAT HU. Using TAT HU and CAT HU, HU difference and HU difference % were calculated as follows: (HU difference) = (TAT HU) − (CAT HU) while (HU difference %) = ((CAT HU) − (TAT HU))/(CAT HU) × 100. Using FDG PET images, we measured two metabolic parameters of primary breast cancer lesion, maximum SUV and MTV. A spheroid-shaped VOI was drawn over the primary cancer lesion on fused PET/CT images including the whole tumor lesion. The maximum SUV of the primary breast cancer lesion was measured. A total volume of voxels that had SUV of 2.50 or greater within VOI was measured and defined as MTV of primary cancer lesion.

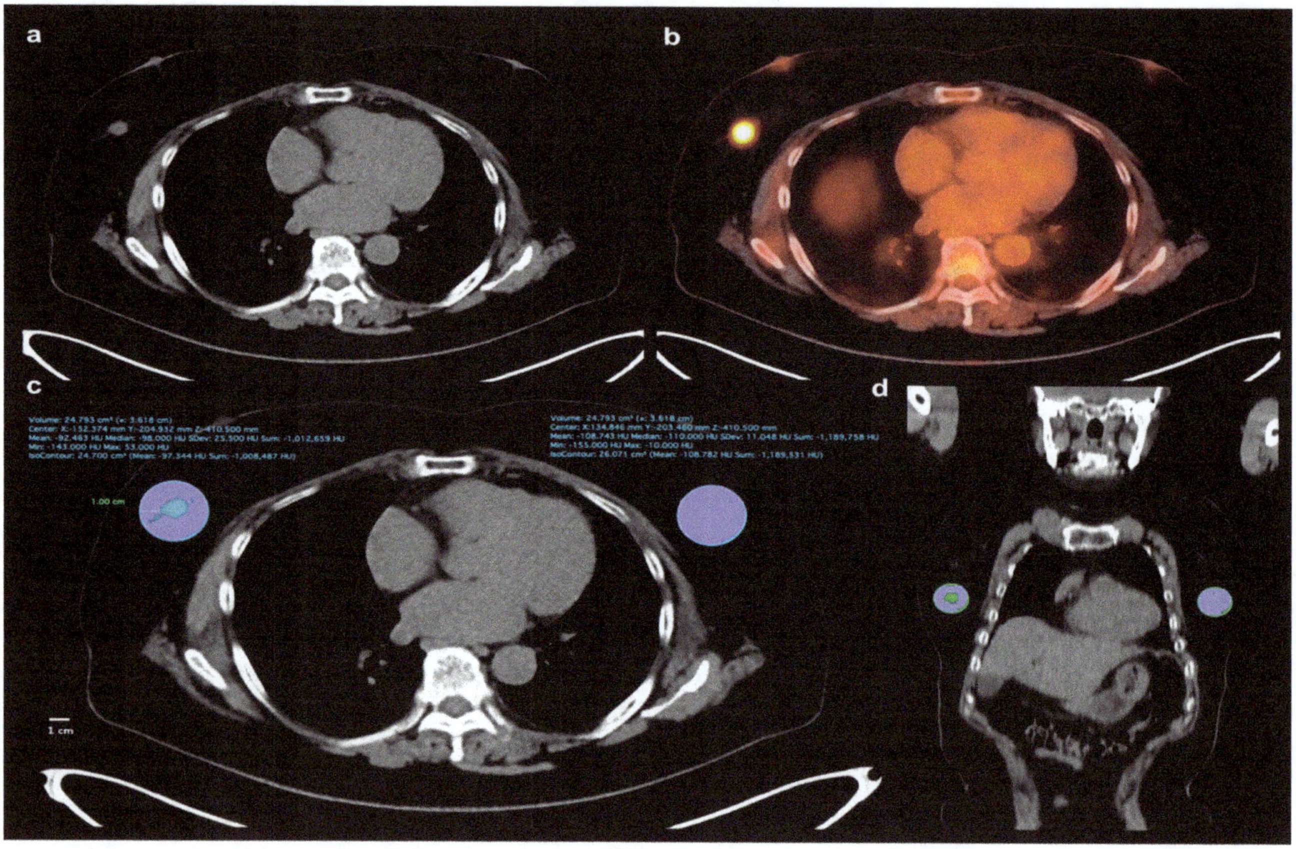

Figure 4. Measurement example of CT-attenuation of tumor-adjacent breast adipose tissue and contralateral breast adipose tissue. A 62-year-old woman underwent FDG PET/CT for staging work-up of right breast cancer, histopathologically confirmed as invasive ductal carcinoma. A mass lesion with intensely increased FDG uptake is observed in outer aspect of right breast, (**a**,**b**), showing maximum SUV of 8.44. A spheroid-shaped volume-of-interest that includes peritumoral breast tissue within a 1-cm distance from the tumor margin was manually drawn over the ipsilateral breast tissue, (**c**,**d**). Another spheroid-shaped volume-of-interest of the same size was drawn over the contralateral breast tissue in the same quadrant of the breast, (c,d). Within the volume-of-interests drawn in bilateral breast tissues, the area of breast adipose tissue defined as an area with CT-attenuation range between −200 and −50 HU was automatically delineated. Mean CT-attenuation value of breast adipose tissue was measured for each VOI (c): −92.463 HU for tumor-adjacent breast adipose tissue and −108.743 for contralateral breast adipose tissue.

4.3. Statistical Analysis

To assess the reproducibility of measurement of TAT HU and CAT HU between the two readers, concordance correlation coefficients for TAT HU and CAT HU were calculated. Paired t test was performed to assess the difference between TAT HU and CAT HU. A Student's *t* test and Kruskal—Wallis test were performed to compare the differences in four breast adipose tissue parameters between groups. After performing the normality test, Spearman rank correlation coefficients were calculated for the breast adipose tissue parameters with regard to BMI and maximum SUV and MTV of the primary breast cancer lesion. The primary endpoint of the present study was RFS. Univariate and multivariate survival analyses using the Cox proportional hazards regression model were performed to assess the association between variables and RFS. Of the four breast adipose tissue parameters, those with a *p*-value of less than 0.10 in univariate analysis were included in multivariate analysis. In the multivariate analysis of breast adipose tissue parameters, three different models with eight different covariates (age, T stage, N stage, ER status, PR status, Ki67 index, maximum SUV, and MTV) were constructed. The significances of the association between breast adipose tissue parameters and RFS were evaluated after adjusting for these eight covariates. For breast adipose tissue parameters that showed statistical significance in univariate survival analysis, the optimal cut-off values were determined using ROC curve analysis, and survival curves for RFS according to the cut-off values were estimated using the Kaplan—Meier method. All statistical analyses were performed using MedCalc Statistical Software version 19.0.3 (MedCalc Software bvba, Ostend, Belgium). A *p*-value of <0.05 was considered statistically significant.

5. Conclusions

TAT HU and HU difference % were independent predictors for RFS in patients with breast cancer, suggesting that qualitative alterations of tumor-adjacent breast adipose tissue may have significant association with tumor recurrence. TAT HU and HU difference % had a significant relationship with T stage and hormone receptor status of breast cancer, and patients with increased CT-attenuation of peritumoral adipose tissue had worse survival. Although further studies are warranted to confirm the results, the results of our study seem to support the close interaction between breast cancer cells and tumor-adjacent adipocytes observed with imaging studies.

Author Contributions: Conceptualization, J.W.L., S.M.L.; methodology, J.W.L., S.Y.K., S.M.L.; formal analysis, J.W.L., S.Y.K., H.J.L., S.M.L.; data curation, H.J.L, S.W.H., J.E.L., S.M.L.; writing—original draft preparation, J.W.L.; writing—review & editing, S.Y.K., H.J.L., S.W.H., J.E.L., S.M.L.; visualization, J.W.L.; supervision, S.W.H, S.M.L.; funding acquisition, J.W.L., S.M.L.

References

1. Duong, M.N.; Geneste, A.; Fallone, F.; Li, X.; Dumontet, C.; Muller, C. The fat and the bad: Mature adipocytes, key actors in tumor progression and resistance. *Oncotarget* **2017**, *8*, 57622–57641. [CrossRef] [PubMed]
2. Vandeweyer, E.; Hertens, D. Quantification of glands and fat in breast tissue: An experimental determination. *Ann. Anat.* **2002**, *184*, 181–184. [CrossRef]
3. Guaita-Esteruelas, S.; Guma, J.; Masana, L.; Borras, J. The peritumoural adipose tissue microenvironment and cancer. The roles of fatty acid binding protein 4 and fatty acid binding protein 5. *Mol. Cell. Endocrinol.* **2018**, *462*, 107–118. [CrossRef] [PubMed]
4. Lehr, S.; Hartwig, S.; Sell, H. Adipokines: A treasure trove for the discovery of biomarkers for metabolic disorders. *Proteom. Clin. Appl.* **2012**, *6*, 91–101. [CrossRef] [PubMed]
5. Divella, R.; De Luca, R.; Abbate, I.; Naglieri, E.; Daniele, A. Obesity and cancer: The role of adipose tissue and adipo-cytokines-induced chronic inflammation. *J. Cancer* **2016**, *7*, 2346–2359. [CrossRef]
6. Engin, A.B.; Engin, A.; Gonul, I.I. The effect of adipocyte-macrophage cross-talk in obesity-related breast cancer. *J. Mol. Endocrinol.* **2019**. [CrossRef] [PubMed]
7. Choi, J.; Cha, Y.J.; Koo, J.S. Adipocyte biology in breast cancer: From silent bystander to active facilitator. *Prog. Lipid. Res.* **2018**, *69*, 11–20. [CrossRef] [PubMed]
8. Dirat, B.; Bochet, L.; Dabek, M.; Daviaud, D.; Dauvillier, S.; Majed, B.; Wang, Y.Y.; Meulle, A.; Salles, B.; Le Gonidec, S.; et al. Cancer-associated adipocytes exhibit an activated phenotype and contribute to breast cancer invasion. *Cancer Res.* **2011**, *71*, 2455–2465. [CrossRef] [PubMed]

9. Fletcher, S.J.; Sacca, P.A.; Pistone-Creydt, M.; Colo, F.A.; Serra, M.F.; Santino, F.E.; Sasso, C.V.; Lopez-Fontana, C.M.; Caron, R.W.; Calvo, J.C.; et al. Human breast adipose tissue: Characterization of factors that change during tumor progression in human breast cancer. *J. Exp. Clin. Cancer Res.* **2017**, *36*, 26. [CrossRef] [PubMed]
10. Murphy, R.A.; Register, T.C.; Shively, C.A.; Carr, J.J.; Ge, Y.; Heilbrun, M.E.; Cummings, S.R.; Koster, A.; Nevitt, M.C.; Satterfield, S.; et al. Adipose tissue density, a novel biomarker predicting mortality risk in older adults. *J. Gerontol. A Biol. Sci. Med. Sci.* **2014**, *69*, 109–117. [CrossRef] [PubMed]
11. Lee, J.W.; Lee, H.S.; Na, J.O.; Lee, S.M. Effect of adipose tissue volume on prognosis in patients with non-small cell lung cancer. *Clin. Imaging* **2018**, *50*, 308–313. [CrossRef] [PubMed]
12. Lee, J.W.; Lee, S.M.; Chung, Y.A. Prognostic value of CT attenuation and FDG uptake of adipose tissue in patients with pancreatic adenocarcinoma. *Clin. Radiol.* **2018**, *73*, 1056.e1–1056.e10. [CrossRef] [PubMed]
13. Lee, J.W.; Ban, M.J.; Park, J.H.; Lee, S.M. Visceral adipose tissue volume and CT-attenuation as prognostic factors in patients with head and neck cancer. *Head Neck* **2019**, *41*, 1605–1614. [CrossRef] [PubMed]
14. Veld, J.; Vossen, J.A.; De Amorim Bernstein, K.; Halpern, E.F.; Torriani, M.; Bredella, M.A. Adipose tissue and muscle attenuation as novel biomarkers predicting mortality in patients with extremity sarcomas. *Eur. Radiol.* **2016**, *26*, 4649–4655. [CrossRef]
15. Yoo, I.D.; Lee, S.M.; Lee, J.W.; Baek, M.J.; Ahn, T.S. Usefulness of metabolic activity of adipose tissue in FDG PET/CT of colorectal cancer. *Abdom. Radiol. (NY)* **2018**, *43*, 2052–2059. [CrossRef]
16. Obeid, J.P.; Stoyanova, R.; Kwon, D.; Patel, M.; Padgett, K.; Slingerland, J.; Takita, C.; Alperin, N.; Yepes, M.; Zeidan, Y.H. Multiparametric evaluation of preoperative MRI in early stage breast cancer: Prognostic impact of peri-tumoral fat. *Clin. Transl. Oncol.* **2017**, *19*, 211–218. [CrossRef]
17. Caresia Aroztegui, A.P.; Garcia Vicente, A.M.; Alvarez Ruiz, S.; Delgado Bolton, R.C.; Orcajo Rincon, J.; Garcia Garzon, J.R.; de Arcocha Torres, M.; Garcia-Velloso, M.J. 18F-FDG PET/CT in breast cancer: Evidence-based recommendations in initial staging. *Tumour Biol.* **2017**, *39*. [CrossRef]
18. Lee, S.S.; Bae, S.K.; Park, Y.S.; Park, J.S.; Kim, T.H.; Yoon, H.K.; Ahn, H.J.; Lee, S.M. Correlation of molecular subtypes of invasive ductal carcinoma of breast with glucose metabolism in FDG PET/CT: Based on the Recommendations of the St. Gallen Consensus Meeting 2013. *Nucl. Med. Mol. Imaging* **2017**, *51*, 79–85. [CrossRef]
19. Kitajima, K.; Yamano, T.; Miyoshi, Y.; Enoki, T.; Yamakado, K. Prognostic value of FDG-PET/CT prior to breast cancer treatment—Comparison with MRS and DWI. *J. Nucl. Med.* **2019**, *60* (Suppl. 1), 603.
20. Onner, H.; Canaz, F.; Dincer, M.; Isiksoy, S.; Sivrikoz, I.A.; Entok, E.; Erkasap, S. Which of the fluorine-18 fluorodeoxyglucose positron emission tomography/computerized tomography parameters are better associated with prognostic factors in breast cancer? *Medicine (Baltimore)* **2019**, *98*, e15925. [CrossRef]
21. Ribeiro, R.J.; Monteiro, C.P.; Cunha, V.F.; Azevedo, A.S.; Oliveira, M.J.; Monteiro, R.; Fraga, A.M.; Principe, P.; Lobato, C.; Lobo, F.; et al. Tumor cell-educated periprostatic adipose tissue acquires an aggressive cancer-promoting secretory profile. *Cell. Physiol. Biochem.* **2012**, *29*, 233–240. [CrossRef] [PubMed]
22. Dirat, B.; Bochet, L.; Escourrou, G.; Valet, P.; Muller, C. Unraveling the obesity and breast cancer links: A role for cancer-associated adipocytes? *Endocr. Dev.* **2010**, *19*, 45–52. [CrossRef] [PubMed]
23. Bochet, L.; Lehuede, C.; Dauvillier, S.; Wang, Y.Y.; Dirat, B.; Laurent, V.; Dray, C.; Guiet, R.; Maridonneau-Parini, I.; Le Gonidec, S.; et al. Adipocyte-derived fibroblasts promote tumor progression and contribute to the desmoplastic reaction in breast cancer. *Cancer Res.* **2013**, *73*, 5657–5668. [CrossRef] [PubMed]
24. Jung, Y.Y.; Lee, Y.K.; Koo, J.S. Expression of cancer-associated fibroblast-related proteins in adipose stroma of breast cancer. *Tumour Biol.* **2015**, *36*, 8685–8695. [CrossRef] [PubMed]
25. Ando, S.; Barone, I.; Giordano, C.; Bonofiglio, D.; Catalano, S. The Multifaceted mechanism of leptin signaling within tumor microenvironment in driving breast cancer growth and progression. *Front. Oncol.* **2014**, *4*, 340. [CrossRef] [PubMed]
26. Huang, C.K.; Chang, P.H.; Kuo, W.H.; Chen, C.L.; Jeng, Y.M.; Chang, K.J.; Shew, J.Y.; Hu, C.M.; Lee, W.H. Adipocytes promote malignant growth of breast tumours with monocarboxylate transporter 2 expression via beta-hydroxybutyrate. *Nat. Commun.* **2017**, *8*, 14706. [CrossRef] [PubMed]
27. McDonald, A.M.; Fiveash, J.B.; Kirkland, R.S.; Cardan, R.A.; Jacob, R.; Kim, R.Y.; Dobelbower, M.C.; Yang, E.S. Subcutaneous adipose tissue characteristics and the risk of biochemical recurrence in men with high-risk prostate cancer. *Urol. Oncol.* **2017**, *35*, 663.e615–663.e621. [CrossRef]

28. Li, Q.; Xia, J.; Yao, Y.; Gong, D.W.; Shi, H.; Zhou, Q. Sulforaphane inhibits mammary adipogenesis by targeting adipose mesenchymal stem cells. *Breast Cancer Res. Treat.* **2013**, *141*, 317–324. [CrossRef]
29. Bochet, L.; Meulle, A.; Imbert, S.; Salles, B.; Valet, P.; Muller, C. Cancer-associated adipocytes promotes breast tumor radioresistance. *Biochem. Biophys. Res. Commun.* **2011**, *411*, 102–106. [CrossRef]
30. Nabavizadeh, N.; Klifa, C.; Newitt, D.; Lu, Y.; Chen, Y.Y.; Hsu, H.; Fisher, C.; Tokayasu, T.; Olshen, A.B.; Spellman, P.; et al. Topographic enhancement mapping of the cancer-associated breast stroma using breast MRI. *Integr. Biol. (Camb.)* **2011**, *3*, 490–496. [CrossRef]
31. Wu, J.; Li, B.; Sun, X.; Cao, G.; Rubin, D.L.; Napel, S.; Ikeda, D.M.; Kurian, A.W.; Li, R. Heterogeneous enhancement patterns of tumor-adjacent parenchyma at MR imaging are associated with dysregulated signaling pathways and poor survival in breast cancer. *Radiology* **2017**, *285*, 401–413. [CrossRef] [PubMed]
32. Kullberg, J.; Brandberg, J.; Angelhed, J.E.; Frimmel, H.; Bergelin, E.; Strid, L.; Ahlstrom, H.; Johansson, L.; Lonn, L. Whole-body adipose tissue analysis: Comparison of MRI, CT and dual energy X-ray absorptiometry. *Br. J. Radiol.* **2009**, *82*, 123–130. [CrossRef] [PubMed]
33. Pescatori, L.C.; Savarino, E.; Mauri, G.; Silvestri, E.; Cariati, M.; Sardanelli, F.; Sconfienza, L.M. Quantification of visceral adipose tissue by computed tomography and magnetic resonance imaging: Reproducibility and accuracy. *Radiol. Bras.* **2019**, *52*, 1–6. [CrossRef] [PubMed]
34. Goo, H.W.; Goo, J.M. Dual-energy CT: New horizon in medical imaging. *Korean J. Radiol.* **2017**, *18*, 555–569. [CrossRef] [PubMed]
35. Toepker, M.; Moritz, T.; Krauss, B.; Weber, M.; Euller, G.; Mang, T.; Wolf, F.; Herold, C.J.; Ringl, H. Virtual non-contrast in second-generation, dual-energy computed tomography: Reliability of attenuation values. *Eur. J. Radiol.* **2012**, *81*, e398–e405. [CrossRef]
36. Jamali, S.; Michoux, N.; Coche, E.; Dragean, C.A. Virtual unenhanced phase with spectral dual-energy CT: Is it an alternative to conventional true unenhanced phase for abdominal tissues? *Diagn. Interv. Imaging* **2019**. [CrossRef]

15

Circulating miRNAs in Untreated Breast Cancer: An Exploratory Multimodality Morpho-Functional Study

Mariarosaria Incoronato [1,*], Anna Maria Grimaldi [1], Peppino Mirabelli [1], Carlo Cavaliere [1], Chiara Anna Parente [1], Monica Franzese [1], Stefania Staibano [2], Gennaro Ilardi [2], Daniela Russo [2], Andrea Soricelli [1,3], Onofrio Antonio Catalano [4,*] and Marco Salvatore [1]

1 IRCCS SDN, 80143 Naples, Italy; agrimaldi@sdn-napoli.it (A.M.G.); pmirabelli@sdn-napoli.it (P.M.); ccavaliere@sdn-napoli.it (C.C.); caparente@sdn-napoli.it (C.A.P.); mfranzese@sdn-napoli.it (M.F.); soricelli@uniparthenope.it (A.S.); direzionescientifica@sdn-napoli.it (M.S.)

2 Department of Advanced Biomedical Sciences, Federico II University, 80131 Naples, Italy; staibano@unina.it (S.S.); gennaro.ilardi@gmail.com (G.I.); danielarusso83@yahoo.it (D.R.)

3 Department of Motor Sciences & Wellness, University of Naples Parthenope, 80133 Naples, Italy

4 Department of Radiology, Athinoula A. Martinos Center for Biomedical Imaging, Massachusetts General Hospital, Harvard Medical School, Charlestown, MA 02129, USA

* Correspondence: mincoronato@sdn-napoli.it (M.I.); onofriocatalano@yahoo.it (O.A.C.)

Abstract: The aim of this study was to identify new disease-related circulating miRNAs with high diagnostic accuracy for breast cancer (BC) and to correlate their deregulation with the morpho-functional characteristics of the tumour, as assessed in vivo by positron emission tomography/magnetic resonance (PET/MR) imaging. A total of 77 untreated female BC patients underwent same-day PET/MR and blood collection, and 78 healthy donors were recruited as negative controls. The expression profile of 84 human miRNAs was screened by using miRNA PCR arrays and validated by real-time PCR. The validated miRNAs were correlated with the quantitative imaging parameters extracted from the primary BC samples. Circulating miR-125b-5p and miR-143-3p were upregulated in BC plasma and able to discriminate BC patients from healthy subjects (miR-125-5p area under the receiver operating characteristic ROC curve (AUC) = 0.85 and miR-143-3p AUC = 0.80). Circulating CA15-3, a soluble form of the transmembrane glycoprotein Mucin 1 (MUC-1) that is upregulated in epithelial cancer cells of different origins, was combined with miR-125b-5p and improved the diagnostic accuracy from 70% (CA15-3 alone) to 89% (CA15-3 plus miR-125b-5p). MiR-143-3p showed a strong and significant correlation with the stage of the disease, apparent diffusion coefficient (ADC_{mean}), reverse efflux volume transfer constant (Kep_{mean}) and maximum standardized uptake value (SUV_{max}), and it might represent a biomarker of tumour aggressiveness. Similarly, miR-125b-5p was correlated with stage and grade 2 but inversely correlated with the forward volume transfer constant ($Ktrans_{mean}$) and proliferation index (Ki67), suggesting a potential role as a biomarker of a relatively more favourable prognosis. In situ hybridization (ISH) experiments revealed that miR-143-3p was expressed in endothelial tumour cells, miR-125-5p in cancer-associated fibroblasts, and neither in epithelial tumour cells. Our results suggested that miR-125-5p and miR-143-3p are potential biomarkers for the risk stratification of BC, and Kaplan-Maier plots confirmed this hypothesis. In addition, the combined use of miR-125-b-5p and CA15-3 enhanced the diagnostic accuracy up to 89%. This is the first study that correlates circulating miRNAs with in vivo quantified tumour biology through PET/MR biomarkers. This integration elucidates the link between the plasmatic increase in these two potential circulating biomarkers and the biology of untreated BC. In conclusion, while miR-143-3b and miR-125b-5p provide valuable information for prognosis, a combination of miR-125b-5p with the tumour marker CA15-3 improves sensitivity for BC detection, which warrants consideration by further validation studies.

Keywords: circulating miRNAs; breast cancer; imaging parameters; PET/MRI; biomarkers

1. Introduction

According to GLOBOCAN 2018, a project of the International Agency for Research on Cancer (IARC), approximately 2.1 million women (1.7 million in 2012) were diagnosed with breast cancer (BC) worldwide, and there were approximately 6.9 million women (6.3 million in 2012) who had been diagnosed with BC in the previous five years [1]. BC is also the most common cause of cancer death among women, with 627,000 deaths in 2018. Early diagnosis plays a major role in fighting BC. However, on a worldwide scale, breast imaging techniques such as screening mammography and ultrasound have intrinsic limitations related to economic costs, limited technology availability in underdeveloped countries, the necessity of well-trained radiologists, and an overall unsatisfactory performance regarding the images. Screening mammography performance indexes vary considerably for sensitivity and specificity, influencing the ability of mammography to reach its full potential for decreasing BC mortality [2]; moreover, ultrasound plus mammography can indicate cancers in high-risk women, but the number of false positives are increased [3].

Circulating biomarkers are biomolecules released into the bloodstream by both tumour cells and other types of neighbouring cells [4]. Their quantification and identification are considered an economical, non-invasive diagnostic method that provides information on the presence and/or absence of the disease as well as its evolution. To date, the carcinoembryonic antigen (CEA) [5] and the soluble form of Mucin 1 (MUC-1) protein (CA15-3) [6] are the most commonly used serum biomarkers for the clinical monitoring of BC patients. Although these biomarkers have been recognized from the international healthcare system as molecules used for the management of BC patients, current guidelines suggest that they fail in the early diagnosis of the disease, having a clinical role only during follow-up [7]. Therefore, there is a compelling need to discover potential biomarkers that might be useful for diagnosing BC. The ideal tumour marker should have high specificity, sensitivity and predictive value and be detectable by an accurate, rapid, simple and inexpensive method that might also be used in countries with less access to expensive technology. In recent decades, non-coding RNA molecules (miRNAs) have emerged as a new class of regulatory genes involved in many cellular processes, such as development, differentiation, proliferation, apoptosis and the response to stress. In their mature form, these single-stranded small molecules are 19 to 25 nucleotides in length and are able to silence gene expression at the post-transcriptional level, thus inhibiting protein translation. They act by recognizing a sequence within the 3′ and/or 5′ untranslated region (UTR) of their mRNA target [8]. miRNAs can exert their action in cancers through both tumour suppression and oncogenic mechanisms [9,10]. Due to their structural characteristics, functions and tissue specificity, miRNAs have been proposed as a new class of biomarkers for the screening of different tumours. Recent discoveries have shown that miRNAs are also present in biological fluids, such as blood [11], urine [12], sputum [13] and saliva [14]; moreover, they were found to be aberrantly expressed in different human cancers and feature unprecedented levels of diagnostic specificity and sensitivity that are associated with tumour burden and malignant progression [15,16]. Additionally, circulating miRNAs are extremely stable against degradation by RNase, easily collected through non-invasive methods (blood sampling), resistant to repeated freeze/thaw cycles and easily identified by nucleic acid amplification techniques (real-time PCR). These factors also make their collection possible in third-world countries and underserved areas. Taken together, these findings highlight the potential usefulness of these molecules as promising biomarkers. To date, many studies have identified different circulating miRNAs as new biomarkers for BC detection; however, the results are discordant [17]. Moreover, they have not been assessed in conjunction with diagnostic imaging, which is used for quantifying the extent of the disease and provides information related to tumour aggressiveness representing an obligatory step for treatment planning. The use of diagnostic imaging to extract quantitative parameters related to the morphology, metabolism and functionality of tumours, as well as to correlate specific imaging parameters with tissue biomarkers, is an emerging research topic [18,19]. The aim of our study was to identify potential new disease-related circulating miRNAs with high diagnostic accuracy for BC and to elucidate the relationship between their circulating deregulation and tumour characteristics, including stage at presentation and the functional quantification of tumour metabolism and perfusion, by using same-day positron emission tomography/magnetic resonance (PET/MR) imaging. Since PET/MR scanners have been approved for use less than 8 years ago, with very few installed worldwide, PET/MR is currently clinically used for BC diagnosis and treatment planning in only an extremely limited number of highly specialized centres that have both the expertise of scanner use and a strong oncologic breast programme. In these centres, PET/MR is used for the whole-body and local staging of newly diagnosed BC cases that are amenable to curative resection, either without or after neoadjuvant treatments, and as problem-solving technology in complicated, more advanced cases. PET/MR is currently not mentioned in the National Comprehensive Cancer Network (NCCN) guidelines or in any other scientific organization/society guidelines despite its higher performances than those of any other non-invasive imaging modality. In fact, the accuracy of PET/MR staging outperformed that of PET/computed tomography (CT) (the most accurate of the routinely clinically approved imaging modalities) on a per patient analysis (98% versus 75%) and was also capable of demonstrating bony metastases not detected by same-day PET/CT in up to 12% of the cases [20,21]. These results have been confirmed by other authors who showed that, in a lesion-per-lesion analysis, PET/MR had higher sensitivity than PET/CT in detecting bony lesions (0.924 and 0.6923, respectively). Moreover, PET/MR also had a better sensitivity than PET/CT in detecting contralateral tumours (1 and 0.25, respectively) and all lesions together (0.89 and 0.77, respectively) [22]. To the best of our knowledge, this is the first study that aimed to correlate the deregulated expression of disease-related circulating miRNAs with the morphological, metabolic and functional parameters of BC lesions (tumour metabolism, cellular density and vascularisation) extracted through a hybrid PET/MR scanner. The plasma samples of BC patients and healthy donors were analysed for miRNA expression, and for each BC patient, PET/MR was used to ascertain the stage of the disease as well as the metabolic, diffusion and perfusion characteristics of the primary cancer. In silico studies and in situ hybridization (ISH) experiments were also performed to better understand miRNA expression in tissue and their cellular localization. Last, we correlated the expression levels of the validated miRNAs with immunohistochemical markers of BC, stage of disease and PET/MR-derived functional and metabolic biomarkers of primary cancer.

2. Results

2.1. Identification and Validation of a Plasma miRNA Signature for Breast Cancer Detection

The study design is illustrated in Figure 1A. The healthy and BC subjects were age-matched (p-value = 0.157), and the clinicopathological characteristics of the study participants are reported in Table 1. By using the miScript miRNA PCR Array, we found that five (miR-125b-5p, miR-143-3p, miR-145-5p, miR-100-5p and miR-23a-3p; Figure 1B–D) out of the 84 miRNAs analysed were significantly (p-value < 0.05) upregulated in the plasma samples of 27 BC patients vs. 14 healthy donors, with a fold change ≥1.5. RT-PCR was conducted to confirm the array results in a study population of 46 healthy donors and 64 naïve BC patients (Supplementary Figure S1). Then, a logistic regression model (Supplementary Table S1A) identified miR-125b-5p and miR-143-3p as the circulating miRNAs able to effectively discriminate affected from unaffected subjects. A logistic stepwise regression model confirmed these results (Supplementary Table S1B). Moreover, the results were corroborated by expanding the case studies to 78 healthy donors and 77 naïve BC patients (Figure 1A, Validation II). In fact, as shown in Figure 2A,B, we confirmed that miR-125b-5p and miR-143-3p were significantly upregulated in the plasma of BC patients with a fold change of 3.3 and 3.2, respectively. These results were confirmed by logistic stepwise regression analysis (Figure 2C).

Table 1. Detailed clinicopathological characteristics of the study participants.

Healthy Control Samples (n = 78)	
Age range	28–84 years
Mean ± S.D.	51.05 ± 11.26
Breast Cancer Samples (n = 77)	
Age range	28–82 years
Mean ± S.D.	53.68 ± 12.02
Subtype	
Luminal A	16
Luminal B	50
HER2+	7
Triple negative	4
Ki67	
Low (1–20%)	21
High (21–100%)	56
Grade	
G1	1
G2	41
G3	35
Stage	
Stage I	1
Stage II	12
Stage III	42
Stage IV	22

S.D.: standard deviation; HER2+: Human epidermal growth factor receptor positive.

A

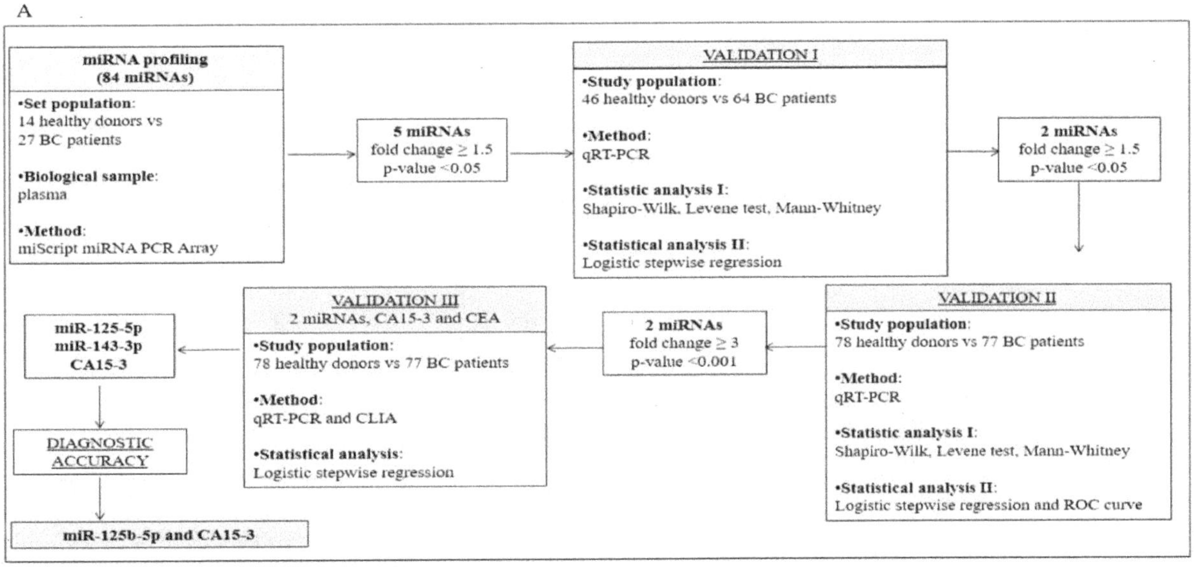

Figure 1. *Cont.*

B

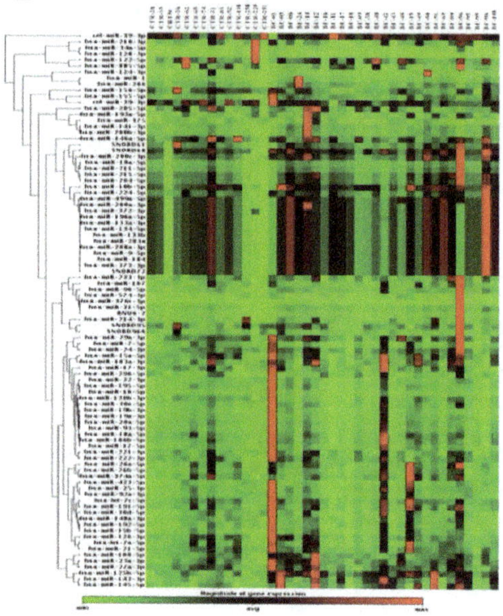

C

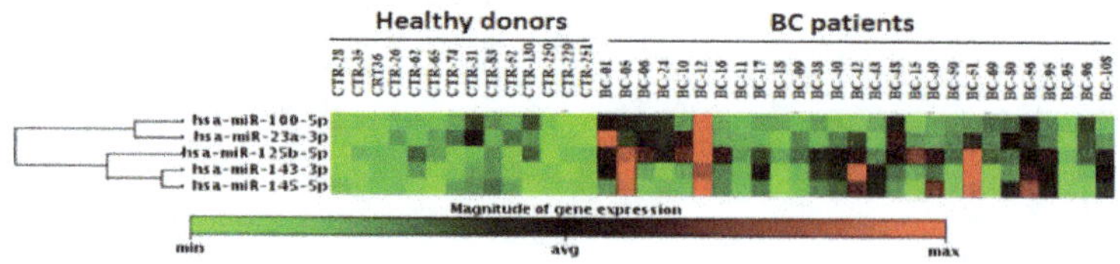

D

miRNAs deregulated in BC patients vs healthy donors		
miRNAs	p-value	fold change
miR-125b-5p	0.000005*	2.81
miR-143-3p	0.0021*	3.03
miR-145-5p	0.01*	2.04
miR-100-5p	0.028*	1.93
miR-23a-3p	0.014*	1.55

Figure 1. Study design for the identification of circulating miRNAs and protein biomarkers able to discriminate breast cancer (BC) patients from healthy donors (**A**). miRNA expression analysis in a set population of 14 healthy donors (CTR) and 27 BC subjects. Expression analysis of 84 miRNAs by using a 96-well miScript miRNA PCR Array (**B**). * miRNAs significantly upregulated ($p < 0.05$) in BC patients vs. healthy donors (**C**,**D**).

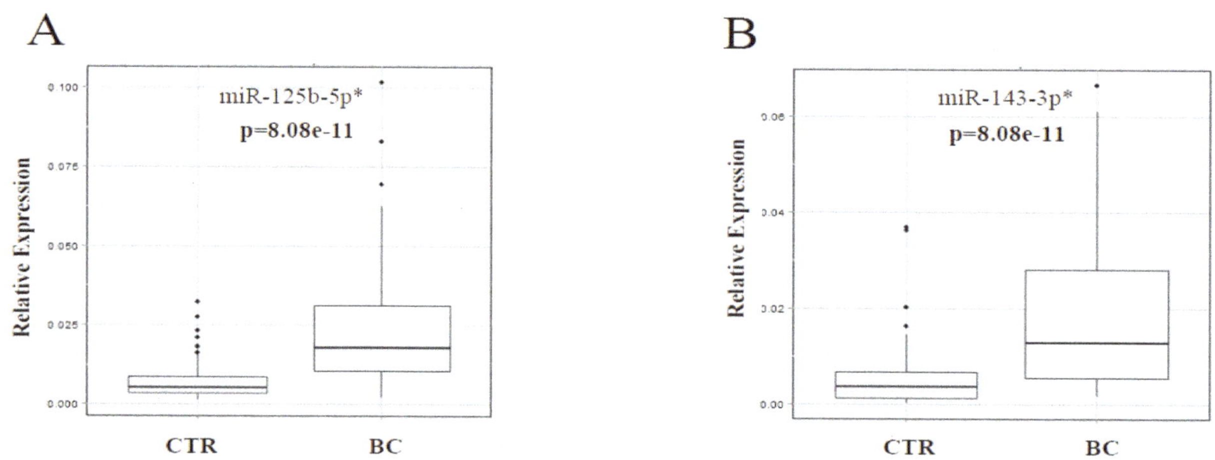

C

miRNAs	Estimate	Std. Error	p-value
miR-125b-5p*	10.73674	2.45984	2.34e-05
miR-143-3p*	9.02322	2.74402	0.00125

Figure 2. Validation II. Relative expression of miRNAs selected in a study population of 78 healthy donors (CTR) and 77 breast cancer (BC) subjects. Box plot analyses performed to show the relative expression of miR-125b-5p (**A**) and miR-143-3p (**B**) in the plasma samples of healthy donors vs. BC patients. Logistic stepwise regression analysis (**C**). * miRNAs that significantly ($p < 0.05$) estimate the probability of having BC.

2.2. *Diagnostic miRNA Signature-Based Model Compared with Established BC Markers*

Receiver operating characteristic (ROC) curve analyses showed that miR-125b-5p (area under the ROC curve (AUC) = 0.85) and miR-143-3p (AUC = 0.80) were able to discriminate BC patients from healthy donors (Figure 3A,B). Then, we compared the AUC value of the selected miRNAs with the AUC value of the traditional BC biomarkers CA15-3 and CEA. As reported in Figure 3C,D, the AUC values of CA15-3 (0.70) and CEA (0.68) were lower than those calculated for miR-125b-5p and miR-143-3p. Based on these results, a logistic stepwise regression analysis was performed considering the miR-125b-5p, miR-143-3p, CA15-3 and CEA molecules as independent variables (Figure 1A, Validation III). According to Table 2, miR-125b-5p, miR-143-3p and CA15-3 were significantly correlated with the disease, although the statistical significance of CA15-3 was lower than that of the miRNAs. Based on these findings, the diagnostic accuracy of each biomarker was evaluated. To this end, the cut-off values of miR-125b-5p and miR-143-3p were calculated, and the clinical cut-off values of CA15-3 and CEA were already known (CA15-3 = 35 UI/mL and CEA = 3 UI/mL). Using the "closest to top-left" method, we defined the cut-off value of miR-125b-5p as 0.0090 and that of miR-143-3p as 0.0064, both related to relative expression. Among the analysed molecules, miR-125b-5p showed the highest diagnostic accuracy (Table 3).

Table 2. Validation III. Logistic stepwise regression on the indicated molecules in a cohort of 78 CTR and 77 BC subjects. * Molecules that significantly ($p < 0.05$) estimate the probability of having a tumour.

Circulating Biomarkers	Estimate	Std. Error	*p*-Value
miR-125b-5p *	9.018	2.401	0.000248
miR-143-3p *	1.017×10^{1}	2.644	0.000179
CA15-3 *	2.123×10^{-3}	8.984×10^{-4}	0.01941
CEA	4.866×10^{-3}	7.095×10^{-3}	0.4939

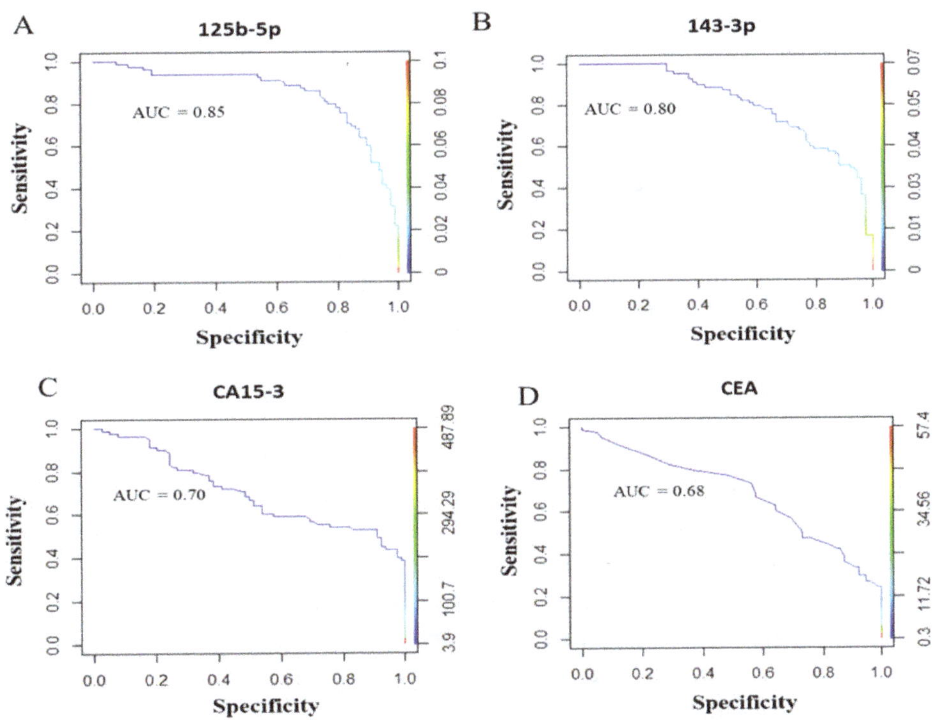

Figure 3. ROC curve analyses and AUC values of miR-125-5p (**A**), miR-143-3p (**B**), CA15-3 (**C**), and CEA (**D**) for discriminating BC patients from healthy controls in 76 BC patients and 78 healthy donors. ROC: Receiver operating characteristic; AUC: area under the ROC curve; CEA: carcinoembryonic antigen.

Table 3. Diagnostic accuracy of the indicated circulating biomarkers.

miR-125b-5p	Disease +	Disease −	Total	Sensitivity	Specificity	Diagnostic Accuracy
Test +	61 (TP)	16 (FP)	77	0.79 (CI 0.68–0.88)	0.79 (CI 0.69–0.88)	0.79 (CI 0.72–0.85)
Test −	16 (FN)	62 (TN)	78			
Total	77	78	155			
miR-143-3p	**Disease +**	**Disease −**	**Total**	**Sensitivity**	**Specificity**	**Diagnostic accuracy**
Test +	53 (TP)	20 (FP)	73	0.69 (CI 0.57–0.79)	0.74 (CI 0.63–0.84)	0.72 (CI 0.64–0.79)
Test −	24 (FN)	58 (TN)	82			
Total	77	78	155			
CA15-3	**Disease +**	**Disease −**	**Total**	**Sensitivity**	**Specificity**	**Diagnostic accuracy**
Test +	29 (TP)	1 (FP)	30	0.38 (CI 0.27–0.50)	0.99 (CI 0.93–1.00)	0.68 (CI 0.60–0.76)
Test −	47 (FN)	75 (TN)	122			
Total	76	76	152			
CEA	**Disease +**	**Disease −**	**Total**	**Sensitivity**	**Specificity**	**Diagnostic accuracy**
Test +	25 (TP)	8 (FP)	73	0.33 (CI 0.23–0.45)	0.89 (CI 0.80–0.95)	0.61 (CI 0.53–0.69)
Test −	51 (FN)	68 (TN)	82			
Total	76	76	152			

CI: confidence interval 95%; Disease +: BC patients, Disease −: healthy donors, TP: True Positive TP, FP: False Positive, FN: False Negative and TN: True Negative. CEA: carcinoembryonic antigen and BC: breast cancer.

2.3. Co-Expression Analysis of Circulating miR-125b-5p, miR-143-3p and miR-145-5p and Their Association with Immunohistochemical Markers of BC

Although miR-145-5p was not able to estimate the probability of pathology (Supplementary Table S1), it is transcribed from a putative miR-143/145 cluster on chromosome 5 in humans (5q33). Therefore, co-expression analyses by Spearman's test were performed not only for miR-125b-5p and miR-143-3p but also for miR-145-5p. As reported in Figure 4A, we found that miR-143-3p and miR-145-5p were strongly co-expressed (ρ: 0.93; p-value $< 2 \times 10^{-16}$) in the plasma samples of BC patients, and the expression levels of miR-125b-5p were significantly correlated with those of miR-143-3p (ρ: 0.57; p-value $= 2 \times 10^{-4}$) and miR-145-5p (ρ: 0.56; p-value $= 6 \times 10^{-6}$), although to a limited extent.

The immunohistochemical (IHC) reports of the enrolled BC patients were used to determine the receptor status (oestrogen, progesterone, and human epidermal growth factor receptor 2), cellular differentiation status (grade) and proliferation index (Ki67) of the tumour lesions. No association was found between the expression levels of miR-125-5p, miR-143-3p and miR-145-5p and the hormonal receptor status of the lesions (Estrogen Receptor positive or negative: ER+/−, Progesteron receptor positive or negative: PR +/− and Human epidermal growth factor receptor positive or negative: HER2 +/−; Supplementary Table S2) or with tumour subtypes (all p-values > 0.05). Nevertheless, only miR-125b-5p was significantly associated with the Ki67 proliferation index (Figure 4B, p-value $= 0.038$) and the differentiation status of tumour cells (Figure 4C, p-value $= 0.003$). Specifically, we found that in the presence of a low Ki67 index and a low grade, the expression levels of miR-125b-5p were increased, suggesting its inverse correlation with the aggressiveness of the disease.

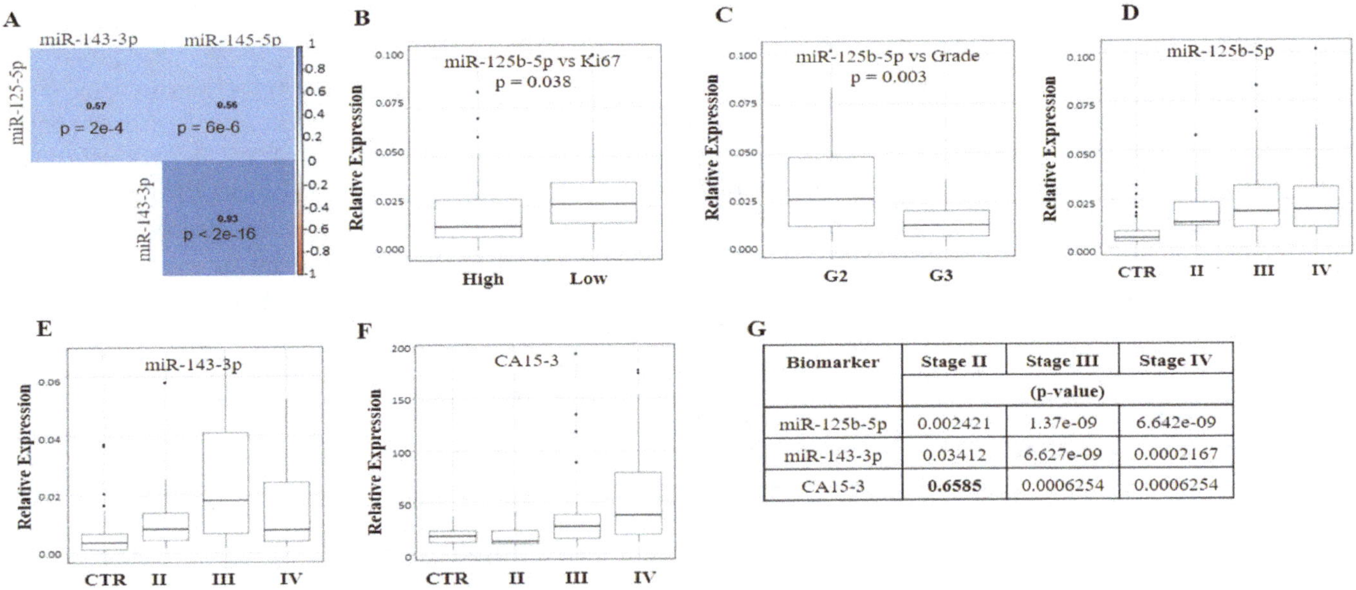

Biomarker	Stage II	Stage III	Stage IV
	(p-value)		
miR-125b-5p	0.002421	1.37e-09	6.642e-09
miR-143-3p	0.03412	6.627e-09	0.0002167
CA15-3	**0.6585**	0.0006254	0.0006254

Figure 4. Correlation studies. Co-expression analyses of miR-125b-5p, miR-143-3p and miR-145-5p (**A**). Expression levels of miR-125b-5p vs. Ki67 (low <20%; high ≥20%) (**B**), and grade (**C**). Expression levels of miR-125b-5p (**D**), miR-143-3p (**E**), and CA15-3 (**F**) vs. stage. Statistical significance (**G**). Non-significant results are reported in bold.

2.4. Correlation Analysis of Circulating miR-125b-5p, miR-143-3p and miR-145-5p with Quantitative Imaging Parameters of Tumour Lesions

The BC patients enrolled in this study underwent same-day contrast-enhanced fluorodeoxyglucose (CE-FDG)-PET/MR and blood collection to better correlate circulating miR-125-5p and miR-143-3p with the morphological, metabolic and functional imaging features of BC (Figure 4). No significant correlations were found between the miRNA expression levels and lesion size (Supplementary Table S2). The plasma levels of miR-125b-5p increased significantly at stage II, reaching higher expression levels at stage III and remained unchanged at stage IV compared to stage III (Figure 4D,G). This trend confirmed that the expression levels of miR-125b-5p were variable and depended on the severity of the disease. Additionally, the expression levels of miR-143-3p (Figure 4E,G) became significantly higher in stage III and drastically decreased in stage IV, reaching expression values close to those of healthy donors. This result suggests that at stage IV, this molecule is not required for the maintenance of the pathology. It is known that CA15-3 levels increase in the late stage of the disease, so its relationship with clinical staging was also evaluated. As reported in Figure 4F,G, in our cohort, CA15-3 was not able to diagnose stage II, but its levels increased significantly at stage III, reaching the maximum concentration at stage IV. This was in agreement with the known performance of CA15-3. In addition, no correlations were found between CA15-3 and grade (p-value = 0.761) or subtypes (p-value = 0.450).

Correlation analyses between miR-125b-5p and miR-143-3p levels and PET/MR-based tumour biomarkers were performed by grouping the data according to staging. Only the statistically significant results were reported (Table 4); we found a strong and significant correlation between circulating miR-143-3p and the mean initial area under the concentration curve ($iAUC_{mean}$) and the mean reverse efflux volume transfer constant (Kep_{mean}) (for both, ρ: 0.943, p-value = 0.005) in the stage II group. Perfusion parameters such as iAUC and Kep are generally correlated with tumour vascularisation [23,24], suggesting that the plasmatic overexpression of miR-143-3p in BC patients might correlate with angiogenesis. The correlation between iAUC and miR-143-3p persisted at stage III but was lost at stage IV, where its relative expression drastically decreased (see Figure 4B). Notably, there was a strong correlation index between miR-143-3p and the maximum standardized uptake value (SUV_{max}) (ρ: 0.829 and p-value = 0.042) at stage II, although the statistical significance was borderline. SUV is a biomarker of tumour metabolism. This result together with those reported above suggest that miR-143-3p could be correlated with tumour aggressiveness. miR-125-5p was significantly inversely correlated with the mean forward volume transfer constant ($Ktrans_{mean}$) and the proliferation index Ki67 at stage IV (Table 4). $Ktrans_{mean}$, like iAUC and Kep, is a perfusion parameter linked to tumour vascularisation [24]. Since the highest plasma concentration of miR-125b-5p was associated with a low Ki67 index (Figure 4B) and grade G2 (Figure 4C) and inversely correlated with $Ktrans_{mean}$ (Table 4), these results suggest that the highest plasma values of miR-125b-5p might predict a better prognosis.

Table 4. Correlation studies among the miRNAs selected and the imaging parameters extracted from tumour lesions. The table reports ρ and p-values ($p < 0.05$ was considered statistically significant).

	Stage II				Stage III		Stage IV	
	$iAUC_{mean}$	**Ki67**	**Kep_{mean}**	**SUV_{max}**	**$iAUC_{mean}$**	**Ki67**	**Ki67**	**$Ktrans_{mean}$**
miR-125-5p	ns	ns	ns	ns	ns	ns	−0.513 p-value 0.029	−0.421 p-value 0.040
miR-143-3p	0.943 p-value 0.005	ns	0.943 p-value 0.005	0.829 p-value 0.042	0.938 p-value 0.044	ns	ns	ns

ns indicates non-significant results. $iAUC_{mean}$: area under the concentration curve; SUV_{max}: maximum standardized uptake value; Kep_{mean}: mean reverse efflux volume transfer constant; $Ktrans_{mean}$: mean forward volume transfer constantin.

2.5. *In Silico Studies*

Large publicly funded projects have generated extensive and freely available multi-assay data resources. To date, The Cancer Genome Atlas (TCGA) represents the largest available resource for multi-assay cancer genomics data that includes ~30000 cases of major primary cancers, including BC (TCGA-BRCA) [25]. To evaluate whether the upregulation of circulating miR-125b-5p, miR-143-3p and miR-145-5p in the plasma samples of BC patients reflected their tumour tissue expression, we performed in silico studies by using the TCGA-BRCA database. We also included miR-145-5p in order to perform co-expression analyses. We found that in BC tissue specimens, the expression of miR-125b-5p, miR-143-3p and miR-145-5p was significantly lower compared to that in normal tissues (Supplementary Figure S2A) and that their downregulation was not correlated with the stage of the disease (Supplementary Figure S2B).

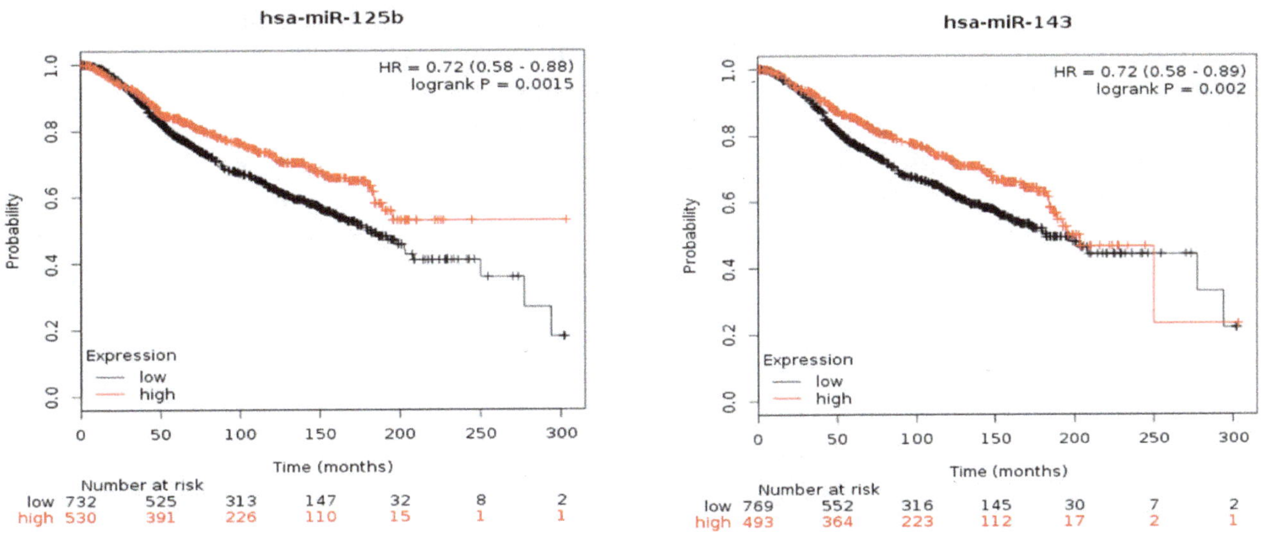

Figure 5. Kaplan-Meier plots, which are based on breast cancer data from the METABRIC database, illustrate the survival probability for patients with low or high miR-125b (upper panel) and miR-143 (lower panel) expression levels in breast cancer. Hazard ratios (HRs) and *p*-values (log-rank test) were generated.

In addition, we found that the downregulation of miR-143-3p and miR-145-5p in BC tissues (Supplementary Figure S2C) showed a lower correlation index compared to that we found in the plasma samples of BC patients (compare Figure 4A with Supplementary Figure S2C: ρ: 0.93 vs. ρ: 0.28). Taken together, these results showed an opposite expression trend of miR-125-5p, miR-143-3p and miR-145-5p in cancer tissue versus plasma.

Since we were unable to monitor patients during follow-up, a survival analysis was performed for both miR-125b-5p and miR-143-3p by using the miRpower software (http://kmplot.com/analysis/index.php?p=service&cancer=breast_mirna). This software uses publicly available BC data from different databases, including data from large databases such as TCGA and Molecular Taxonomy of Breast Cancer International Consortium (METABRIC). To generate Kaplan-Meier curves, we selected the option to auto select the best cut-off for defining high and low groups. The algorithm computes all possible cut-off values between the lower and upper quartiles and uses the best performing threshold. The hazard ratios (HRs) and *p*-values (log-rank test) were calculated. By using the TCGA dataset, the Kaplan-Meier plots were not statistically significant for miR-125b-5p or miR-143-3p (data not shown), so the METABRIC dataset was used. As reported in Figure 5, we found that high tissue expression levels of miR-125b-5p were associated with the best prognosis (upper panel), and this result was in agreement with those obtained correlating this miRNA with grade, Ki67 and $Ktrans_{mean}$. The effect of high expression levels of miR-143 on the survival of BC patients varied with age, and higher values contributed to worse prognoses starting at 250 months (lower panel). This result was in part in agreement with those obtained correlating this miRNA with the imaging parameters linked with tumour aggressiveness. It is necessary to point out that the miRpower software did not discriminate miR-143-3p from miR-143-5p, grouping them in miR-143, and miR-125b-5p from miR-125b-3p, grouping them in miR-125b.

2.6. Cellular Origin of miR-125b-5p, miR-143-3p and miR-145-5p in Normal and BC Tissues

To corroborate the obtained results and confirm the in silico data, we performed ISH experiments. We hypothesized that release of miR-125b-5p, miR-143-3p and miR-145-5p into the bloodstream did not originate from tumour cells. As reported in Figure 6, the results confirmed that the expression of miR-143-3p (B) and miR-145-5p (C) was low or absent in epithelial tumour tissue (right) but high in endothelial cells, highlighting their vascular origin, as anticipated by correlation studies among miRNAs with image biomarkers. In addition, in benign breast tissue, miR-143-3p stained in glandular epithelial and endothelial cells (Figure 6B, left), and miR-145-5p was expressed with the strongest staining intensity in myoepithelial cells and endothelial cells (Figure 6C, left panel). Moreover, miR-125b-5p was weakly expressed in normal tissue (Figure 6D, left) and low-to-absent in neoplastic cells (Figure 6D, right). This supported the hypothesis that miR-125b-5p could have a stromal origin. This hypothesis was further confirmed by the result shown in Figure 6E, in which miR-125b-5p expression occurred in cancer-associated fibroblasts. Taken together, these results confirmed that the BC plasma upregulation of miR-125-5p and miR-143-3p could be related to their overexpression in endothelial and fibroblast cells and not in tumour epithelial cells.

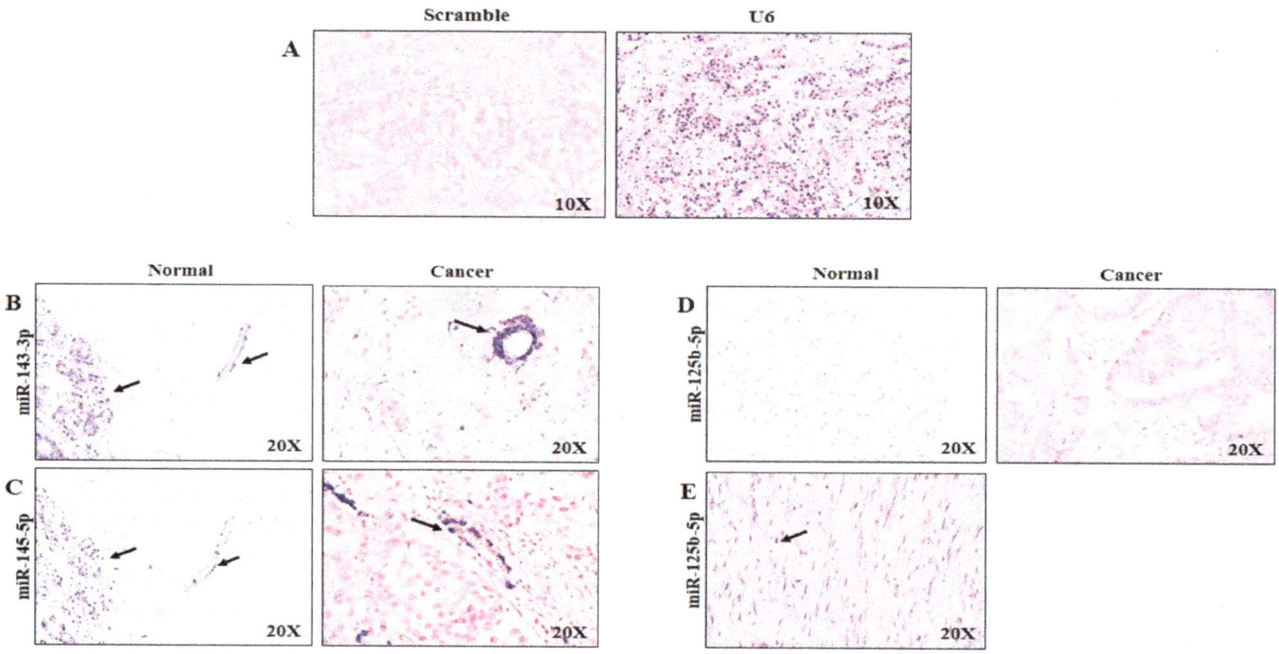

Figure 6. In situ hybridization staining patterns in benign and malignant breast tissues. Scrambled miR negative control probe and U6 positive control probe (**A**). miR-143-3p in normal (left) and BC tissues (right) (**B**). miR-145-5p in normal (left) and BC tissues (right) (**C**). miR-125b-5p in normal (left) and BC tissues (right) (**D**). miR-125b-5p in stromal tumour tissue (**E**). BC: breast cancer.

2.7. Combining Diagnostic test Results to Increase Accuracy

Since the relationship between upregulated circulating miRNA expression and the functional characteristics of tumour lesions was clarified, we next sought to optimize their diagnostic role by evaluating a combined detection of miR-125b-5p and miR-143-3p with CA15-3. As reported in Figure 7A, we found that combining the diagnostic test results of miR-125b-5p and CA15-3 improved the accuracy (AUC = 0.89) compared to the same molecules analysed individually (see Figure 3: miR-125-5p, AUC = 0.85; CA15-3, AUC = 0.68). In contrast, combining miR-143-3p and CA15-3 reduced the diagnostic accuracy (data not shown). Additionally, the combined analysis of miR-125b-5p and miR-143-3p did not improve the accuracy (Figure 7B, AUC = 0.85) in comparison to the same molecules analysed individually (see Figure 3: miR-125-5p, AUC = 0.85; miR-143-3p, AUC = 0.80).

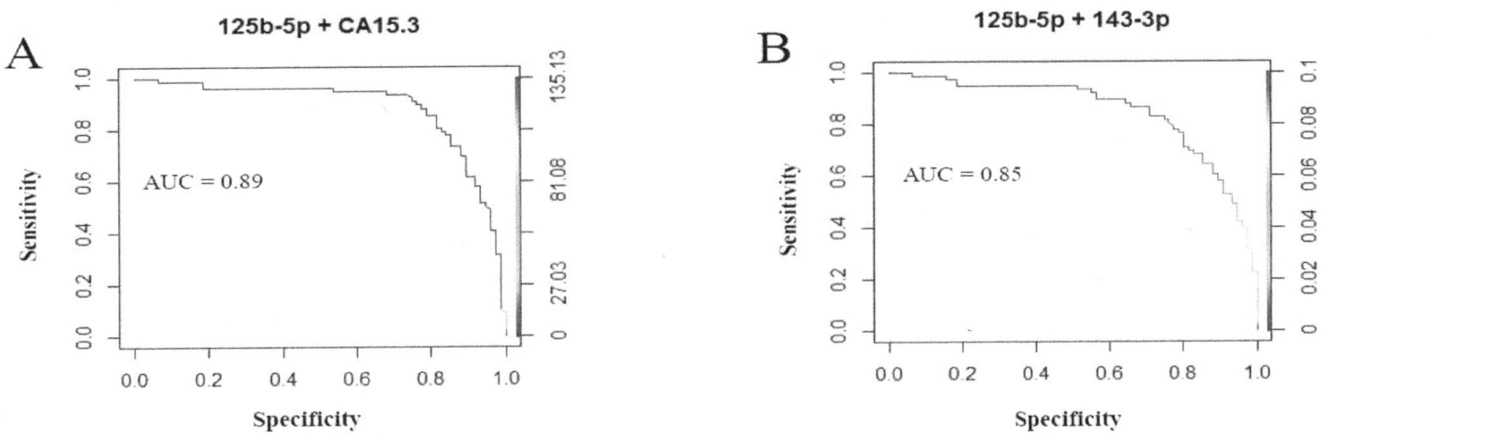

Figure 7. ROC curve analyses and AUC values combining the profiles of miR-125b-5p and CA15-3 (**A**) and miR-125-5p and miR-143-3p (**B**) for discriminating BC patients from healthy patients. ROC: Receiver operating characteristic; AUC: area under the ROC curve; BC: breast cancer.

3. Discussion

The detection of BC is pivotal for proper patient management, especially at an early stage. However, the currently utilized technology, which is heavily based on screening mammography and ultrasound (in specific patient populations), is imperfect, with limited accessibility in underdeveloped/underserved areas and might be economically challenging. Therefore, there is a compelling need to identify new biomarkers that might be diagnostically advantageous. Due to their structural and functional characteristics, microRNAs have been proposed as a new class of biomarkers for cancer screening; in fact, they are stable, deregulated, and found in different biological fluids, including blood that can be easily withdrawn in the field and subsequently processed in centralized laboratories. To date, circulating biomarkers that are able to diagnose BC with high specificity and sensitivity are lacking, so our study aimed to (i) identify new circulating miRNAs for the diagnosis of BC; (ii) to elucidate the relationship between their circulating deregulation and the functional characteristics of tumour lesions for in vivo investigation through PET/MR; and (iii) understand the link between circulating miRNA deregulation and their origin in the primary tumour.

By using the miScript miRNA PCR Array, we found that five miRNAs (miR-125b-5p, miR-143-3p, miR-145-5p, miR-100-5p and miR-23a-3p) were significantly ($p \leq 0.0005$) overexpressed in the plasma samples of BC patients compared to healthy subjects and defined miR-125b-5p and miR-143-3p as the best molecules able to estimate the probability of having the disease. The circulating levels of miR-125b-5p and miR-143-3p are of intense debate in the scientific literature, especially in BC. Matamala et al. [26] found that circulating miR-143 was upregulated in BC patients; on the contrary, some studies showed a downregulation of circulating miR-143 in BC patients [27–30], and others found no significant deregulation of circulating miR-125b and miR-143 in BC patients [30]. These discrepancies could be explained by the usage of serum rather than plasma [31]. Regardless of whether the choice of the biological sample can affect the result, different studies reported the upregulation of miR-125b in the serum samples of BC patients [32–34]. These discrepancies highlight the need to standardize protocols, including sample collection, storage, choice of the starting biological material, and processing. To better understand the biological basis and clinical implications of miR-125b-5p and miR-143-3p, we performed a correlation analysis between the circulating expression of the deregulated disease-related miRNAs and the metabolic and functional characteristics of the primary tumour, also taking into consideration the TNM (Tumour Lymph Nodes Metastasis) classification of malignant tumours stage of the disease. For this purpose, we employed biomarkers extracted from a hybrid clinically approved PET/MR scanner. We decided to use PET/MR since it couples two modalities (FDG-PET and MR) capable of sampling different biological features of cancers in vivo, specifically glucose metabolism through PET and cellular density plus tissue perfusion through MR. The advantages arising from the simultaneous acquisition of PET- and MR-derived biomarkers in investigating BC biology have been shown by some exploratory studies that demonstrated the capability of PET/MR to predict BC subtypes, including those with a better prognosis [19,35]. In this study, we found that the expression of circulating miR-143-3p was strongly and significantly correlated with $iAUC_{mean}$ at stage II (ρ: 0.943, p-value = 0.005) and at stage III (ρ: 0.938, p-value = 0.044) and with Kep_{mean} at stage II (ρ: 0.943, p-value = 0.005). Both $iAUC_{mean}$ and Kep_{mean} are perfusion parameters that provide information on tumour vascularisation, suggesting that miR-143-3p overexpression in the plasma samples of BC patients could be linked to tumour angiogenesis. Our hypothesis was in agreement with the editorial comment of Almeida and Calin [36] that argued the possible critical role of these miRNAs in the neoangiogenesis of lung cancer. To confirm this hypothesis and to further validate our results, we performed ISH experiments on BC and normal breast tissue specimens and found that miR-143-3p had a clear vascular endothelial origin. In addition, we also found that miR-143-3p was correlated with SUV_{max} at stage II (ρ: 0.829, p-value = 0.042). The SUV parameter reflects the metabolic activity of tumours, so we speculate that miR-143-3p could have a role in neoangiogenesis and that its overexpression in the plasma samples of BC patients could be correlated with the aggressiveness of the disease, both in terms of tumour vascularisation and metabolic activity. This hypothesis was in part corroborated by the survival analysis performed *in silico* by using the miRpower software.

Another interesting result correlated the expression levels of miR-125b-5p with IHC biomarkers and imaging parameters. We concluded that miR-125b-5p was inversely associated with the proliferation index Ki67 (p-value = 0.038), grading (p-value = 0.003) and the perfusion imaging parameter $Ktrans_{mean}$ (ρ: −0.421, p-value = 0.040) and that its expression occurred in cancer-associated fibroblasts. These findings suggest that the highest concentration of miR-125b-5p could be correlated with a better prognosis, and the survival analysis confirmed this hypothesis. This is in agreement with the "seed and soil" hypothesis, which postulates that different components of the tumour microenvironment (the soil) may have stimulatory or inhibitory effects on tumour progression (the seed) [37], and with recent studies showing that miR-125b-5p overexpression in BC cell lines could inhibit cell proliferation, migration and invasion [38,39].

One of the limitations of this study is the sample size (n = 77 BC patients). In fact, the heterogeneity and complexity of BC make it challenging to find a unique circulating signature of pathology with high diagnostic accuracy. Each circulating biomarker released in the blood of affected patients exists as a consequence of genetic and/or epigenetic alterations linked to the pathology. Breast carcinoma is divided into different subtypes with different genetic characteristics [40,41], which can affect the release of specific miRNAs in the blood. Moreover, the variety of biomarkers and the difference in concentration in the blood might be influenced by the stage, so the analysis of a cohort not homogeneous for staging could be a limitation, and the BC patients included in this cohort are lacking stage I and grade 1 (one patient for each condition). Therefore, a limitation of our study is the paucity of stage I and II cancers. However, this is unavoidable in studies that recruit clinically justified PET acquisition since, as per the Clinical Practice Guidelines in Oncology (NCCN guidelines), PET is not indicated in the initial work-up of clinical stage I, II, or operable stage III (NCCN Guidelines Version 1.2019, accessed on 22th May 2019).

This staging group heterogeneity might lead to different results in different cohorts. Another limitation was the inability of monitoring patients during follow-up to better understand the prognostic and predictive role of miR-125b-5p and miR-143-3p. Nevertheless, the strengths of this study included the analysis performed on naïve patients as well as the availability of the same-day imaging parameters that provided information related to the morpho-functional characteristics of the primary cancers to correlate circulating miRNAs with in vivo quantified tumour biology. We performed a combined detection of miR-125b-5p and miR-143-3p with CA15-3 to improve the diagnostic accuracy. As suggested by guidelines, CA15-3 is not recommended for BC diagnosis [42,43], and our result ($CA15\text{-}3_{AUC}$ = 0.70) was in agreement with those of Liu and colleagues ($CA15\text{-}3_{AUC}$ = 0.71 [44]), Zaleski and colleagues ($CA15\text{-}3_{AUC}$ = 0.72 [45]) and Zajkowska and colleagues ($CA15\text{-}3_{AUC}$ = 0.70 [46]). Nevertheless, the coupled analysis of miR-125b-5p and CA15-3 increased the diagnostic accuracy up to AUC = 0.89. To the best of our knowledge, this is one of the best results published so far and the first study that combines the expression of a circulating miRNA with the expression of an established BC tumour marker. The combined detection of plasma miR-125b-5p and serum CA15-3 improved the diagnostic accuracy of BC detection up to ~90%, suggesting that this signature could be used for the diagnosis of BC. In addition, for stage II, the expression levels of CA15-3 were not correlated with the pathology (p-value = 0.658), whereas those of miR-125b-5p were (p-value = 0.002). The combined analysis of miR-125b-5p and CA 15-3 not only improved diagnostic accuracy in its entirety but also provided additional diagnostic information at less advanced pathological stages, suggesting the use of miRNAs as potential diagnostic circulating biomarkers that warrants consideration by further validation studies.

4. Materials and Methods

4.1. Participants and Study Design

This Health Insurance Portability and Accountability Act–compliant prospective study was approved by the institutional review board. All procedures performed in studies involving human participants were in accordance with the ethical standards of the institutional and/or national research committee and with the principles of the 1964 Declaration of Helsinki and its later amendments or comparable ethical standards. Informed consent was obtained from all individual participants included in the study. For study enrolment, all participants provided written informed consent before undergoing imaging PET/MR and blood collection. Between September 2012 and November 2015 at the IRCCS SDN Institute, 221 female Caucasian patients with BC who underwent a clinically indicated same-day CE-FDG-PET/MR and blood collection were evaluated for inclusion in this study. Plasma haemolysation was evaluated as described by Kirschner MB and colleagues [47]. The inclusion criteria for BC patients were as follows: (i) diagnosis of BC by core biopsy report; (ii) absence of any prior surgical or pharmacological treatment for BC (naïve); (iii) negative previous personal oncological history; (iv) age > 18 years; (v) CE-FDG-PET/MR and blood collection were performed on the same day; and (vi) fasting for at least 8 hours. The exclusion criteria for BC patients were as follows: (i) pregnancy; (ii) blood glucose levels > 140 mg/dL (7.77 mmol/L); (iii) artefacts affecting PET/MR images; (iv) standard contraindications for MR; (v) performance of CE-FDG-PET/MR and blood collection on different days; and (vi) plasma haemolysation. Blood samples of age-matched healthy donors were collected; their inclusion criteria were as follows: (i) >18 years of age; (ii) negative previous personal oncological history; (iii) absence of suspected BC as confirmed by ultrasound and/or mammography during the last 6 months from enrolment; iv) absence of a family history of BC; and (v) fasting for at least 8 hours. The exclusion criteria for healthy donors were the presence of one or more of the criteria reported above, including haemolysed plasma. We recruited 77 BC patients and 78 healthy donors for a total of 155 plasma/serum samples. The clinicopathological characteristics of the enrolled patients are reported in Table 1, and the whole study design is shown in Figure 1A.

This study was approved by the institutional Ethics Committee (Protocol Number: Prot2-11, approved 06/07/2011 by Ethical Committee IRCCS Fondazione SDN). This article does not describe any studies with animals performed by any of the authors

4.2. PET/MR Data Acquisition

PET/MR was performed with a Biograph mMR imager (Siemens Healthiness, Erlangen, Germany). First, a whole-body protocol was used to assess the overall extent of cancer and provide the NM stage. Thereafter, a dedicated breast protocol to provide both metabolic and functional biomarkers of primary cancer and its T stage was acquired. For total body acquisition, we used a 16-channel head-neck coil and three or four 12-channel body coils depending on the patient's height; for breast acquisition, a 4-channel breast coil was employed. Acquisitions were performed according to previously described protocols [19,20,35,48,49]. All patients fasted for at least 8 h before the procedure. They received

401 ± 32 MBq (mean ± standard deviation) of 18F-FDG intravenously. After a 60-min incubation time, PET and MR data were acquired simultaneously. The mean total time for the PET/MR examination was 107.87 ± 18.92 min [19].

4.3. Data Processing and Multiparametric Analysis

The PET data obtained from the PET/MR examinations were processed with comparable reconstruction and correction algorithms. Emission data were corrected for randomness, dead time, scatter, and attenuation.

Lymph node involvement and distant metastases were assessed on the entire dataset of PET/MR sequences for the purpose of NM staging. The primary tumour size and infiltration of neighbouring structures were evaluated on the dedicated breast PET/MR protocol for T staging [50].

The dynamic contrast-enhanced (DCE)-MRI images were processed through commercially available and clinically approved software for estimating tissue perfusion (Tissue 4D, Siemens Healthiness) according to the same established procedures provided by the manufacturer manual and widely used in the published literature. The pharmacokinetic modelling is based on a two-compartment Toft's model that allows for the calculation of the following: the transfer constant between vascular, extravascular, and extracellular space (EES) (Ktrans); volume of EES (Ve); constant reflux between EES and blood plasma (kep); initial area under the concentration curve (iAUC) [51,52]. Ktrans is a parameter related to vessel permeability and tissue blood flow. The volume of the extravascular extracellular space Ve is a marker of cell density, kep is a transfer constant from the extracellular/extravascular space to plasma, and iAUC is related to the blood volume in the tissue of interest [51].

After automatic motion correction and registration of the pre- and post-contrast acquisitions, T1 mapping was automatically obtained from the multiple flip angle pre-contrast part of the DCE-MRI sequence. Arterial input function (AIF) was related to the gadolinium dose injected and automatically modelled by a bi-exponential function using an intermediate population-derived mode provided by the software. On each single slice, a region-of-interest (ROI) was manually plotted around the tumour excluding the neighbouring vessels (internal mammary arteries and heart chambers) to compute the MR perfusion biomarker maps that were stored in the system.

For the subsequent tumour ROI analysis, PET/MR datasets (PET acquisition, dynamic axial T1 weighted post-contrast, dynamic axial T1 weighted subtracted contrast-enhanced images, axial T2 weighted sequences, axial apparent diffusion coefficient (ADC) map, and perfusion maps for Ktrans, Ve, kep and iAUC) were simultaneously evaluated on a clinically approved hybrid imaging workstation (Syngo.via, Siemens Healthiness) allowing the visual and quantitative comparison of the multiparametric data.

The maximum standardized uptake value (SUVmax) was automatically calculated by using an iso-contour automatic volume-of-interest (VOI) method of tissue delineation that selected a fixed threshold fraction (40%) of the peak activity in the tumour.

To obtain Ktrans, Ve, Kep and iAUC, the subtracted dynamic post-contrast T1-weighted series that best visualized the tumour was chosen. ROIs were manually drawn around the tumour on each image of that series, copied and then pasted on the corresponding Ktrans, Ve, Kep and iAUC maps. The values of all the ROIs were averaged. To obtain the ADC values, the ROIs were drawn on each image of the high-b value (800 s/mm^2) diffusion-weighted imaging (DWI), copied and then pasted on the ADC maps. The values of all the ROIs were averaged.

While the ROIs were drawn around the tumours, care was taken to avoid including large feeding vessels and areas of frank necrosis, as seen on T2 weighted and subtracted dynamic post-contrast T1-weighted images.

The maximal diameter of the tumour was measured on every single slice of the reference subtracted dynamic post-contrast T1-weighted images. The measurements were performed by a radiologist and a nuclear medicine physician with more than 5 years of experience. The whole-body and breast PET/MR protocols were derived from the published literature [20,35].

4.4. Plasma Sampling, RNA Extraction and Reverse Transcription

Blood samples were collected immediately before FDG injection. For each patient, a total of 10.5 mL of venous blood was collected in BD Vacutainer® 3 mL ethylenediaminetetraacetic acid (EDTA) tubes (Becton Dikinson, Franklin Lakes, NJ, USA) and 7.5 mL serum separating tubes. Blood was processed within 1 h of harvest. Plasma and serum were obtained from the whole blood samples by centrifugation at 1900× g for 10 min at 4 °C. The supernatant was further centrifuged at 16,000× g for 10 min at 4 °C and stored in aliquots of 0.5 mL at −80 °C until analysis. The samples were stored at −80 °C at the SDN Biobank (IRCCS DSN, Naples, Italy) [53]. The extraction of total RNA from 200 µL of plasma was performed within 1 year of storage at −80 °C using an miRNeasy Serum/Plasma Kit (Qiagen, Hilden, Germany) according to the manufacturer's instructions. Briefly, 3.5 µL of *Caenorhabditis elegans* miR-39 (cel-miR-39, 1.6 × 108 copies/µL) was added as the spike-in control after the denaturing solution. Total RNA (including miRNAs) was eluted in 14 µL of RNase-free water. Reverse transcription was performed using the miScript II RT Kit (Qiagen, Hilden, Germany) according to the manufacturer's instructions. Because extracellular miRNAs are less than 1% of the total RNA recovered [54] their concentration is often under the detection limits of spectrophotometric devices, so we decided to use a fixed volume rather than a fixed miRNA amount for qRT-PCR. To this aim, 1.5 µL of total RNA was added to the HiSpect Buffer (Qiagen, Hilden, Germany), nucleic acid mix and reverse transcriptase in a final volume of 20 µL. Reactions were incubated for 60 min at 37 °C and then for 5 min at 95 °C to inactivate the miScript Reverse Transcriptase mix (Qiagen, Hilden, Germany). At the end of the reactions, the resulting cDNAs were stored undiluted at −20 °C. The cycling conditions for real-time PCR were as follows: 15 min at 95 °C as the initial activation step, followed by 3-step cycling including denaturation (15 s at 94 °C), annealing (30 s at 55 °C) and extension (30 s at 70 °C) for a total of 40 cycles.

4.5. miRNA Microarray and Validation by Real-Time PCR (qRT-PCR)

By using the miScript miRNA PCR Array (Qiagen; MIHS-106Z), the expression profile of 84 human miRNAs (Supplementary Table S3) from the plasma samples of naïve BC patients and healthy donors were screened according to the manufacturer's protocol. The miScript miRNA PCR Array profiles the expression of 84 human miRNAs known to be deregulated in different cancers and are best characterized in miRBase. miRNA profiles were initially checked against a set population of 41 plasma samples (14 plasma samples from healthy donors and 27 from BC patients at diagnosis) on a MyiQ PCR system (Bio-Rad, Hercules, CA, USA). To identify interindividual variability, we did not pool plasma samples from each group (BC patients and healthy donors), but each sample was individually analysed by miRNA PCR arrays. The 96-well array also included n = 2 miRNA isolation controls, n = 6 "Housekeeping" snRNAs, n = 2 miRNA Reverse Transcription Controls (miRTC) and n = 2 Positive PCR Controls (PPC). Briefly, 200 µL of RNase-free water was added to each 20 µL of reverse transcription reaction, and 100 µL of diluted cDNA was used to prepare a reaction mix according to the manufacturer's protocol. For data analysis, the Baseline and Threshold settings, which were the same across all PCR runs, were from cycle 2 to cycle 15 for Baseline and 20 for Threshold. By using a data analysis tool (GeneGlobe Data Analysis Center, Qiagen, Hilden, Germany), the threshold cycle (CT) values were exported, and the steps performed by the software were as follows: any CT value ≥ 33 was considered negative; if the RNA sample was of high quality, the cycling programme was correctly run and the threshold was correctly defined, the value of the positive PCR control wells from the CT samples (CTPPC) should be 19 ± 2 or 15 ± 2; if the CT values of the reverse transcription control are less than 7, no inhibition of the reverse transcription reaction is apparent; the ΔCT value for each mature miRNA profiled is calculated using the formula ΔCT = CTmiRNA - CTnormalizer. The relative expression for each miRNA was calculated as $2^{-\Delta CT}$, and the criteria for the selection of miRNAs differentially expressed between the two populations with a statistical significance were a fold change ≥1.5 and a p-value < 0.05. Data validations were performed by qRT-PCR screening for only the following molecules: miR-125b-5p, miR-143-3p, miR-145-5p, miR-100-5p and miR-23a-3p. The Qiagen miScript SYBR Green PCR Kit was used for qPCR according to the manufacturer's protocol on the

Bio-Rad MyiQ PCR system. To determine the best standard genes to normalize our data, BestKeeper software was used [55]. By analysing $n = 41$ plasma samples, we found that the best normalizer included in the miScript miRNA PCR Array was the exogenous cel-mir 39. The MiScript Primers Assay was purchased from Qiagen (Qiagen, Hilden, Germany).

4.6. TCGA Data Processing

TCGA Breast Invasive Carcinoma (TCGA-BRCA project, February 2018) transcriptome profiling data (miRNA Expression Quantification) and clinical metadata were extracted from the Genomic Data Commons (GDC) portal (https://portal.gdc.cancer.gov/) for primary tumour ($n = 1096$ files for 1078 BC cases) and normal solid tissue ($n = 104$ files for 104 normal cases) using the open source R software and the TCGAbiolinks R package [56]. For the miRNA datasets, we selected the level-3 miRNA-Seq data, which were produced on Illumina HiSeq 2000 sequencers (Illumina Ventures, San Diego, CA, USA) The miRNA-Seq expression level-3 data contains raw read counts ($n = 1881$ miRNAs). The miRNA raw counts were filtered as follows: we calculated the mean value for duplicated BC cases and filtered out miRNA counts with null expression values on both conditions (tumour/normal) for a total of 1625 filtered counts. We considered only 1625 filtered miRNAs for the normalization step. Filtered raw counts were normalized using the Upper Quartile approach, and the patients with "−Inf" normalized values were removed for a total of 1076 tumours. The normalized counts were used to evaluate miR-125b-5p, miR-143-3p and miR-145-5p expression levels (tumour vs. normal) as log2-transformed relative expression values. We performed a Wilcoxon test to assess the statistical significance between tumour and normal conditions and calculated the adjusted p-value for each selected miRNA profile. We also reported miRNA tumour expression profiles based on the American Joint Committee on Cancer (AJCC) TNM staging. We grouped the clinical stages into four categories: (1) stage I; (2) stage II; (3) stage III; and (4) stage IV. We filtered out data with unassessed stage (stage x) or unreported information. Finally, we carried out a Spearman correlation analysis among the selected miRNA profiles and reported the associated p-values.

4.7. In Situ Hybridization

ISH was performed on formalin-fixed and paraffin-embedded tissue specimens surgically resected from patients diagnosed with BC. For each case analysed (a total of 22 breast tissues), we selected a block of tissue fixed in formalin and embedded in paraffin representative of the tumour and used it to obtain 4 μm-thick sections mounted on Superfrost Plus slides (Thermo Fisher Scientific, Waltham, MA, USA). The paraffin sections were placed in an oven at 60 °C for 45 min the day before ISH was performed and were stored overnight at 4 °C. Double digoxigenin (DIG)-labelled miRCURY LNA™ microRNA detection probes (Exiqon, Vedbæk, Denmark) were employed in this study. Specifically, we used 60 nM miR-145-5p target probe (Exiqon, Cat #619865-360), 60 nM miR-143-3p target probe (Exiqon, Cat #619872-360), 60 nM miR-125-5p target probe (Exiqon, Cat #611756-360), 40 nM scramble miR negative control probe (Exiqon, Cat #90-001) and 10 nM U6 positive control probe (Exiqon, Cat #90-002). The detection of microRNA by ISH was performed using the Enhanced miRCURY LNA microRNA ISH Optimization Kit (Exiqon, Vedbæk, Denmark) according to the manufacturer's protocol. Briefly, formalin-fixed paraffin-embedded sections were deparaffinized in xylene, rehydrated through solutions of ethanol to phosphate-buffered saline (PBS, pH 7.4) and pre-treated by enzymatic digestion (Proteinase K at 20 μg/mL for 30 min at 37 °C). Hybridization was performed by adding 60 nM LNA detection probes diluted in Exiqon hybridization buffer (Exiqon, Vedbæk, Denmark, Cat #90000) to each slide and incubating for 1 h at 60 °C in a hybridizer oven. After hybridization, the sections were washed under stringent conditions. Stringent washes were performed in pre-heated saline-sodium citrate (SSC) buffers in 5-min washes at 60 °C: once in 5× SSC, twice in 1× SSC and twice in 0.2× SSC. Then, the slides were placed in 0.2× SSC at room temperature and washed in PBS with 0.1% Tween-20. The sections were blocked against the unspecific binding of the detection antibody using a blocking solution according to the manufacturer's recommendations at room temperature for 15 min. The chromogenic detection of the miRNA LNA-ISH probe was performed with anti- anti-digoxygenin -alkaline phosphatase conjugate (1:800 dilution of the conjugate in blocking reagent, Roche Diagnostics GmbH, Mannheim, Germany) and incubated at room temperature for 1 h. Enzymatic development was performed by incubating the slides with 4-nitro-blue tetrazolium (NBT) and 5-bromo-4-chloro-3′-indolyl phosphate (BCIP) substrate (Roche) at 30 °C overnight to allow the formation of dark-blue 4-nitro-blue tetrazolium formazan precipitate. The following day, the sections were washed twice for 5 min in KTBT buffer (50 mM Tris–HCl, 150 mM NaCl, 10 mM KCl) and then shortly twice in water. Counterstaining using ISH nuclear fast red was performed for 1 min at room temperature. The sections were rinsed in tap water for 10 min, dehydrated through an increasing gradient of ethanol solutions and mounted with Eukitt mounting medium (VWR, Herlev, Denmark). A scrambled probe and U6 small nuclear RNA-specific probe were used as controls.

4.8. Measurement of CA 15-3

The CA15-3 serology test was performed in accordance with the manufacturer's protocols and reference intervals. Specifically, this tumour marker was measured in 155 serum samples ($n = 78$ healthy donors and $n = 77$ BC patients) on a Dimension Vista®1500 System (Siemens Healthcare Diagnostics Inc., Tarrytown, NY, USA) that uses the LOCI method (Siemens Healthcare Diagnostics, Eschborn, Germany), a homogeneous sandwich chemiluminescent immunoassay-based LOCI® technology (Siemens Healthcare Diagnostics, Eschborn, Germany). The threshold value provided by the supplying company for CA15-3 was 35 UI/mL. For serum tumour marker determination, when its level exceeded a threshold value, the samples were considered to be positive; otherwise, they were considered to be negative.

4.9. Statistical Analysis

Statistical analyses were performed using the open source R Statistical Software. All p-values were two-sided, and $p < 0.05$ was considered statistically significant. We used Shapiro–Wilk analysis and the Levene test to assess the normality and homoscedasticity of the distribution of the data, respectively. We performed the Mann-Whitney non-parametric test to compare the expression of the selected miRNAs between the two groups (BC and healthy controls). Furthermore, stepwise logistic regression was implemented to assess the association between miRNA expression and the probability of pathology. ROC curves were constructed for each miRNA, CA15-3 and CEA, and AUC values with 95% confidence intervals were calculated to evaluate the predictive power of the selected molecules for detecting BC. We evaluated the diagnostic accuracy of each circulating miRNA, CA15-3 and CEA, and their combination. The non-parametric Spearman's rank-order correlation and Mann-Whitney U test were performed to verify the correlations/associations among the biological markers and imaging parameters. To assess the association between the molecular and imaging parameters, the data were grouped according to positive or negative expression of ER, PR and HER2 receptors, low or high expression of Ki67 (low $\leq$20% and high >20%), grading, and staging as I, II, III, and IV, according to BC guidelines.

5. Conclusions

Our study highlighted that the addition of PET/MR biomarkers led to a better understanding of the relationships between circulating miRNAs and tumour biology in our BC population. Nevertheless, further studies with larger samples and a more homogeneous distribution of tumour subtypes and staging are needed to confirm our results.

Author Contributions: Conception and design: M.I. and O.A.C.; development of methodology: M.I., O.A.C., A.S. and S.S.; acquisition of data: M.I., O.A.C., P.M., C.C., G.I. and D.R.; analysis and interpretation of data: M.I., A.M.G., C.C., C.A.P. and M.F.; writing, review, and/or revision of the manuscript: M.I., A.M.G., O.A.C., C.C. and P.M.; study supervision: M.S.

Acknowledgments: We would like to thank Silvia Varricchio for technical support on the ISH assay.

References

1. Bray, F.; Ferlay, J.; Soerjomataram, I.; Siegel, R.L.; Torre, L.A.; Jemal, A. Global cancer statistics 2018: GLOBOCAN estimates of incidence and mortality worldwide for 36 cancers in 185 countries. *CA A Cancer J. Clin.* **2018**, *68*, 394–424. [CrossRef] [PubMed]
2. Carney, P.A.; Sickles, E.A.; Monsees, B.S.; Bassett, L.W.; Brenner, R.J.; Feig, S.A.; Smith, R.A.; Rosenberg, R.D.; Bogart, T.A.; Browning, S.; et al. Identifying Minimally Acceptable Interpretive Performance Criteria for Screening Mammography. *Radiology* **2010**, *255*, 354–361. [CrossRef] [PubMed]
3. Berg, W.A.; Blume, J.D.; Cormack, J.B.; Mendelson, E.B.; Lehrer, D.; Bohm-Velez, M.; Pisano, E.D.; Jong, R.A.; Evans, W.P.; Morton, M.J.; et al. Combined screening with ultrasound and mammography vs. mammography alone in women at elevated risk of breast cancer. *JAMA J. Am. Med Assoc.* **2008**, *299*, 2151–2163. [CrossRef] [PubMed]
4. Maric, P.; Ozretic, P.; Levanat, S.; Oreskovic, S.; Antunac, K.; Beketic-Oreskovic, L. Tumor Markers in Breast Cancer—Evaluation of their Clinical Usefulness. *Coll. Antropol.* **2011**, *35*, 241–247. [PubMed]
5. Duffy, M.J. Serum tumor markers in breast cancer: Are they of clinical value? *Clin. Chem.* **2006**, *52*, 345–351. [CrossRef]
6. Kufe, D.W. MUC1-C oncoprotein as a target in breast cancer: Activation of signaling pathways and therapeutic approaches. *Oncogene* **2013**, *32*, 1073–1081. [CrossRef] [PubMed]
7. Lin, N.U.; Thomssen, C.; Cardoso, F.; Cameron, D.; Cufer, T.; Fallowfield, L.; Francis, P.A.; Kyriakides, S.; Pagani, O.; Senkus, E.; et al. International guidelines for management of metastatic breast cancer (MBC) from the European School of Oncology (ESO)-MBC Task Force: Surveillance, staging, and evaluation of patients with early-stage and metastatic breast cancer. *Breast* **2013**, *22*, 203–210. [CrossRef]
8. Lytle, J.R.; Yario, T.A.; Steitz, J.A. Target mRNAs are repressed as efficiently by microRNA-binding sites in the 5′ UTR as in the 3′ UTR. *Proc. Natl. Acad. Sci. USA* **2007**, *104*, 9667–9672. [CrossRef]
9. Esquela-Kerscher, A.; Slack, F.J. Oncomirs—MicroRNAs with a role in cancer. *Nat. Rev. Cancer* **2006**, *6*, 259–269. [CrossRef]
10. Kent, O.A.; Mendell, J.T. A small piece in the cancer puzzle: MicroRNAs as tumor suppressors and oncogenes. *Oncogene* **2006**, *25*, 6188–6196. [CrossRef]
11. Schwarzenbach, H.; Hoon, D.S.B.; Pantel, K. Cell-free nucleic acids as biomarkers in cancer patients. *Nat. Rev. Cancer* **2011**, *11*, 426–437. [CrossRef] [PubMed]
12. Hanke, M.; Hoefig, K.; Merz, H.; Feller, A.C.; Kausch, I.; Jocham, D.; Warnecke, J.M.; Sczakiel, G. A robust methodology to study urine microRNA as tumor marker: MicroRNA-126 and microRNA-182 are related to urinary bladder cancer. *Urol. Oncol. Semin. Orig. Investig.* **2010**, *28*, 655–661. [CrossRef] [PubMed]
13. Xie, Y.; Todd, N.W.; Liu, Z.Q.; Zhan, M.; Fang, H.B.; Peng, H.; Alattar, M.; Deepak, J.; Stass, S.A.; Jiang, F. Altered miRNA expression in sputum for diagnosis of non-small cell lung cancer. *Lung Cancer* **2010**, *67*, 170–176. [CrossRef] [PubMed]
14. Michael, A.; Bajracharya, S.D.; Yuen, P.S.T.; Zhou, H.; Star, R.A.; Illei, G.G.; Alevizos, I. Exosomes from human saliva as a source of microRNA biomarkers. *Oral Dis.* **2010**, *16*, 34–38. [CrossRef] [PubMed]
15. Amorim, M.; Salta, S.; Henrique, R.; Jeronimo, C. Decoding the usefulness of non-coding RNAs as breast cancer markers. *J. Transl. Med.* **2016**, *14*. [CrossRef] [PubMed]
16. Madhavan, D.; Cuk, K.; Burwinkel, B.; Yang, R. Cancer diagnosis and prognosis decoded by blood-based circulating microRNA signatures. *Front. Genet.* **2013**, *4*, 116. [CrossRef] [PubMed]
17. Leidner, R.S.; Li, L.; Thompson, C.L. Dampening Enthusiasm for Circulating MicroRNA in Breast Cancer. *PLoS ONE* **2013**, *8*. [CrossRef] [PubMed]
18. Sala, E.; Mema, E.; Himoto, Y.; Veeraraghavan, H.; Brenton, J.D.; Snyder, A.; Weigelt, B.; Vargas, H.A. Unravelling tumour heterogeneity using next-generation imaging: Radiomics, radiogenomics, and habitat imaging. *Clin. Radiol.* **2017**, *72*, 3–10. [CrossRef]
19. Incoronato, M.; Grimaldi, A.M.; Cavaliere, C.; Inglese, M.; Mirabelli, P.; Monti, S.; Ferbo, U.; Nicolai, E.; Soricelli, A.; Catalano, O.A.; et al. Relationship between functional imaging and immunohistochemical markers and prediction of breast cancer subtype: A PET/MRI study. *Eur. J. Nucl. Med. Mol. Imaging* **2018**. [CrossRef]
20. Catalano, O.A.; Daye, D.; Signore, A.; Iannace, C.; Vangel, M.; Luongo, A.; Catalano, M.; Filomena, M.;

Mansi, L.; Soricelli, A.; et al. Staging performance of whole-body DWI, PET/CT and PET/MRI in invasive ductal carcinoma of the breast. *Int. J. Oncol.* **2017**, *51*, 281–288. [CrossRef]

21. Catalano, O.A.; Nicolai, E.; Rosen, B.R.; Luongo, A.; Catalano, M.; Iannace, C.; Guimaraes, A.; Vangel, M.G.; Mahmood, U.; Soricelli, A.; et al. Comparison of CE-FDG-PET/CT with CE-FDG-PET/MR in the evaluation of osseous metastases in breast cancer patients. *Br. J. Cancer* **2015**, *112*, 1452–1460. [CrossRef] [PubMed]
22. Botsikas, D.; Bagetakos, I.; Picarra, M.; Barisits, A.C.D.C.A.; Boudabbous, S.; Montet, X.; Giang Thanh, L.; Mainta, I.; Kalovidouri, A.; Becker, M. What is the diagnostic performance of 18-FDG-PET/MR compared to PET/CT for the N- and M- staging of breast cancer? *Eur. Radiol.* **2019**, *29*, 1787–1798. [CrossRef] [PubMed]
23. Ma, Z.S.; Wang, D.W.; Sun, X.B.; Shi, H.; Pang, T.; Dong, G.Q.; Zhang, C.Q. Quantitative analysis of 3-Tesla magnetic resonance imaging in the differential diagnosis of breast lesions. *Exp. Ther. Med.* **2015**, *9*, 913–918. [CrossRef] [PubMed]
24. Li, L.; Wang, K.; Sun, X.L.; Wang, K.Z.; Sun, Y.Y.; Zhang, G.F.; Shen, B.Z. Parameters of Dynamic Contrast-Enhanced MRI as Imaging Markers for Angiogenesis and Proliferation in Human Breast Cancer. *Med. Sci. Monit.* **2015**, *21*, 376–382. [PubMed]
25. Ma, C.X.; Ellis, M.J. The Cancer Genome Atlas: Clinical Applications for Breast Cancer. *Oncology (New York)* **2013**, *27*, 1263–1269.
26. Matamala, N.; Vargas, M.T.; Gonzalez-Campora, R.; Minambres, R.; Arias, J.I.; Menendez, P.; Andres-Leon, E.; Gomez-Lopez, G.; Yanowsky, K.; Calvete-Candenas, J.; et al. Tumor MicroRNA Expression Profiling Identifies Circulating MicroRNAs for Early Breast Cancer Detection. *Clin. Chem.* **2015**, *61*, 1098–1106. [CrossRef] [PubMed]
27. Ng, E.K.O.; Li, R.F.N.; Shin, V.Y.; Jin, H.C.; Leung, C.P.H.; Ma, E.S.K.; Pang, R.; Chua, D.; Chu, K.M.; Law, W.L.; et al. Circulating microRNAs as Specific Biomarkers for Breast Cancer Detection. *PLoS ONE* **2013**, *8*. [CrossRef]
28. Thakur, S.; Grover, R.K.; Gupta, S.; Yadav, A.K.; Das, B.C. Identification of Specific miRNA Signature in Paired Sera and Tissue Samples of Indian Women with Triple Negative Breast Cancer. *PLoS ONE* **2016**, *11*. [CrossRef]
29. Kodahl, A.R.; Lyng, M.B.; Binder, H.; Cold, S.; Gravgaard, K.; Knoop, A.S.; Ditzel, H.J. Novel circulating microRNA signature as a potential non-invasive multi-marker test in ER-positive early-stage breast cancer: A case control study. *Mol. Oncol.* **2014**, *8*, 874–883. [CrossRef]
30. Chan, M.; Liaw, C.S.; Ji, S.M.; Tan, H.H.; Wong, C.Y.; Thike, A.A.; Tan, P.H.; Ho, G.H.; Lee, A.S.G. Identification of Circulating MicroRNA Signatures for Breast Cancer Detection. *Clin. Cancer Res.* **2013**, *19*, 4477–4487. [CrossRef]
31. Wang, K.; Yuan, Y.; Cho, J.H.; McClarty, S.; Baxter, D.; Galas, D.J. Comparing the MicroRNA Spectrum between Serum and Plasma. *PLoS ONE* **2012**, *7*. [CrossRef] [PubMed]
32. Wang, H.J.; Tan, G.; Dong, L.; Cheng, L.; Li, K.J.; Wang, Z.Y.; Luo, H.F. Circulating MiR-125b as a Marker Predicting Chemoresistance in Breast Cancer. *PLoS ONE* **2012**, *7*. [CrossRef] [PubMed]
33. Mar-Aguilar, F.; Mendoza-Ramirez, J.A.; Malagon-Santiago, I.; Espino-Silva, P.K.; Santuario-Facio, S.K.; Ruiz-Flores, P.; Rodriguez-Padilla, C.; Resendez-Perez, D. Serum circulating microRNA profiling for identification of potential breast cancer biomarkers. *Dis. Mark.* **2013**, *34*, 163–169. [CrossRef]
34. Liu, B.Q.; Su, F.; Chen, M.W.; Li, Y.; Qi, X.Y.; Xiao, J.B.; Li, X.M.; Liu, X.C.; Liang, W.T.; Zhang, Y.F.; et al. Serum miR-21 and miR-125b as markers predicting neoadjuvant chemotherapy response and prognosis in stage II/III breast cancer. *Hum. Pathol.* **2017**, *64*, 44–52. [CrossRef] [PubMed]
35. Catalano, O.A.; Horn, G.L.; Signore, A.; Iannace, C.; Lepore, M.; Vangel, M.; Luongo, A.; Catalano, M.; Lehman, C.; Salvatore, M.; et al. PET/MR in invasive ductal breast cancer: Correlation between imaging markers and histological phenotype. *Br. J. Cancer* **2017**, *116*, 893–902. [CrossRef] [PubMed]
36. Almeida, M.I.; Calin, G.A. The miR-143/miR-145 cluster and the tumor microenvironment: Unexpected roles. *Genome Med.* **2016**, *8*. [CrossRef]
37. Berindan-Neagoe, I.; Calin, G.A. Molecular Pathways: MicroRNAs, Cancer Cells, and Microenvironment. *Clin. Cancer Res.* **2014**, *20*, 6247–6253. [CrossRef]
38. Li, Y.; Wang, Y.; Fan, H.; Zhang, Z.; Li, N. miR-125b-5p inhibits breast cancer cell proliferation, migration and invasion by targeting KIAA1522. *Biochem. Biophys. Res. Commun.* **2018**, *504*, 277–282. [CrossRef]
39. Feliciano, A.; Castellvi, J.; Artero-Castro, A.; Leal, J.A.; Romagosa, C.; Hernandez-Losa, J.; Peg, V.; Fabra, A.; Vidal, F.; Kondoh, H.; et al. miR-125b Acts as a Tumor Suppressor in Breast Tumorigenesis via Its Novel Direct Targets ENPEP, CK2-alpha, CCNJ, and MEGF9. *PLoS ONE* **2013**, *8*. [CrossRef]

40. Koboldt, D.C.; Fulton, R.S.; McLellan, M.D.; Schmidt, H.; Kalicki-Veizer, J.; McMichael, J.F.; Fulton, L.L.; Dooling, D.J.; Ding, L.; Mardis, E.R.; et al. Comprehensive molecular portraits of human breast tumours. *Nature* **2012**, *490*, 61–70. [CrossRef]
41. Parker, J.S.; Mullins, M.; Cheang, M.C.U.; Leung, S.; Voduc, D.; Vickery, T.; Davies, S.; Fauron, C.; He, X.; Hu, Z.; et al. Supervised Risk Predictor of Breast Cancer Based on Intrinsic Subtypes. *J. Clin. Oncol.* **2009**, *27*, 1160–1167. [CrossRef] [PubMed]
42. Molina, R.; Barak, V.; van Dalen, A.; Duffy, M.J.; Einarsson, R.; Gion, M.; Goike, H.; Lamerz, R.; Nap, M.; Soletormos, G.; et al. Tumor markers in breast cancer—European Group on Tumor Markers recommendations. *Tumor Biol.* **2005**, *26*, 281–293. [CrossRef] [PubMed]
43. Mirabelli, P.; Incoronato, M. Usefulness of Traditional Serum Biomarkers for Management of Breast Cancer Patients. *Biomed Res. Int.* **2013**. [CrossRef] [PubMed]
44. Liu, C.; Sun, B.; Xu, B.; Meng, X.; Li, L.; Cong, Y.; Liu, J.; Wang, Q.; Xuan, L.; Song, Q.; et al. A panel containing PD-1, IL-2R alpha, IL-10, and CA15-3 as a biomarker to discriminate breast cancer from benign breast disease. *Cancer Manag. Res.* **2018**, *10*, 1749–1761. [CrossRef] [PubMed]
45. Zaleski, M.; Kobilay, M.; Schroeder, L.; Debald, M.; Semaan, A.; Hettwer, K.; Uhlig, S.; Kuhn, W.; Hartmann, G.; Holdenrieder, S. Improved sensitivity for detection of breast cancer by combination of miR-34a and tumor markers CA 15-3 or CEA. *Oncotarget* **2018**, *9*, 22523–22536. [CrossRef] [PubMed]
46. Zajkowska, M.; Glazewska, E.K.; Bedkowska, G.E.; Chorazy, P.; Szmitkowski, M.; Lawicki, S. Diagnostic Power of Vascular Endothelial Growth Factor and Macrophage Colony-Stimulating Factor in Breast Cancer Patients Based on ROC Analysis. *Mediat. Inflamm.* **2016**. [CrossRef]
47. Kirschner, M.B.; Edelman, J.J.B.; Kao, S.C.H.; Vallely, M.P.; van Zandwijk, N.; Reid, G. The Impact of Hemolysis on Cell-Free microRNA Biomarkers. *Front. Genet.* **2013**, *4*, 94. [CrossRef] [PubMed]
48. Catalano, O.A.; Rosen, B.R.; Sahani, D.V.; Hahn, P.F.; Guimaraes, A.R.; Vangel, M.G.; Nicolai, E.; Soricelli, A.; Salvatore, M. Clinical Impact of PET/MR Imaging in Patients with Cancer Undergoing Same-Day PET/CT: Initial Experience in 134 Patients-A Hypothesis-generating Exploratory Study. *Radiology* **2013**, *269*, 857–869. [CrossRef]
49. Pace, L.; Nicolai, E.; Luongo, A.; Aiello, M.; Catalano, O.A.; Soricelli, A.; Salvatore, M. Comparison of whole-body PET/CT and PET/MRI in breast cancer patients: Lesion detection and quantitation of 18F-deoxyglucose uptake in lesions and in normal organ tissues. *Eur. J. Radiol.* **2014**, *83*, 289–296. [CrossRef]
50. Veronesi, U.; Zurrida, S.; Viale, G.; Galimberti, V.; Arnone, P.; Nole, F. Rethinking TNM: A Breast Cancer Classification to Guide to Treatment and Facilitate Research. *Breast J.* **2009**, *15*, 291–295. [CrossRef]
51. Inglese, M.; Cavaliere, C.; Monti, S.; Forte, E.; Incoronato, M.; Nicolai, E.; Salvatore, M.; Aiello, M. A multi-parametric PET/MRI study of breast cancer: Evaluation of DCE-MRI pharmacokinetic models and correlation with diffusion and functional parameters. *NMR Biomed.* **2018**, e4026. [CrossRef] [PubMed]
52. Monti, S.; Aiello, M.; Incoronato, M.; Grimaldi, A.M.; Moscarino, M.; Mirabelli, P.; Ferbo, U.; Cavaliere, C.; Salvatore, M. DCE-MRI Pharmacokinetic-Based Phenotyping of Invasive Ductal Carcinoma: A Radiomic Study for Prediction of Histological Outcomes. *Contrast Media Mol. Imaging* **2018**. [CrossRef] [PubMed]
53. Mirabelli, P.; Incoronato, M.; Coppola, L.; Infante, T.; Parente, C.A.; Nicolai, E.; Soricelli, A.; Salvatore, M. SDN biobank: Bioresource of human samples associated with functional and/or morphological bioimaging results for the study of oncological, cardiological, neurological, and metabolic diseases. *Open J. Bioresour.* **2017**, *4*. [CrossRef]
54. Bellingham, S.A.; Coleman, B.M.; Hill, A.F. Small RNA deep sequencing reveals a distinct miRNA signature released in exosomes from prion-infected neuronal cells. *Nucleic Acids Res.* **2012**, *40*, 10937–10949. [CrossRef] [PubMed]
55. Pfaffl, M.W.; Tichopad, A.; Prgomet, C.; Neuvians, T.P. Determination of stable housekeeping genes, differentially regulated target genes and sample integrity: BestKeeper—Excel-based tool using pair-wise correlations. *Biotechnol. Lett.* **2004**, *26*, 509–515. [CrossRef] [PubMed]
56. Colaprico, A.; Silva, T.C.; Olsen, C.; Garofano, L.; Cava, C.; Garolini, D.; Sabedot, T.S.; Malta, T.M.; Pagnotta, S.M.; Castiglioni, I.; et al. TCGAbiolinks: An R/Bioconductor package for integrative analysis of TCGA data. *Nucleic Acids Res.* **2016**, *44*. [CrossRef] [PubMed]

Permissions

All chapters in this book were first published by MDPI; hereby published with permission under the Creative Commons Attribution License or equivalent. Every chapter published in this book has been scrutinized by our experts. Their significance has been extensively debated. The topics covered herein carry significant findings which will fuel the growth of the discipline. They may even be implemented as practical applications or may be referred to as a beginning point for another development.

The contributors of this book come from diverse backgrounds, making this book a truly international effort. This book will bring forth new frontiers with its revolutionizing research information and detailed analysis of the nascent developments around the world.

We would like to thank all the contributing authors for lending their expertise to make the book truly unique. They have played a crucial role in the development of this book. Without their invaluable contributions this book wouldn't have been possible. They have made vital efforts to compile up to date information on the varied aspects of this subject to make this book a valuable addition to the collection of many professionals and students.

This book was conceptualized with the vision of imparting up-to-date information and advanced data in this field. To ensure the same, a matchless editorial board was set up. Every individual on the board went through rigorous rounds of assessment to prove their worth. After which they invested a large part of their time researching and compiling the most relevant data for our readers.

The editorial board has been involved in producing this book since its inception. They have spent rigorous hours researching and exploring the diverse topics which have resulted in the successful publishing of this book. They have passed on their knowledge of decades through this book. To expedite this challenging task, the publisher supported the team at every step. A small team of assistant editors was also appointed to further simplify the editing procedure and attain best results for the readers.

Apart from the editorial board, the designing team has also invested a significant amount of their time in understanding the subject and creating the most relevant covers. They scrutinized every image to scout for the most suitable representation of the subject and create an appropriate cover for the book.

The publishing team has been an ardent support to the editorial, designing and production team. Their endless efforts to recruit the best for this project, has resulted in the accomplishment of this book. They are a veteran in the field of academics and their pool of knowledge is as vast as their experience in printing. Their expertise and guidance has proved useful at every step. Their uncompromising quality standards have made this book an exceptional effort. Their encouragement from time to time has been an inspiration for everyone.

The publisher and the editorial board hope that this book will prove to be a valuable piece of knowledge for researchers, students, practitioners and scholars across the globe.

List of Contributors

Taye Girma Debelee
Artificial Intelligence Center, 40782 Addis Ababa, Ethiopia
College of Electrical and Mechanical Engineering, Addis Ababa Science and Technology University, 120611 Addis Ababa, Ethiopia

Samuel Rahimeto Kebede
Artificial Intelligence Center, 40782 Addis Ababa, Ethiopia
Department of Electrical and Computer Engineering, Debreberhan University, 445 Debre Berhan, Ethiopia

Friedhelm Schwenker
Institute of Neural Information Processing, University of Ulm, 89081 Ulm, Germany

Zemene Matewos Shewarega
Artificial Intelligence Center, 40782 Addis Ababa, Ethiopia

Yan Jin and James W. Randall
Department of Radiation Oncology, the University of Texas MD Anderson Cancer Center, Houston, TX 77030, USA
The University of Texas Medical Branch, Galveston, TX 77555, USA

Hesham Elhalawani, Karine A. Al Feghali, Andrew M. Elliott, Lara Lacerda, Benjamin L. Tran, Abdallah S. Mohamed, Clifton D. Fuller and Caroline Chung
Department of Radiation Oncology, the University of Texas MD Anderson Cancer Center, Houston, TX 77030, USA

Brian M. Anderson and Kristy K. Brock
Department of Imaging Physics, the University of Texas MD Anderson Cancer Center, Houston, TX 77030, USA

Lauren A. Baldwin, Edward J. Pavlik, Emma Ueland, Hannah E. Brown, Kelsey M. Ladd, Christopher P. DeSimone, John R. van Nagell, Frederick R. Ueland and Rachel W. Miller
Division of Gynecologic Oncology, Department of Obstetrics and Gynecology, The University of Kentucky Chandler Medical Center and the Markey Cancer Center, 800 Rose Street, Lexington, KY 40536-0293, USA

Giulia Polverari
Division of Nuclear Medicine, Department of Medical Sciences, University of Turin, AOU Città della Salute e della Scienza, 10126 Turin, Italy
PET/CT Center, Affidea IRMET, 10135 Turin, Italy

Francesco Ceci, Roberto Passera, Virginia Liberini and Désirée Deandreis
Division of Nuclear Medicine, Department of Medical Sciences, University of Turin, AOU Città della Salute e della Scienza, 10126 Turin, Italy

Valentina Bertaglia, Maria Lucia Reale and Silvia Novello
Department of Oncology, University of Turin, San Luigi Gonzaga Hospital, Orbassano, 10043 Torino, Italy

Osvaldo Rampado and Elena Gallio
Medical Physics Unit, S.C. Fisica Sanitaria, A.O.U. Città della Salute e della Scienza, 10135 Turin, Italy

Paola Scapoli and Manuela Racca
Nuclear Medicine, Istituto per la Ricerca e la Cura del Cancro (IRCC), 10060 Candiolo, Italy

Vincenzo Arena
PET/CT Center, Affidea IRMET, 10135 Turin, Italy

Andrea Veltri
Radiology Unit, Department of Oncology, University of Turin, San Luigi Gonzaga Hospital, Orbassano, 10043 Torino, Italy

Natalia Samolyk-Kogaczewska
Department of Radiotherapy, Comprehensive Cancer Center, 15-027 Bialystok, Poland

Ewa Sierko
Department of Radiotherapy, Comprehensive Cancer Center, 15-027 Bialystok, Poland
Department of Oncology, Medical University of Bialystok, 15-027 Bialystok, Poland

Dorota Dziemianczyk-Pakiela
Department of Otolaryngology and Maxillofacial Surgery, Jedrzej Sniadecki Memorial Regional Hospital, 15-950 Bialystok, Poland

Klaudia Beata Nowaszewska
Department of Maxillofacial and Plastic Surgery, Medical University of Bialystok, 15-276 Bialystok, Poland

Malgorzata Lukasik and Joanna Reszec
Department of Medical Pathology, Medical University of Bialystok, 15-089 Bialystok, Poland

Robert N. Ore
The Division of Gynecologic Oncology, Department of Obstetrics and Gynecology, The University of Kentucky College of Medicine, 800 Rose Street, 330 Whitney-Hendrickson Building, Lexington, KY 40536, USA

Quan Chen
Division of Cancer Biostatistics, College of Public Health & Biostatistics Shared Resource Facility, Markey Cancer Center, University of Kentucky, Lexington, KY 40506, USA

Bin Huang
Division of Gynecologic Oncology, Department of Obstetrics and Gynecology, The University of Kentucky Chandler Medical Center and the Markey Cancer Center, 800 Rose Street, Lexington, KY 40536-0293, USA
Division of Cancer Biostatistics, College of Public Health & Biostatistics Shared Resource Facility, Markey Cancer Center, University of Kentucky, Lexington, KY 40506, USA

Thomas C. Tucker
Department of Epidemiology, College of Public Health & Kentucky Cancer Registry, Markey Cancer Center, University of Kentucky, Lexington, KY 40506, USA

Connie G. White
Kentucky Department for Public Health, Frankfort, KY 40601, USA

Michael A. Andrykowski
Department of Behavioral Science, University of Kentucky College of Medicine, Lexington, KY 40536-0086, USA

Manuela Andrea Hoffmann
Department of Occupational Health & Safety, Federal Ministry of Defense, 53123 Bonn, Germany
Clinic of Nuclear Medicine, Johannes Gutenberg-University, 55101 Mainz, Germany

Hans-Georg Buchholz, Matthias Miederer, Stefanie Pektor and Mathias Schreckenberger
Clinic of Nuclear Medicine, Johannes Gutenberg-University, 55101 Mainz, Germany

Helmut J. Wieler
Clinic of Nuclear Medicine, Bundeswehr Central Hospital, 56072 Koblenz, Germany

Florian Rosar
Clinic of Nuclear Medicine, Johannes Gutenberg-University, 55101 Mainz, Germany
Department of Nuclear Medicine, Saarland University Medical Center, 66421 Homburg, Germany

Nicolas Fischer
Department of Urology, Helios Kliniken Krefeld, 47805 Krefeld, Germany

Jonas Müller-Hübenthal
Practice of Radiology and Nuclear Medicine, Praxis im KölnTriangle, 50679 Köln, Germany

Ludwin Trampert
Clinic of Nuclear Medicine, Klinikum Mutterhaus der Borromäerinnen, 54290 Trier, Germany

Katsuo Usuda, Shun Iwai, Aika Funasaki, Atsushi Sekimura, Nozomu Motono and Hidetaka Uramoto
Department of Thoracic Surgery, Kanazawa Medical University, Ishikawa 920-0293, Japan

Munetaka Matoba and Mariko Doai
Department of Radiology, Kanazawa Medical University, Ishikawa 920-0293, Japan

Sohsuke Yamada
Department of Pathology and Laboratory Medicine, Kanazawa Medical University, Ishikawa 920-0293, Japan

Yoshimichi Ueda
Department of Pathophysiological and Experimental Pathology, Kanazawa Medical University, Ishikawa 920-0293, Japan

Matteo Bauckneht and Selene Capitanio
Nuclear Medicine Unit, IRCCS Ospedale Policlinico San Martino, 16132 Genoa, Italy

Maria Isabella Donegani, Alberto Miceli, Stefano Raffa and Martina Vitti
Department of Health Sciences (DISSAL), University of Genova, 16132 Genoa, Italy

Elisa Zanardi and Francesco Boccardo
Academic Unit of Medical Oncology, IRCCS Ospedale Policlinico San Martino, 16132 Genoa, Italy
Department of Internal Medicine and Medical Specialties (DIMI), University of Genoa, 16132 Genoa, Italy

Roberto Murialdo
Internal Medicine Unit, IRCCS Ospedale Policlinico San Martino, 16132 Genoa, Italy

Laura Tomasello
Academic Unit of Medical Oncology, IRCCS Ospedale Policlinico San Martino, 16132 Genoa, Italy

Alessia Cavo and Manlio Mencoboni
Oncology Unit, Villa Scassi Hospital, 16149, Genova, Italy

Fabio Catalano and Giuseppe Fornarini
Medical Oncology Unit, IRCCS Ospedale Policlinico San Martino, 16132 Genoa, Italy

Marcello Ceppi
Clinical Epidemiology Unit, IRCCS Ospedale Policlinico San Martino, 16132 Genoa, Italy

Cecilia Marini
Department of Health Sciences (DISSAL), University of Genova, 16132 Genoa, Italy
CNR Institute of Molecular Bioimaging and Physiology (IBFM), 20090 Segrate (MI), Italy

Gianmario Sambuceti and Silvia Morbelli
Nuclear Medicine Unit, IRCCS Ospedale Policlinico San Martino, 16132 Genoa, Italy
Department of Health Sciences (DISSAL), University of Genova, 16132 Genoa, Italy

Christopher G. Smith
Department of Obstetrics & Gynecology, University of Kentucky Medical Center, 800 Rose Street, Lexington, KY 40536-0293, USA

Stefano Fanti
Department of Experimental, Diagnostic and Specialty Medicine – DIMES, University of Bologna, and Nuclear Medicine Division, Policlinico S.Orsola, 40138 Bologna, Italy

Wim Oyen
Department of Radiology and Nuclear Medicine, Rijnstate Hospital, 6815 Arnhem, The Netherlands
Department of Biomedical Sciences, Humanitas University and Department of Nuclear Medicine, Humanitas Clinical and Research Center, 20126 Milan, Italy

Elisabetta Lalumera
Psychology Department, Milano-Bicocca University, 20126 Milan, Italy

Wouter Froyman, Chiara Landolfo and Dirk Timmerman
Department of Development and Regeneration, KU Leuven, Leuven, Belgium
Department of Obstetrics and Gynecology, University Hospitals Leuven, Leuven 3000, Belgium

Laure Wynants and Ben Van Calster
Department of Development and Regeneration, KU Leuven, Leuven, Belgium

Tom Bourne
Department of Development and Regeneration, KU Leuven, Leuven, Belgium
Department of Obstetrics and Gynecology, University Hospitals Leuven, Leuven 3000, Belgium
Queen Charlotte's and Chelsea Hospital, Imperial College, London W12 0HS, UK

Lil Valentin and Povilas Sladkevicius
Department of Obstetrics and Gynecology, Skåne University Hospital Malmö, Lund University, Malmö 20502, Sweden

Antonia Testa
Department of Oncology, Catholic University of the Sacred Heart, Rome 00168, Italy

Dorella Franchi
Preventive Gynecology Unit, Division of Gynecology, European Institute of Oncology, Milan 20141, Italy

Daniela Fischerova
Gynecological Oncology Center, Department of Obstetrics and Gynecology, Charles University, Prague 12108, Czech Republic

Luca Savelli
Department of Obstetrics and Gynecology, S. Orsola-Malpighi Hospital, University of Bologna, Bologna 40138, Italy

Jeong Won Lee
Department of Nuclear Medicine, International St. Mary's Hospital, Catholic Kwandong University College of Medicine, 25 Simgok-ro 100 beon-gil, Seo-gu, Incheon 22711, Korea

Sung Yong Kim, Sun Wook Han and Jong Eun Lee
Department of Surgery, Soonchunhyang University Cheonan Hospital, 31 Suncheonhyang 6-gil, Dongnam-gu, Cheonan, Chungcheongnam-do 31151, Korea

Hyun Ju Lee
Department of Pathology, Soonchunhyang University Cheonan Hospital, 31 Suncheonhyang 6-gil, Dongnam-gu, Cheonan, Chungcheongnam-do 31151, Korea

Sang Mi Lee
Department of Nuclear Medicine, Soonchunhyang University Cheonan Hospital, 31 Suncheonhyang 6-gil, Dongnam-gu, Cheonan, Chungcheongnam-do 31151, Korea

Mariarosaria Incoronato, Anna Maria Grimaldi, Peppino Mirabelli, Carlo Cavaliere, Chiara Anna Parente, Monica Franzese and Marco Salvatore
IRCCS SDN, 80143 Naples, Italy

Stefania Staibano, Gennaro Ilardi and Daniela Russo
Department of Advanced Biomedical Sciences, Federico II University, 80131 Naples, Italy

Andrea Soricelli
IRCCS SDN, 80143 Naples, Italy
Department of Motor Sciences & Wellness, University of Naples Parthenope, 80133 Naples, Italy

Onofrio Antonio Catalano
Department of Radiology, Athinoula A. Martinos Center for Biomedical Imaging, Massachusetts General Hospital, Harvard Medical School, Charlestown, MA 02129, USA

Index

www.ingramcontent.com/pod-product-compliance
Lightning Source LLC
LaVergne TN
LVHW061513220926
848485LV00018B/1026
* 9 7 8 1 6 3 9 2 7 6 3 4 9 *